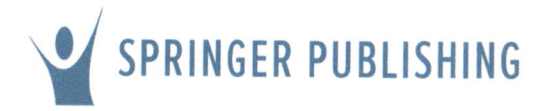

GET THE MOST FROM YOUR BOOK

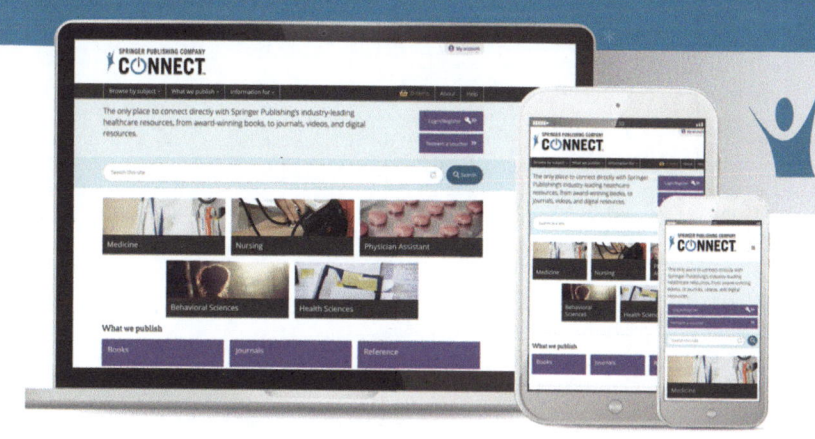

VOUCHER CODE:

K0YCXXT6

Online Access

Your print purchase of *Population-Based Nursing: Concepts and Competencies for Advanced Practice, Fourth Edition,* includes **online access via Springer Publishing Connect**™ to increase accessibility, portability, and searchability.

Insert the code at http://connect.springerpub.com/content/book/978-0-8261-4377-8 or scan the QR code and insert the voucher code today!

Having trouble? Contact our customer service department at **cs@springerpub.com**

Instructor Resource Access for Adopters

Let us do some of the heavy lifting to create an engaging classroom experience with a variety of instructor resources included in most textbooks SUCH AS:

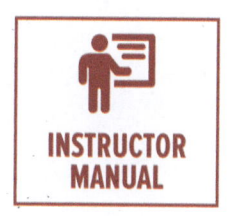

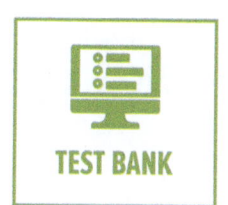

INSTRUCTOR MANUAL	POWERPOINTS	TEST BANK

Visit **https://connect.springerpub.com/** and look for the **"Show Supplementary"** button on your **book homepage** to see what is available to instructors! First time using Springer Publishing Connect?

Email **textbook@springerpub.com** to create an account and start unlocking valuable resources.

POPULATION-BASED NURSING

ANN L. CUPP CURLEY, PhD, RN, is retired from her position as the Nurse Research Specialist at Capital Health in Trenton, New Jersey, where she was responsible for promoting and guiding the development of nursing research and evidence-based practice. She has an extensive background in nursing education at the undergraduate, graduate, and doctoral levels and more than 10 years' experience in community and public health nursing. Dr. Curley has been principal or co-principal investigator of many research projects and served as an advisor on many DNP project committees. She received a BSN from Boston College, an MSN in community health/clinical nurse specialist track from the University of Pennsylvania, and a PhD in urban planning and policy development from Rutgers, The State University of New Jersey.

BARBARA A. NIEDZ, PhD, RN, CPHQ, has been a nurse for 50+ years and has held leadership positions in New Jersey hospitals and managed care organizations, as well as holding an extensive academic background. Dr. Niedz has taught at the undergraduate, graduate, and doctoral levels. She is presently a Senior Contributing Faculty Member at Walden College of Nursing in the doctoral program on a part-time basis and a full-time Assistant Professor in the Advanced Practice Division at Rutgers, The State University of New Jersey. Her roles provide support to students as they craft their capstone DNP project using quality improvement methods and tools and particularly managing data to demonstrate a change in practice. All three of Dr. Niedz' nursing degrees, BSN, MS, and PhD, are from Rutgers, The State University of New Jersey. She has held CPHQ certification in quality improvement since 1992 and provides consulting in quality and research methods through Quality Outcomes, LLC.

ALYSSA E. ERIKSON, PhD, MSN, RN, CNE, currently serves as Chair and Professor in the Department of Nursing at California State University Monterey Bay. She has taught in undergraduate and graduate nursing programs for the past 15 years. She holds the position of Campus Faculty Director for the Shiley Haynes Institute for Palliative Care and works toward improving community awareness and access to palliative care services and education. Her research and publications are in the areas of bereavement care and palliative care training for healthcare providers. Dr. Erikson received her BSN from California State University Chico and her MSN and PhD from University of California San Francisco.

POPULATION-BASED NURSING

CONCEPTS AND COMPETENCIES FOR ADVANCED PRACTICE

Fourth Edition

Ann L. Cupp Curley, PhD, RN

Barbara A. Niedz, PhD, RN, CPHQ

Alyssa E. Erikson, PhD, MSN, RN, CNE

Editors

SPRINGER PUBLISHING

Copyright © 2025 Springer Publishing Company, LLC

All rights reserved.

First Springer Publishing edition 9780826106711, 2012; 2016, 2020.

No part of this publication may be reproduced, stored in a retrieval system, or transmitted in any form or by any means, electronic, mechanical, photocopying, recording, or otherwise, without the prior permission of Springer Publishing Company, LLC, or authorization through payment of the appropriate fees to the Copyright Clearance Center, Inc., 222 Rosewood Drive, Danvers, MA 01923, 978-750-8400, fax 978-646-8600, info@copyright.com or at www.copyright.com.

Springer Publishing Company, LLC
www.springerpub.com
connect.springerpub.com

Acquisitions Editor: Joseph Morita
Content Development Editor: Lucia Gunzel
Production Editor: Joseph Stubenrauch
Compositor: Thomson Digital

ISBN: 978-0-8261-4376-1
ebook ISBN: 978-0-8261-4377-8
DOI: 10.1891/9780826143778

SUPPLEMENTS:

A robust set of instructor resources designed to supplement this text is located at http://connect.springerpub.com/content/book/978-0-8261-4377-8. Qualifying instructors may request access by emailing textbook@springerpub.com.

Instructor Materials:
LMS Common Cartridge With All Instructor Resources and Instructions for Use ISBN: 978-0-8261-4382-2
Instructor Manual ISBN: 978-0-8261-4378-5
Instructor PowerPoint Presentations ISBN: 978-0-8261-4379-2
Mapping to AACN Essentials: Core Competencies for Professional Nursing Education ISBN: 978-0-8261-4393-8
Transition Guide: Third Edition to Fourth Edition ISBN: 978-0-8261-4383-9

24 25 26 27 / 5 4 3 2 1

The author and the publisher of this Work have made every effort to use sources believed to be reliable to provide information that is accurate and compatible with the standards generally accepted at the time of publication. Because medical science is continually advancing, our knowledge base continues to expand. Therefore, as new information becomes available, changes in procedures become necessary. We recommend that the reader always consult current research and specific institutional policies before performing any clinical procedure or delivering any medication. The author and publisher shall not be liable for any special, consequential, or exemplary damages resulting, in whole or in part, from the readers' use of, or reliance on, the information contained in this book. The publisher has no responsibility for the persistence or accuracy of URLs for external or third-party Internet websites referred to in this publication and does not guarantee that any content on such websites is, or will remain, accurate or appropriate.

Cataloging information is available from the Library of Congress.

Contact sales@springerpub.com to receive discount rates on bulk purchases.

Publisher's Note: **New and used products purchased from third-party sellers are not guaranteed for quality, authenticity, or access to any included digital components.**

Printed in the United States of America.

This book is dedicated to all the nurses who worked on the front line of the COVID-19 pandemic, providing care and compassion in often treacherous conditions. Thank you.

ALCC, BAN, AEE

CONTENTS

Contributors xi
Foreword Linda Flynn, PhD, RN, FAAN xiii
Preface xv
Acknowledgments xxi
Springer Publishing Resources xxiii

1. **Introduction to Population-Based Nursing**   *1*
   Ann L. Cupp Curley
       Introduction   1
       Background   2
       Defining Populations   6
       Using Data to Target Populations and Aggregates at Risk   7
       Alcohol   7
       Obesity   8
       Health and the Social Environment   10
       Population Strategies in Acute Care   12
       Suicide   12
       Chronic Conditions   13
       Summary   15
       Exercises   17
       References   18

2. **Principles of Public and Community Health**   *21*
   Karen T. D'Alonzo
       Introduction   21
       Background   22
       Social Determinants of Health   24
       Objectives of Public Health   25
       Cost-Saving or Cost-Effective?   28
       Public Health Ethics   29
       Public Health Methods   35
       Summary   35
       Exercises and Discussion Questions   37
       References   38

3. **Identifying Outcomes in Population-Based Nursing**   *40*
   Alyssa E. Erikson
   - Introduction   40
   - Identifying and Defining Population Outcomes   41
   - National Healthcare Objectives   53
   - Summary   62
   - Exercises and Discussion Questions   63
   - References   64
   - Internet Resources   68

4. **Epidemiological Methods and Measurements in Population-Based Nursing Practice: Part I**   *69*
   Ann L. Cupp Curley
   - Introduction   69
   - The Natural History of Disease   70
   - Prevention   73
   - Causation   75
   - Methods of Analysis   76
   - Descriptive Studies   90
   - Analytic Epidemiology   92
   - Summary   100
   - Exercises and Discussion Questions   101
   - References   104

5. **Epidemiological Methods and Measurements in Population-Based Nursing Practice: Part II**   *107*
   Ann L. Cupp Curley
   - Introduction   107
   - Errors in Measurement   107
   - Confounding   112
   - Interaction   114
   - Randomization   114
   - Data Collection   115
   - Causality   116
   - Scientific Misconduct (Fraud)   118
   - Study Designs   119
   - Databases   123
   - Summary   124
   - Exercises and Discussion Questions   126
   - References   128

6. **Applying Evidence at the Population Level**   *130*
   Vera Kunte
   - Introduction   130
   - Asking the Clinical Question   131

The Literature Review   *135*
  Assessing the Evidence   *137*
  Integration of Evidence Into Practice   *149*
  Summary   *154*
  Exercises and Discussion Questions   *155*
  References   *155*

7. **Using Information Technology to Improve Population Outcomes**   **159**
  Laura P. Rossi and Alyssa E. Erikson
  Introduction   *159*
  Using Technology in Care Delivery for Populations   *160*
  Using Technology to Improve Care Delivery Processes   *162*
  Using Technology to Obtain Health Information   *165*
  Opportunities and Barriers to Using New Technology   *167*
  Electronic Resources That Support Population-Based Nursing   *173*
  Summary   *177*
  Exercises and Discussion Questions   *179*
  References   *179*

8. **Concepts in Program Design and Development**   **183**
  Laura P. Rossi
  Introduction   *183*
  Models for Program Design and Implementation   *183*
  Program Planning: Where to Start   *191*
  Sources of Data   *192*
  Program Design and Implementation   *200*
  Implementation   *203*
  Overcoming Barriers and Challenges   *206*
  Summary   *207*
  Exercises and Discussion Questions   *208*
  References   *208*

9. **Evaluation of Practice at the Population Level**   **211**
  Barbara A. Niedz
  Introduction   *211*
  Monitoring Healthcare Quality   *212*
  Summary   *237*
  Exercises and Discussion Questions   *238*
  References   *239*
  Internet Resources   *243*

10. **The Role of Accreditation and Certification in Validating Population-Based Practice/Programs**   **245**
  Gail M. Johnson
  Introduction   *245*
  Governmental Programs   *248*

Nongovernmental Programs   253
The Role of Advanced Practice Registered Nurses in Program Accreditation   258
Summary   259
Exercises   261
References   261
Internet Resources   262

11. Building Relationships and Engaging Communities Through Collaboration   **264**
Sonda M. Oppewal
Introduction   264
Foundation for Collaboration and Community Engagement   265
Community Health Assessment   269
Assessment Tools and Methods   271
Building Relationships   280
Summary   284
Exercises and Discussion Questions   285
References   286

12. Challenges in Program Implementation   **289**
Barbara A. Niedz
Introduction   289
Implementation Science   290
Lewin's Stages of Change   291
Rogers' Diffusion of Innovations Theory   293
The Reach, Adoption, Implementation, and Maintenance Model and the Practical Robust Implementation and Sustainability Model   295
Summary   300
Exercises   301
References   302

13. Implications of Global Health in Population-Based Nursing   **304**
Suzanne Willard and Vera Kunte
Core Competencies in Global Health   304
The United Nations Millennium Development Goals   324
Summary   331
Exercises   332
References   332

Index   337

CONTRIBUTORS

Ann L. Cupp Curley, PhD, RN, (Retired) Nurse Research Specialist, Capital Health, Trenton, New Jersey

Karen T. D'Alonzo, PhD, RN, APN-c, FAAN, Associate Professor, School of Nursing, Rutgers, The State University of New Jersey, New Brunswick, New Jersey

Alyssa E. Erikson, PhD, MSN, RN, CNE, Professor, Department of Nursing, California State University Monterey Bay, Seaside, California

Gail M. Johnson, EdD, RN, Director, Regulatory Affairs, Clinical Education, and Infection Prevention, Capital Health, Trenton, New Jersey

Vera Kunte, DNP, APN-C, CNE, Assistant Professor, California State University, Dominguez Hills, Carson, California

Barbara A. Niedz, PhD, RN, CPHQ, Assistant Professor, School of Nursing, Rutgers, The State University of New Jersey, Newark, New Jersey

Sonda M. Oppewal, PhD, MSN, RN, Professor Emeritus, The University of North Carolina at Chapel Hill School of Nursing, Chapel Hill, North Carolina

Laura P. Rossi, RN, PhD, Assistant Professor, Simmons University College of Natural, Behavioral, and Health Sciences, Boston, Massachusetts

Suzanne Willard, PhD, APN, FAAN, Professor Emeritus, School of Nursing, Rutgers, The State University of New Jersey, New Brunswick, New Jersey

FOREWORD

Nursing has a long and distinguished history of providing care to groups of people who, due to shared characteristics, are at risk for compromised health outcomes. Whether those groups of people were veterans suffering from chronic pain and posttraumatic stress disorders, lonely elders at risk for falls and medication errors, young mothers unsure of how to care for their newborns, or sedentary office workers whose lifestyles were silently shortening their lifespans, nurses have traditionally intervened with these and other populations to improve health and reduce health risks.

Fast forward to the 21st century in which advanced practice nurses are critical to the delivery of primary care across even broader sets of diverse populations. Hence, the union of population health and primary care presents the need for today's advanced practice nurse to acquire even more knowledge, more skills, more tools, more data, and more collaborations to design, implement, and evaluate population-specific, health-promoting interventions and programs. In short, today's advanced practice nurses need even more knowledge and tools to ensure that that they are effectively practicing population-based nursing.

Fortunately, the fourth edition of *Population-Based Nursing: Concepts and Competencies for Advanced Practice* provides a one-stop shop for today's advanced practice nurse. Starting with foundational principles of public health, community heath, and population-based nursing, chapters sequentially move to the more advanced principles of epidemiological methods and measures, population-level evidence, program design and evaluation, use of information technology, and the development of collaborative community-based relationships that can positively influence health policies.

This latest edition of *Population-Based Nursing: Concepts and Competencies for Advanced Practice* is a "must have" for seasoned advanced practice nurses and students, alike. The time is now; people and populations await; and advanced practice nurses must answer the call to provide primary care while working to improve health outcomes and reduce health risks for all.

Linda Flynn, PhD, RN, FAAN
Dean and Professor
Rutgers School of Nursing
Newark and New Brunswick, New Jersey

PREFACE

The original inspiration for this book grew out of the experience of teaching an epidemiology course for students enrolled in a doctorate in nursing practice (DNP) program. It was difficult to find a textbook that both addressed the course objectives and was relevant to nursing practice. The intention behind the first edition was to write a population-based nursing textbook, targeted for use as a primary course textbook in a DNP program or as a supplement to other course materials in a graduate community health nursing program. The chapters in the first through the third edition address the essential areas of content for a DNP program as recommended by the American Association of Colleges of Nursing (AACN), with a focus on the AACN core competencies for population-based nursing.

Nursing is an evolving profession, and the materials used to educate nurses must also evolve in order to address the needs of students. In this book, the fourth edition, we address the domains and competencies for advanced-level nursing education as recommended by the AACN, with a focus on Domain 3: Population Health. Our goals were to not only update the content of the existing chapters but also to add content that recognizes the broad role of advanced practice registered nurses (APRNs) in today's challenging healthcare environment. Two chapter authors have taken on the additional role of book editor for this edition; Barbara A. Niedz and Alyssa E. Erikson bring with them a wealth of knowledge and experience. A new chapter on the principles of public and community health has been added. In order to make it easier for readers to enhance their knowledge of the information that is covered in the book, we also decided to add case studies to the chapters. We use the title "advanced practice registered nurse" (APRN) which is the title used in *The Consensus Model for APRN Regulation, Licensure, Accreditation, Certification, and Education* (APRN Consensus Workgroup & National Council of State Boards of Nursing APRN Advisory Committee, 2008). This document is the product of the APRN Consensus Work Group and the National Council of State Boards of Nursing (NCSBN).

Several events covering a wide range of issues in the healthcare field have occurred over the past few years. One of those events stands out as an example of how the interconnected world in which we live can cause a global health emergency. The first indication that a new infectious disease had surfaced occurred in China in December of 2019. On January 20, 2020, the U.S. Centers for Disease Control and Prevention (CDC) reported the first laboratory-confirmed case of the 2019 Novel Coronavirus in the United States. In March 2020, the World Health Organization declared the COVID-19 outbreak a global pandemic. By April 2020, more than 1 million cases of COVID-19 had been confirmed worldwide. As of May 3, 2023, there were a reported 764,413,623 confirmed cases of COVID-19 in the United States and 6,915,273 deaths (CDC, 2023). The pandemic wreaked havoc in healthcare systems, global economies, and people's lives. It placed a spotlight on the problem of health disparities, as the disease disproportionately affected Black, Indigenous, Hispanic, and socially disadvantaged communities. It also revealed the danger of disinformation spread widely and rapidly through social media, which makes it difficult for many people to differentiate fact from fiction. This edition addresses the pandemic as well as other current issues in population-based nursing.

As in the first three editions, this textbook includes successful strategies that nurses have used to improve population outcomes and reinforces high-level application of activities that require the synthesis and integration of information learned. The goal is to provide readers with information that will help them to identify healthcare needs at the population level and improve population outcomes. In particular, Chapter 1, "Introduction to Population-Based Nursing," introduces the concept of population-based nursing and discusses examples of successful approaches and interventions to improve population health. Chapter 2, "Principles of Public and Community Health," is new to this edition. It introduces the reader to the basic principles of public health and community health nursing, explains the overall purpose of public health interventions, the ethical principles underlying such interventions, and, lastly, the various methods that APRNs can use to improve public health.

In order to design, implement, and evaluate interventions that improve the health of populations and aggregates, APRNs need to be able to identify and target outcome measures. Chapter 3, "Identifying Outcomes in Population-Based Nursing," explains how to define, categorize, and identify population outcomes using specific examples from practice settings. The identification of outcomes or key health indicators is an essential first step in planning effective interventions and is a requirement for evaluation. The chapter includes a discussion of nurse-sensitive indicators, *Healthy People 2030*, national health objectives, and health disparities. Emphasis is on the identification of healthcare disparities and approaches that can be used to eliminate or mitigate them. APRNs can advocate needed change at local, regional, state, or national levels by identifying areas for improvement in practice, by comparing evidence needed for effective practice, and by better understanding health disparities. APRNs have an important collaborative role with professionals from other disciplines and community members to work toward eliminating health disparities.

Epidemiology is the basic science of prevention (Celentano & Szklo, 2018). Evidence-based practice, as it relates to population-based nursing, combines clinical practice and public health using population health sciences in clinical practice (Heller & Page, 2002). Programs or interventions that are designed by APRNs should be evaluated and assessed for their effectiveness and ability to change or improve outcomes. This is true at an individual or population level. Data from these programs should be collected systematically and in such a manner that can be replicated in future programs. Data collection must be organized and analyzed using clearly defined outcomes developed early in the planning process. Best practice requires that data are not just collected; data must also be analyzed, interpreted correctly, and, if significant, put into practice. Understanding how to interpret and report data accurately is critical as it sets up the foundation for evidence-based practice. With that said, it is important to understand the basics of how to measure disease or outcomes, how to present these measures, and to know what types of measures are needed to analyze a project or intervention.

Chapter 4, "Epidemiological Methods and Measurements in Population-Based Nursing Practice: Part I," describes the natural history of disease and concepts that are integral to the prevention and recognition (e.g., screening) of disease. Basic concepts that are necessary to understand how to measure disease and design studies that are used in population-based research are discussed. Disease measures, such as incidence, prevalence, and mortality rates, are covered, and their relevance to practice is discussed. This chapter also includes information on primary, secondary, and tertiary prevention, and the concept of causality is introduced. A section on survival and prognosis is included. This material broadens the knowledge of readers with information necessary for advanced practice and interpretation of survival data. The basics of data analysis, including the calculation of relative risk, attributable risk, and odds ratio, are presented with examples of how to use these measures. Study design selection is an important part of the planning process for implementing a program. A portion of Chapter 4, "Epidemiological Methods and Measurements in Population-Based Nursing Practice: Part I," is dedicated to introducing the most common study designs because correct design selection is an essential part of sound methodology, successful program implementation, and overall success.

For APRNs to lead the field of evidence-based practice, it is critical that they possess skills in analytic methods to identify population trends and evaluate outcomes and systems of care (American Association of Colleges of Nursing [AACN], 2021). They need to carry out studies with strong methodology and be cognizant of factors that can affect study results. Identification and early recognition of factors that can affect the results or outcomes of a study, such as systematic errors (e.g., bias), should be acknowledged because they cannot always be prevented. In Chapter 5, "Epidemiological Methods and Measurements in Population-Based Nursing Practice: Part II," the APRN is introduced to the elements of bias with a comprehensive discussion of the complexities of data collection. More in-depth discussion of study designs is covered, as well as a comprehensive review of ways to report on randomized and nonrandomized studies. Critical components of data analysis are discussed, including causality, confounding, and interaction.

In order to provide care at an advanced level, nurses must incorporate the concepts and competencies of advanced practice into their daily practice. This requires that APRNs acquire the knowledge, tools, and resources to know when and how to integrate them into practice. In Chapter 6, "Applying Evidence at the Population Level," the APRN learns how to integrate and synthesize information in order to design interventions that are based on evidence to improve population outcomes. Nurses require several skills to become practitioners of evidence-based care. In this chapter, they learn how to identify clinical problems, recognize patient safety issues, compose clinical questions that provide a clear direction for study, conduct a search of the literature, appraise and synthesize the available evidence, and successfully integrate new knowledge into practice.

Information technologies are transforming the way that information is learned and shared. Online communities provide a place for people to support each other and share information. Online databases contain knowledge that can be assessed for information on populations and aggregates, and many websites provide up-to-date information on health and healthcare. Chapter 7, "Using Information Technology to Improve Population Outcomes," describes how technology can be used to enhance population-based nursing. It identifies websites that are available and how to evaluate them for quality. It also describes potential ways that technology can be used to improve population outcomes and how to incorporate technology into the development of new and creative interventions. APRNs use data to make decisions that lead to program development, implementation, and evaluation. In Chapter 8, "Concepts in Program Design and Development," the APRN learns how to design new programs using organizational theory. Nursing care delivery models that address organizational structure, process, and outcomes are described.

Oversight responsibilities for clinical outcomes at the population level are a critical part of advanced practice nursing. The purpose of Chapter 9, "Evaluation of Practice at the Population Level," is to identify ways and means to evaluate population outcomes and systems changes, as well as to address issues of effectiveness and efficiency and trends in care delivery across the continuum. Strategies to monitor healthcare quality are addressed, as are factors that lead to success. These concepts are explored within the role and competencies of the APRN.

The healthcare marketplace is extremely competitive. Administrators are constantly on the lookout to identify opportunities to differentiate and validate their organization. Achieving accreditation helps to validate programs and organizations in the context of national and professional standards. Chapter 10, "The Role of Accreditation and Certification in Validating Population-Based Practice/Programs," describes the role of the APRN in the accreditation process.

In order for APRNs to make decisions at the community level, APRNs who work in the community need to be part of the higher level of care management and policymaking and decision-making, in partnership with the community-based consortium of healthcare policymakers. Chapter 11, "Building Relationships and Engaging Communities Through Collaboration," describes the tools for successful community collaboration and project development. Emphasis is placed on identifying community needs and assessment of their resources. Specific examples are given to guide APRNs in developing their own community projects.

Chapter 12, "Challenges in Program Implementation," identifies barriers to change within communities and the importance of developing and sustaining community partnerships. Specific strategies for program implementation are discussed, as well as the methods to empower the community to advocate for themselves. Specific examples are given in order to guide APRNs in executing a project that has community acceptance and sustainability.

Finally, Chapter 13, "Implications of Global Health in Population-Based Nursing," explores the implications of global health for the APRN. Theories of global health, population health, and public/community health are differentiated and compared, to further the understanding of how environmental conditions (e.g., poverty, housing, access to care) affect the health status of individuals and groups. Recent patterns in international interdisciplinary collaborations are reviewed, including the global health competencies developed by the Association of Schools of Public Health (ASPH) and the AACN.

Ann L. Cupp Curley

REFERENCES

American Association of Colleges of Nursing. (2021). *AACN Essentials*. AACN. Retrieved 2/22/2023 from https://www.aacnnursing.org/DNP/DNP-Essentials

APRN Consensus Workgroup & National Council of State Boards of Nursing APRN Advisory Committee. (2008). *The consensus model for APRN regulation, licensure, accreditation, certification and education*. Retrieved from Report of the APRN Joint Dialogue Group Based on the Work of the APRN Consensus Group and the NCSBN APRN Committee

Celentano, D. D., & Szklo, M. (Eds.). (2018). *Gordis epidemiology* (6th ed.). Elsevier.

Centers for Disease Control and Prevention. (2023). *COVID data tracker*. Retrieved from CDC COVID Data Tracker: Home

Heller, R., & Page, J. (2002). A population perspective to evidence-based medicine: "Evidence for population health." *Journal of Epidemiology & Community Health*, 56(1), 45–47. https://doi.org/10.1136/jech.56.1.45

ACKNOWLEDGMENTS

We wish to express our thanks to those professional colleagues who provided direction, guidance, and assistance in writing this book. Thank you also to our family and friends for their support throughout this process. We give a very special thank you to our spouses for their unending patience and excellent advice. Thank you to our team at Springer Publishing Company, especially Lucia Gunzel, Senior Content Development Editor, for her valuable advice, assistance, and infinite patience; and to Joe Morita, Executive Content Strategist. Finally, a nod of appreciation goes to Erika Moncrief, MS, Director of Library Services at the Health Services Library of Capital Health, for her valuable assistance.

SPRINGER PUBLISHING RESOURCES

A robust set of instructor resources designed to supplement this text is located at http://connect.springerpub.com/content/book/978-0-8261-4377-8. Qualifying instructors may request access by emailing textbook@springerpub.com.

INSTRUCTOR RESOURCES

Available resources include:

- LMS Common Cartridge With All Instructor Resources and Instructions for Use
- Instructor Manual
    - Chapter Exercises and Discussion Questions/Answers
- Instructor PowerPoint Presentations
- Mapping to AACN Essentials: Core Competencies for Professional Nursing Education
- Transition Guide: Third Edition to Fourth Edition

SPRINGER PUBLISHING

Visit https://connect.springerpub.com/ and look for the **"Show Supplementary"** button on the book **homepage**.

CHAPTER 1

INTRODUCTION TO POPULATION-BASED NURSING

ANN L. CUPP CURLEY

INTRODUCTION

Some of the most significant figures in the history of nursing made their reputations by providing population-based care. Their influence on nursing has been such that their names live on, and their achievements continue to be recognized because of their important contributions to nursing and to healthcare. A brief look at the stories of some of these nurses helps to provide a background for understanding population health.

Although she started her career as a teacher, Clarissa (Clara) Barton won her greatest acclaim as a nurse. Horrified by the suffering of wounded soldiers in the American Civil War (many of them were former neighbors and students) and struck by the lack of supplies needed to care for them, she worked to obtain various supplies and put herself at great risk by nursing soldiers on the front lines of several major battles. Her experience would eventually lead to her becoming the founder and first president of the American Red Cross (Evans, 2003).

During the Crimean War, Florence Nightingale used statistical analysis to plot the incidence of preventable deaths among British soldiers. She used a diagram to dramatize the unnecessary deaths of soldiers caused by unsanitary conditions and lobbied political and military leaders in London for the need to reform. She worked to promote the idea that social phenomena could be objectively measured and subjected to mathematical analysis. Along with William Farr, she was one of the earliest healthcare practitioners to collect and analyze data in order to persuade people of the need for change in healthcare practices (Dossey, 2000; Lipsey, 1993).

Mary Breckinridge started the Frontier Nursing Service (FNS) in Kentucky in 1925 and remained its director until her death in 1965. Educated as a nurse and midwife, she devoted her life to improving health in rural areas, especially among women and children.

She believed in working with the communities that were served by the FNS and formed and worked with committees composed of community members to help plan and provide care. Similar to Florence Nightingale, she believed in the use of statistics to measure outcomes. From its onset, the FNS was so successful that there was an immediate drop in infant and maternal deaths in the communities served by the FNS (Martin, 2023).

These three nurses all worked to improve the health of at-risk populations. They met with political leaders to advocate changes in policies to benefit those populations, and both Nightingale and Breckinridge used statistical analysis to support the need for change and to evaluate their interventions. Breckinridge was an early advocate of engaging communities to help address community health issues. They were all pioneers of nursing and, although perhaps not in name, certainly in fact, among the first nurses working in advanced practice.

For decades, community health nurses have recognized the importance and the impact of population-based care, but large segments of nursing practice focused primarily on caring for individual patients. Nursing remains, and should remain, a practice-based and caring profession, but nursing practice has evolved. There is an awareness of the need to provide evidence-based care and to design interventions that have a broad impact on the populations that nursing serves, no matter the setting. Population health obligates healthcare professionals to implement standard interventions, based on the best research evidence, to improve the health of targeted groups of people. It also obligates nurses to discover new and effective strategies for providing care and promoting health. Although clinical decision-making related to individual patients is important, it has little impact on overall health outcomes for populations. Interventions at the population level have the potential to improve overall health across communities.

This book addresses the domains and competencies for advanced-level nursing education as recommended by the American Association of Colleges of Nursing (AACN), with a focus on Domain 3: Population Health. The goal is to provide readers with information that will help them to identify healthcare needs at the population level and to improve population outcomes. The intent is to broadly address practice issues that should be the concern of any nurse in an advanced practice role.

This chapter introduces the reader to the concept of population-based nursing. The reader learns how to identify population parameters, the potential impact of a population-based approach to care, and the importance of designing nursing interventions at the population level in advanced nursing practice.

BACKGROUND

For all the scare tactics out there, what's truly scary—truly risky—is the prospect of doing nothing.

—President Barack Obama, The New York Times, August 16, 2009

The first 2 decades of the 21st century were witness to a growing and contentious debate on healthcare reforms. President Barack Obama's stated goals in pushing for reforming health insurance were to extend healthcare coverage to the millions who lacked health insurance, stop the insurance industry's practice of denying coverage on the basis of preexisting conditions, and cut overall healthcare costs. Driven by a need for change in how healthcare is paid for, the Patient Protection and Affordable Care Act (ACA) was signed into law by President Obama in 2010. It went into effect over the span of 4 years, beginning in 2011. Currently, there are three different "markets" for insurance through the ACA. The federal marketplace is run solely by the federal government. The state marketplace is run solely by the state, and in partnership marketplaces, states run many of the important functions and make key decisions but the marketplace is operated by the federal government. The ACA includes an option that allows states to expand Medicaid eligibility to uninsured adults and children whose incomes are at or below 138% of the federal poverty level (there is also a provision for people living with mental illness).

Initial reaction to the ACA was mixed. A 2010 survey revealed that 40% of the American public held a favorable view of the legislation and 46% held an unfavorable view. In 2023, those numbers changed to 62% (favorable) and 36% (unfavorable) (KFF, 2023). The increase in the favorability response has been largely attributed to two very popular provisions of the ACA legislation: the provision that allows dependents, mostly children, to remain on their parents' insurance plan until their 26th birthday and the provision that insurers are prohibited from denying coverage to people with preexisting conditions. There have been several challenges to the ACA since its passage. Most recently (March 30, 2023), a judge in the U.S. District Court in the Northern District of Texas issued a final judgment in the case of Braidwood Management v. Becerra that challenged the provision of the ACA that requires the coverage of preventive care service. Because of an ACA requirement, most private health plans are required to cover a range of preventive services and cannot impose deductibles or co-pays for them. The ruling imposes new limits on the government's ability to enforce those requirements nationwide and applies specifically to services recommended by the U.S. Preventive Services Task Force (USPSTF) that were made after 2010 when the ACA was enacted. The ruling would not overturn all coverage requirements. For example, the ruling will not affect coverage for vaccines recommended by the Advisory Committee on Immunization Practices (ACIP), women's preventive health services (such as contraception, well women care, and prenatal care) recommended by the Health Resources and Services Administration (HRSA), or services for children and young adults recommended by Bright Futures, although that decision could be appealed. The ruling only applies to updates or new USPSTF recommendations. Any service that was first recommended by USPSTF after March 2010 (and is not also recommended by another group like HRSA or ACIP) would no longer be required to be covered without out-of-pocket costs (Levitt et al., 2023). It will take time to understand the full extent of the impact of this ruling. The contentious debate surrounding healthcare legislation and reform in the United States continues.

There is ample evidence of a need for healthcare reform in the United States. The *gross domestic product* (GDP) is the total market value of the output of labor and property located in the United States. It reflects the contribution of the healthcare sector relative to all other production in the United States. In 1960, the health sector's proportion (national health expenditure [NHE]) of the GDP was at 5% (i.e., $5 of every $100 spent in the United States went to pay for healthcare services). By 1990, this figure had grown to 12% and by 2021, 18.3%. The Centers for Medicare and Medicaid Services (CMS) published its forecast of healthcare costs for 2021 to 2030. The report projects that annual growth in national health spending will average 5.1% from 2021 to 2030 and will reach nearly $6.8 trillion by 2030. Growth in the nation's GDP is also projected to be 5.1% annually over the same period. As a result, the health share of GDP is expected to rise from 17.9% in 2017 to 19.4% by 2027 (CMS, 2023).

The Organization for Economic Cooperation and Development (OECD) provides a global picture of healthcare spending. It reports that U.S. expenditures for healthcare, as reflected by the GDP, are the highest among OECD countries; they are 8% higher than the average (with the GDP range for OECD countries spanning from a low of 8.7% for Italy to 11.7% for Germany). One interesting fact is that administrative costs in the United States are five times the average of other OECD countries (OECD, 2022).

The rising cost of healthcare is reflected in the insurance industry. According to the Henry J. Kaiser Family Foundation (KFF) (2022), the average annual premium for employer-sponsored family health coverage in 2017 was $18,687. This figure rose to $22,463 in 2022. The average annual contribution from employees was $5,218 in 2017 and $6,106 in 2022.

Unfortunately, although the United States ranks first in spending on healthcare among industrialized nations, it ranks lower than most industrialized countries in some important health indicators. The United States is one of 13 members of the OECD that are ranked as high-income countries. There are several commonly used indicators for measuring a country's health; two of these are infant mortality and life expectancy at birth. Of the 13 high-income OECD nations, the United States ranks last for life expectancy at birth (life expectancy at birth in the United States is 77 years) and last for infant mortality (infant mortality rate in the United States is 5.4 per 1,000 live births) (The Commonwealth Fund, 2023). Readers can refer to Chapter 13, "Implications of Global Health in Population-Based Nursing," for a more detailed description of how the United States ranks among other countries in relation to health indicators.

Health insurance is an important factor in any discussion about healthcare. The United States is the only industrialized country in the world without universal care. People who are uninsured are less likely than those who are insured to receive preventive care (KFF, 2019). The Commonwealth Fund, a private foundation whose stated mission is to promote a high-performing healthcare system, commissioned a survey of U.S. adults that was conducted by Princeton Survey Research Associates (Collins et al., 2011). The survey looked at the effect of health insurance coverage on healthcare-seeking behaviors. They found that among uninsured women aged 50 to 64, 48% say they did not see a doctor when they were sick, did not fill a prescription, or skipped a test, treatment, or follow-up visit because they could not afford it. The survey results also showed that only 67% of uninsured adult respondents had their blood pressure checked within the past year, compared to 91% of insured adults. Additionally, only 31% of uninsured women aged 50 to 64 reported having a mammogram in the past 2 years, compared to 79% of women with health insurance.

TABLE 1.1 Breakdown on Insurance Coverage for Children and Adults in 2022

	UNINSURED	PRIVATE COVERAGE	PUBLIC COVERAGE
Adults (18–64 years)	12.2%	67.8%	22%
Children (0–17 years)	4.2%	54.3%	43.7%

Source: Data from Cohen, R. A., & Cha, A. E. (2022, November). Health insurance coverage: Early release of estimates from the National Health Interview Survey, January–June 2022. National Center for Health Statistics. DOI: dx.doi.org/10.15620/cdc:121909

The ACA has had an impact on insurance rates. The National Health Interview Survey (NHIS) estimates the extent and quality of health insurance coverage for the U.S. civilian noninstitutionalized population. The number of uninsured adults decreased from 19.3% in 2013 to 18.4% during the first quarter of 2014 and to 8.4% in 2022. The 2022 results reveal that, for the most part, fewer adults are uninsured today compared to 2010, and the duration of coverage gaps people experience has shortened significantly. Table 1.1 provides a breakdown on insurance coverage for children and adults. For complete results of the survey, go to the Centers for Disease Control and Prevention's (CDC) Health Insurance Coverage: Estimates from the National Health Interview Survey at www.cdc.gov/nchs/nhis/healthinsurancecoverage.htm.

Differences in insurance rates are being observed based on the choices made by states as they relate to the ACA. In Medicaid expansion states, the percentage of uninsured adults decreased from 18.4% in 2013 to 6.6% in 2021. In non-expansion states, the percentage of uninsured adults decreased from 22.7% in 2013 to 12.7% in 2021 (Conway & Mykyta, 2022).

Enough time has passed since the enactment of the ACA that researchers have been able to examine the impact of Medicaid expansion on health outcomes. As of 2023, 41 states, including the District of Columbia, have opted to expand Medicaid (Massachusetts and Wisconsin, which are included in these numbers, expanded Medicaid before enactment of the ACA). Constantin and Wehby (2023) examined the effects of the 2014 ACA Medicaid expansion on infant mortality by race and ethnicity over the first 6 years. They compared expansion to non-expansion states and found that Medicaid expansions were associated with an overall decline in infant mortality by 0.37 deaths per 1,000 live births in 2019 in expansion states. They also identified a statistically significant decline in mortality of both Black and Hispanic infants in these states. Mazurenko et al. (2018) analyzed 77 published, peer-reviewed studies. They found expansion of Medicaid under the ACA was linked to increases in health coverage, use of health services, and quality of care. Among their findings was that health insurance gains were largest for adults without a college degree; use of primary care, mental health services, and preventive care among Medicaid enrollees went up; and reliance on EDs decreased. In another study, researchers found that counties in states where Medicaid expanded had four fewer deaths per 100,000 residents each year from cardiovascular causes after expansion, compared with counties in non-expansion states (Khatana et al., 2019).

A literature review is available from the KFF that summarizes evidence from 197 studies published between February 2020 and March 2021 on the impact of state Medicaid expansions under the ACA (Guth & Ammula, 2021). The authors report that overall findings generally show positive effects of Medicaid expansion, while a smaller number of studies find no impact of expansion on specific outcomes for specific populations. Very few studies suggest any negative effects. Among the positive effects they mention is that recent research finds largely positive impacts of expansion on coverage and access to care among populations with cancer, chronic disease, and/or disabilities. They also discovered a growing body of research that finds that Medicaid expansion has improved overall mortality rates, as well as mortality rates associated with some specific health conditions. For the complete report, go to Building on the Evidence Base: Studies on the Effects of Medicaid Expansion, February 2020 to March 2021 at files.kff.org/attachment/Report-Building-on-the-Evidence-Base-Studies-on-the-Effects-of-Medicaid-Expansion.pdf.

Our healthcare system is complex, and there is no simple solution to lowering costs and improving access. The goal of this textbook is not to provide an overarching solution to the issues of cost but to propose that nurses can contribute to improving the cost-effectiveness and efficiency of care, through the provision of evidence-based treatment guidelines to identified populations with shared needs and by advocating for policies that address the underlying factors that impact health and healthcare. To do this, we must change the way that we deliver healthcare and become politically active. In an ideal world, healthcare policies are created based on valid and reliable evidence and population need and demand. The ideal premise is that there is equitable distribution of healthcare services and that the appropriate care is given to the right people at the right time and at a reasonable cost. For more than 20 years, the American Nurses Association (ANA) has been advocating for healthcare reforms that would guarantee access to high-quality healthcare for all. It is a function of individual choice to either support or not support healthcare reforms. The actions of professional organizations are driven by membership. Regardless of your political alliance, involvement in professional organizations as well as in local, state, and national political activities (even if only minimally as a registered, active, and informed voter) is part of the professional responsibility of advanced practice registered nurses (APRNs).

DEFINING POPULATIONS

The AACN (2021) specifies that "population health spans the healthcare delivery continuum, including public health, acute care, ambulatory care, and long term care" (p. 33) and that graduates of advanced-level nursing education programs should collaborate with others to strive for equity in population health outcomes. Regardless of whether APRNs practice with a focus on clinical prevention or population health, the ability to define, identify, and analyze outcomes is imperative for improving the health status of individuals and populations.

The goal of population-based nursing is to provide evidence-based care to targeted groups of people with similar needs in order to improve outcomes. Population-based nursing uses a defined population or aggregate as the organizing unit for care. The Merriam-Webster Dictionary ("Population," 2019, para. 1) defines a *population* as "the whole number of people or inhabitants in a country or region." A second definition is given as "a body of persons or individuals having a quality or characteristic in common" (para. 1).

Subpopulations may be referred to as *aggregates*. Many different parameters can be used to identify or categorize subpopulations or aggregates. They may be defined by ethnicity (e.g., Black or Hispanic), religion (e.g., Roman Catholic or Muslim), or geographical location (e.g., Boston or San Diego). Aggregates can also be defined by age or occupation. People with a shared diagnosis (e.g., diabetes mellitus [DM]) or a shared risk factor (e.g., smoking) comprise other identifiable aggregates. Sometimes people may choose to describe themselves as members of a particular group (e.g., conservative or liberal). One person may belong to more than one such group (e.g., White, younger than 18 years, current smoker).

A community is composed of multiple aggregates. The most common aggregate used in population-based nursing is the high-risk aggregate. A high-risk aggregate is a subgroup or subpopulation of a community that shares a high-risk factor among its members, such as a high-risk health condition (e.g., congestive heart failure [CHF]) or a shared high-risk factor (e.g., living in a location with poor air and/or water quality). The aggregate concept can be used to target interventions to specific aggregates or subpopulations within a community. The implementation of standard or proven (evidence-based) strategies to prevent illness and/or improve the health of targeted groups of people can have the effect of ameliorating health problems at the population and/or aggregate level. Making change at the population level may impact the health of a community, not only in the present but also for generations to come. As we learn how to approach and target populations using evidence, we improve our chance of long-term success and can strive to make lifelong changes in the health of a group of people.

USING DATA TO TARGET POPULATIONS AND AGGREGATES AT RISK

The collection and analysis of data provides healthcare professionals and policymakers with a starting point for identifying, selecting, and implementing interventions that target specific populations and aggregates. Many of the leading causes of death in the United States are preventable. Cardiovascular disease (CVD) has been the leading cause of death among both men and women in the United States since 1950. On the basis of data from 2021, the CDC has identified, in descending order, the ten leading causes of death in the United States. They are heart disease, cancer, COVID-19, accidents (unintentional injuries), stroke (cerebrovascular diseases), chronic lower respiratory diseases, Alzheimer's disease, DM, chronic liver disease and cirrhosis, and renal diseases (CDC, 2023a). Several factors, such as the physical environment, healthcare systems, personal behaviors, and the social environment, can have a deleterious impact on individual and community health. The negative consequences of these factors are researched and well-documented.

ALCOHOL

Being informed about risky behaviors is of primary importance for APRNs to be effective in planning and delivering evidence-based education and in lobbying for changes to protect the public's health. Alcohol use disorder (AUD) is the fifth leading root cause of death in the United States. Excessive alcohol use was responsible for more than 140,000 deaths in the United States each year from 2015 to 2019 or more than 380 deaths per day. These deaths were mostly due to the health effects from drinking too much over time, such as various types of cancer, liver disease, and heart disease (CDC, 2022a). Alcohol consumption is linked to cancers of the mouth, esophagus, liver, breast, and colon. From 2013 to 2016, drinking alcohol was tied to more than 75,000 new diagnoses of cancer and almost 19,000 deaths from cancer each year (Goding Sauer et al., 2021). Alcohol abuse is also a drain on the U.S. economy. It is estimated that excessive alcohol consumption causes an annual loss of $249 billion (CDC, 2022a). From a global perspective, alcohol kills 3 million people annually (5.9% of all deaths) (WHO, 2023a).

Less than half of Americans recognize that alcohol is a leading cause of cancer (American Institute for Cancer Research [AICR], 2019). The link between alcohol consumption and cancer is dose related. The more alcohol is consumed, the higher the risk of cancer. To reduce the risk of developing these cancers, the American Cancer Society (ACS) recommends that men limit themselves to two alcoholic beverages per day and women to one. One drink is equivalent to 12 ounces of beer, 5 ounces of wine, or 1.5 ounces of distilled alcohol.

Wiseman et al. (2022) carried out a study to assess how often U.S. adults report discussions with their clinicians about the risks of alcohol and to examine the association between such discussions and awareness of alcohol as a risk factor for cancer. Less than half of adults reported discussing the harms of alcohol with a clinician seen during the year prior to the study. The authors report that discussing alcohol and its risks with patients was associated with higher awareness of the carcinogenic nature of alcohol, independent of other known correlates of awareness and irrespective of cancer status. Their results support the need to increase counseling about alcohol as a cancer risk factor in the general population.

As with any potential threat to health, education of our youth and adult populations regarding the deleterious effects of alcohol is paramount to reducing the potential alcohol-related morbidity and mortality. It is a health behavior that an APRN can attempt to modify by evidence-based prevention education. There is huge potential for cost savings by preventing alcohol-related illnesses, and it is important to recognize not only the direct effects of alcohol on health but also the indirect effects on family members, coworkers, friends, and society.

While education is an effective primary prevention strategy, APRNs should be aware of and support legislation that is designed to decrease alcohol abuse. The CDC lists several evidence-based legislative strategies that target excessive alcohol consumption. Among these are enhanced enforcement of laws prohibiting sales to minors, limiting days and hours of sales, and regulation of alcohol outlet density. For more information on preventing excessive alcohol use, go to the CDC's Preventing Excessive Alcohol Use at www.cdc.gov/alcohol/fact-sheets/prevention.htm.

OBESITY

In 2009, researchers published their analysis of the cost of obesity in the United States, taking into account separate categories for inpatient, outpatient, and prescription drug spending. They estimated that the medical costs of obesity may have been as high as

$147 billion/year by 2008 (including $7 billion in Medicare prescription drug costs). According to their findings, the annual medical costs for people who are obese were $1,429 higher than those for normal-weight people (Finkelstein et al., 2009). As the prevalence of obesity has increased in the United States, so too have the costs. In 2022, the CDC estimated that obesity costs the U.S. healthcare system nearly 173 billion dollars yearly (CDC, 2022b). A study conducted by Cawley et al. (2021) revealed that the annual medical care expenditures of adults with obesity ($5,010) were double that of people with normal weight ($2,504).

As part of *Healthy People 2030*, the United States has set a goal to reduce overweight and obesity by helping people eat healthy and get physical activity. There are a number of related objectives, such as reduce the proportion of children and adolescents with obesity (U.S. Department of Health and Human Services [HHS], 2023). *Healthy People 2030* uses the baseline of 17.8%, which was the percentage of persons aged 2 to 19 years of age who were obese in 2013 to 2016. The most recent data for this age group (2017–2020) shows this figure has increased to 19.7%. The 2030 goal is 15.5%. The baseline for adults is 38.6% (2013–2016). The most recent data for adults reveals that 41.8% are obese (2017–2020). This represents an increase from the *Healthy People* baseline. The 2030 target for adults is 36%. The highest rates were found among non-Hispanic Black adults (41.7%), followed by non-Hispanic Native American or Alaska Native adults (38.4%), Hispanic adults (36.1%), non-Hispanic White adults (31.0%), and non-Hispanic Asian adults (11.7%) (CDC, 2022b).

Obesity is associated with increased morbidity and mortality rates. Abdelaal et al. (2017) have summarized the most important comorbidities of obesity. They point out that obesity can cause both psychosocial (depression) and metabolic (DM) dysfunction and identified 13 specific domains that account for morbidity and mortality in obesity. CVD and cancer account for the greatest mortality risk associated with obesity even when controlling for demographic and behavioral characteristics. Although people are familiar with the association between heart disease and obesity, many are just learning about the relationship between obesity and cancer. Obesity is associated with an increased risk for many cancers, including esophageal, pancreatic, colon and rectal, breast (after menopause), endometrial, kidney, thyroid, and gallbladder. According to research from the AICR (2019), excess body weight is thought to be responsible for about 8% of all cancers in the United States, as well as about 7% of all cancer deaths.

One cannot talk about the epidemic of obesity and not mention its concomitant relationship to DM. The number of American adults treated for DM more than doubled between 1996 and 2007 (from about 9 to 19 million). According to the CDC (2023a), in 2019, 37.3 million Americans (about one in ten) had DM. About 1.4 million new cases of DM were diagnosed during that 1-year time period. For people aged 10 to 19 years, new cases of type 2 DM increased for all racial and ethnic minority groups, especially Black teens. DM was highest among Black and Hispanic/Latino adults, in both men and women. In the United States, medical costs and lost work and wages amounted to an estimated $327 billion. This information highlights the importance of tracking morbidity rates and the need to be aware of trends in order to target groups for intervention.

The rise in both incidence and prevalence rates for DM is closely tied to rising obesity levels, which is a preventable risk factor. This upward trend in the incidence rate for DM provides a clear direction for targeting prevention measures toward younger populations. There is, in fact, a huge potential for improving the health of populations by targeting children using primary prevention measures that go well beyond reducing DM rates. Implications for early interventions beginning in pregnancy and continuing through infancy and early childhood are clear. Evidence is increasing that early feeding patterns (e.g., breastfeeding versus formula feeding), as well as parental obesity and parental eating patterns, are linked to the increased likelihood of developing obesity in children, which puts them at an increased risk for type 2 DM (Dubois et al., 2022; Webber-Ritchey et al., 2023). There are many opportunities for APRNs to apply evidence-based, primary prevention interventions to improve the long-term outcomes of children at the beginning of pregnancy and at birth and thereafter. This approach may include targeting high-risk aggregates (e.g., parents with obesity and type 2 DM) and then expanding to communities through educational campaigns or changes in health policy.

HEALTH AND THE SOCIAL ENVIRONMENT

Most of the information discussed earlier exemplifies the biological and environmental factors that contribute to poor health in adults. However, it is becoming more apparent that social (e.g., psychological) factors starting as early as conception (e.g., maternal stress) may play a more significant role in adult health than was once thought. Having a comprehensive understanding of the underlying causes of adult diseases (including social, psychological, biological, and environmental) is necessary to successfully approach the problems seen in populations. Without this comprehensive understanding, it may be difficult to successfully implement a primary prevention program (the goal of which is to prevent disease before it occurs).

Stress is a regular part of day-to-day life, and small amounts of stress are normal and necessary for developing coping skills. However, exposure to prolonged and severe stressors, such as abuse, neglect, or being a witness to or victim of violence, can lead to changes that occur in the brain and can lead to short-term and even long-term poor health outcomes. This type of stress is termed *toxic stress*. The effects of toxic stress are being rigorously studied, and in particular, studies looking at adverse childhood experiences (ACEs) were some of the first to show a correlation between toxic stress exposures and high-risk behaviors and poor health outcomes in adults. The ACE study is an ongoing, joint project of the CDC and Kaiser Permanente that looks retrospectively at the relationships among several categories of childhood trauma. Childhood trauma exposures are broken down into three categories: abuse (e.g., physical or sexual), neglect (e.g., emotional or physical), and household dysfunction (e.g., having an incarcerated household member, family member with mental health issue and/or drug and alcohol problems, domestic violence, or parental divorce or separation). An ACE score is calculated based on past exposures to the subparts of each of the aforementioned categories.

The higher the ACE score, the stronger the relationship to high-risk behaviors and/or poor health outcomes (CDC, 2021). In the original ACE study (Felitti et al., 1998), people who experienced a score of four or more categories of ACEs, compared with those who had no history of exposure, had a four- to twelvefold increased risk for alcoholism, drug abuse, depression, and suicide attempts. They also experienced a two- to fourfold increase in smoking and self-reported poor health. Subsequent research provides additional evidence to support the link between childhood trauma and adverse events and poor health outcomes. For additional information on the effects of childhood stress, as well as strategies to prevent toxic stress, refer to the CDC publication at www.cdc.gov/violenceprevention/aces/fastfact.html.

Many additional studies have been conducted that demonstrate the destructive effects of exposure to toxic stress. Seon et al. (2021) completed a study of college students at seven universities. They examined the relationships among ACEs, intimate partner violence (IPV) victimization, and three adulthood health outcomes: perceived physical and mental health and depression. Their findings suggest that exposure to toxic stress in childhood influences young adult physical and mental health through IPV victimization. The study highlights the impact of childhood trauma on different health consequences, including intimate partner relationships, perceived physical and mental health, and depression. Childhood adverse events have also been linked to drug abuse and dependence (van Zyl et al., 2023) and to chronic pain and mood disorders (Antoniou et al., 2023). McKelvey et al. (2019) examined the associations between ACEs in infancy and toddlerhood and obesity and related health indicators in middle childhood. Across all outcomes examined, children with four or more ACEs had the poorest health and were more likely to be obese when compared to children with no ACE exposure.

Researchers have identified similar outcomes in studies carried out with populations in other countries. A study conducted in Saudi Arabia, where beating and insults are often an acceptable parenting style, identified a correlation between beating and insults (once or more per month) and an increased risk for cancer, cardiac disease, and asthma (Hyland et al., 2012). A large-scale, cross-sectional study of college students in China revealed a relationship between childhood sexual abuse, post-traumatic stress disorder (PTSD), and other psychiatric symptoms (Jin et al., 2022). A descriptive cross-sectional study conducted in Nepal revealed that emotional neglect during childhood and depression were independent predictors of poor quality of life (Dhungana et al., 2022).

More and more studies are being conducted to look at the relationship of sustained exposure to toxic stress to a variety of poor health outcomes and high-risk behaviors. These behaviors include such things as cutting, hypervigilance, promiscuity, eating disorders, poor school performance, depression, violence, suicidal ideation/attempts, and justice system involvement. These are just a few of the many behaviors found to be associated with sustained exposure to toxic stress. Studies such as these illustrate the importance of understanding the social determinants of poor health and the potential for doing good and preventing harm to aggregates and populations by targeting exposures to such things as child abuse and neglect for prevention, early recognition, and intervention. They also provide evidence of the importance of supporting public policies and legislation designed to prevent child abuse.

POPULATION STRATEGIES IN ACUTE CARE

Targeting evidence-based interventions toward aggregates in the acute care population also has the potential to improve health outcomes broadly. How can we improve the quality of care for our acute care patients by taking a population-based approach? When nurses apply evidence-based interventions to identified aggregates, they can improve outcomes more effectively than when interventions are designed on a case-by-case (individualized) basis.

Healthcare organizations, whether they are hospitals or more broadly based systems, have prided themselves on the use of evidence that can result in improved outcomes. AACN's fourth domain is entitled *Scholarship for the Nursing Discipline* (AACN, 2023) and advances the use of research in practice. The domains are intended to pervade nursing education from the Baccalaureate to the Doctor of Nursing Practice (DNP) and the Doctor of Philosophy (PhD). All levels have responsibility with regard to shaping nursing practice based on the highest form of evidence, nursing research. The advent of the American Nurses Credentialing Center's (ANCC) Magnet award, which demonstrates excellence in nursing practice (ANCC, 2023) for hospitals, requires a similar demonstration. Organizations must demonstrate *exemplary professional practice, new knowledge, innovation, and improvement* as well *as empirical quality results*. Thus, the influence of research to craft evidence-based interventions ultimately informs nursing practice and results in better outcomes for patients. See also Chapter 9, "Evaluation of Practice at the Population Level," and Chapter 10, "The Role of Accreditation in Validating Population-Based Practice/Programs," for more specific examples of how research influences practice to reduce error and to improve outcomes.

SUICIDE

Suicide is the 11th leading cause of death in the United States and the third leading cause of death for Americans aged 15 to 24. The highest rates (per 100,000) are among White males (26.4%), Native American/Alaska Native males (23%), and Black males (14.1%). Among age groups, the highest suicide rate is for people 85 and older (22.4%). Firearms are the most common method used (more than 50%). One suicide attempt is made in the United States every 26.2 seconds. It is estimated that one death occurs for every five attempts (SAVE, 2023). Suicide rates in the United States increased almost every year between 2001 (10.7) and 2021 (14.1) (CDC, 2023c). In 2021, for every suicide death, there were three hospitalizations for self-harm and eight emergency room visits (CDC, 2023d). Suicide and suicide attempts impact the emotional and physical health of survivors as well as their family, friends, coworkers, and community. It also has an economic cost. Suicides and suicide attempts cost the nation almost $70 billion per year in medical and work-related costs alone (CDC, 2023d).

Suicide prevention is an objective of *Healthy People 2023* and a National Patient Safety Goal (#15) of The Joint Commission (TJC). Betz et al. (2016) identify ED as prime locations for identifying individuals at risk for suicide and for initiating effective interventions. They present several recommendations including the universal or targeted screening of ED patients and the training of ED providers. A study by Dunlap et al. (2019) was carried out to determine whether the increased costs of implementing screening and intervention in hospital (EDs) are justified by improvements in patient outcomes (decreased attempts and deaths by suicide). Their findings revealed that the average cost per patient for a participating ED of universal screening plus intervention was $1,063 per month, approximately $500 more than universal screening added to treatment as usual. Universal screening plus intervention was more effective in preventing suicides compared to no screening and treatment as usual.

Identifying patients at risk for suicide and designing evidence-based interventions to prevent suicide are a way for APRNs to improve patient care and outcomes. Two excellent resources are the CDC at www.cdc.gov/suicide/prevention/index.html and the Suicide Prevention Resource Center, located at www.sprc.org/edguide.

CHRONIC CONDITIONS

Noncommunicable diseases (NCDs) are the main cause of illness and disability in the United States and are responsible for the greater part of healthcare costs according to the CDC. About 60% of U.S. adults have at least one chronic condition, and 40% have two or more chronic conditions. Most chronic conditions result from preventable risk factors such as smoking, poor diet, sedentary behavior, and excessive alcohol consumption (CDC, 2023e). The National Center for Chronic Disease Prevention and Health Promotion (NCCDPHP) falls under the purview of the CDC. The goal of the NCCDPHP is to reduce the risk factors for chronic diseases, especially for groups affected by health disparities which are differences in health across different geographical, racial, ethnic, and socioeconomic groups (CDC, 2023f). To this end, the NCCDPHP works to:

- Find out how chronic diseases affect populations in the United States
- Study interventions to find out what works best to prevent and control chronic diseases
- Fund and guide states, territories, cities, and tribes to use interventions that work
- Share information to help Americans understand risk factors for chronic diseases and how to reduce them

The problem of chronic diseases is not restricted to the United States. Chronic diseases, such as heart disease, stroke, cancer, chronic respiratory diseases, and DM, are the leading causes of global mortality. The World Health Organization (WHO) estimates that NCDs kill 41 million people each year and account for 71% of deaths worldwide. Nearly 15 million people between the ages of 30 and 69 die each year from NCDs; of these, 85% are from low-income counties (WHO, 2023b). Modifiable risk factors such as smoking, sedentary behavior, alcohol consumption, and unhealthy diets increase the risk of NCDs. Food insecurity, lack of clean water, poverty, and air pollution are contributing factors that, while modifiable, are out of the control of individuals. The WHO promotes several actions to reduce NCD, including banning smoking in public places, enforcing tobacco advertising bans, restricting access to alcohol, and reducing added sugars in foods as well as salt in food. All these actions require a population approach to be effective (WHO, 2023b).

Various surveys lend an interesting perspective to this issue. The American Heart Association (AHA) surveyed 1,000 people in the United States and found that only 30% of respondents knew the AHA's recommended limits for daily wine consumption. Drinking too much alcohol of any kind can increase blood pressure and lead to heart failure. The survey results also found that most respondents do not know the source of sodium content in their diets and are confused by low-sodium food choices. A majority of the respondents (61%) believe that sea salt is a low-sodium alternative to table salt when in fact it is chemically the same (AHA, 2011). A survey conducted in 2019 by the American Institute for Cancer Research (AICR) revealed that less than 50% of Americans recognize that alcohol; diets high in red meat; diets low in vegetables, fruits, and fiber; and insufficient physical activity are all linked to cancer (AICR, 2019). These surveys reinforce the idea that people require more understanding of nutrition and the relationship between nutrition and health. They also reinforce the argument that interventions to improve health must be addressed at the community or population level.

Interventions that are evidence based and population appropriate can reduce the underlying causes of chronic disease. This approach has the potential to lower the mean level of risk factors and shift outcomes in a favorable direction. An example that receives a lot of attention is sodium intake. Excess sodium in the diet can put people at risk for stroke and heart disease. The CDC has reported that nine of ten Americans consume more salt than is recommended. Only 5.5% of adults follow the recommendation to limit sodium intake to less than 2,300 mg a day. Most sodium does not come from salt added to foods at the table but from processed foods. These foods include grain-based frozen meals, soup, and processed meat. Sodium content can vary across brands, making it difficult to monitor intake. A cheeseburger from a fast-food restaurant, for example, can have between 370 mg and 730 mg of sodium. Reducing dietary salt could greatly reduce the yearly number of U.S. cases of coronary heart disease, stroke, and heart attacks, with a savings of up to $18 billion in healthcare costs each year (CDC, 2023g).

This discussion illustrates the need to promulgate laws and develop policies that can affect positive health outcomes. It also illustrates the difficulty involved in planning interventions when evidence is sometimes contradictory, and causation is not only multifactorial but sometimes outside of the control of the people whose health is compromised. Changing individual behavior is difficult and has little impact on population health. Using the power of legislation and regulation to make changes in the environment, such as banning smoking in public places, improving air quality, and reducing the amount of sodium in processed foods, has enormous potential for improving the overall health of populations.

The basic sciences of public health (particularly epidemiology and biostatistics) provide tools for the APRN working with specialized populations and the means to find evidence for effective and efficient interventions. The care of specialized groups is the core of advanced practice. The ANA (2023) provides a simple but straightforward definition of evidence-based practice: "Evidence-based practice in nursing involves providing holistic, quality care based on the most up-to-date research and knowledge rather than traditional methods, advice from colleagues, or personal beliefs" (para. 1).

Population-based nursing requires APRNs to plan, implement, and evaluate care in the population of interest. The evaluation of outcome measures in populations begins with an identification of the health problems, the needs of defined populations, and the differences among groups. The rates calculated from these numbers can help the APRN to identify risk factors, target populations at risk, and lay the foundation for designing interventions. Prevention is best carried out at the population level, whether at the level of direct care or through the support and promotion of policies. For example, an evidence-based program to prevent hospital readmissions for CHF can lead to improved health and decreased health-related costs. The promulgation of policies and regulations to support primary prevention measures, such as decreased sodium in prepared foods, could potentially lead to decreased rates of hypertension and heart disease. Interventions that are appropriate at the individual level and applied at the population level can result in a far-reaching effect.

Outcomes research in APRN practice is research that focuses on the effectiveness of nursing interventions. Outcomes measurement in population-based care begins with the identification of the population and the problem, followed by the generation of a clinical question related to outcomes. It is a measure of the process of care. An outcomes measure should be clearly quantifiable, be relatively easy to define, and lend itself to standardization.

In outcomes measurement, the APRN is ultimately concerned with whether a population benefits from an intervention. The APRN also needs to be concerned with the question of quality, efficacy (i.e., does the intervention work under ideal conditions?), and effectiveness (i.e., does it work under real-life situations?). Other important considerations are efficiency (cost benefit), affordability, accessibility, and acceptability.

SUMMARY

The Robert Wood Johnson Foundation and the Institute of Medicine (IOM) issued a report to respond to the need to transform the nursing profession. The committee developed four key messages:

1. Nurses should practice to the full extent of their education and should achieve higher levels of education and training.
2. The education system for nurses should be improved so that it provides seamless academic progression.
3. Nurses should be full partners with physicians and other healthcare professionals.
4. Healthcare in the United States should be redesigned for effective workforce planning and policymaking. (IOM, 2011)

To improve population health, APRNs need to practice to the full extent of their education, be active in the political arena, and work collaboratively with other healthcare professionals. To promote health, APRNs can use epidemiological methods to identify aggregates at risk, analyze problems of highest priority, design evidence-based interventions, and evaluate the results. An important concept in the field of population health is attention to the multiple determinants of health outcomes and the identification of their distribution throughout the population. These determinants include medical care, public health interventions, characteristics of the social environment (e.g., income, education, employment, social support, culture), physical environment (e.g., housing, air, and water quality), genetics, and individual behavior. A final note about the use of "APRN" in this book: *The Consensus Model for APRN Regulation: Licensure, Accreditation, Certification and Education* was completed and published in 2008 by the APRN Consensus Work Group and the National Council of State Boards of Nursing (NCSBN) APRN Advisory Committee. The title "APRN" is used throughout this book to refer to certified nurse anesthetists, certified nurse midwives, clinical nurse specialists, and certified nurse practitioners. The model was created through a collaborative effort of more than 40 organizations. The original goal for implementation of the model was 2015. As of 2023, many states have adopted portions of the model but there are variations from state to state. APRNs can check the status of the model in their state by going to www.nursecompact.com (NCSBN, 2023).

END-OF-CHAPTER RESOURCES

EXERCISES

EXERCISE 1.1 Using Table 1.2 as an example, list the parameters that describe the population(s) to whom you provide care.

EXERCISE 1.2 PolitiFact is a website created by the *St. Petersburg Times* (now the *Tampa Bay Times*) and a winner of the 2009 Pulitzer Prize (www.politifact.com). It was created to help people find the truth in American politics. PolitiFact is owned by the nonprofit Poynter Institute for Media Studies. In 2018, ownership of PolitiFact was transferred from the *Times* to Poynter, which is the newspaper's parent company. The move allows PolitiFact to function fully as a not-for-profit national news organization. Reporters and editors from across the United States check statements by members of Congress, the White House, lobbyists, and interest groups and rate them on a *Truth-O-Meter*. Find a statement that is being circulated about COVID-19, and then check the Truth-O-Meter to determine the veracity of the statement.

EXERCISE 1.3 Identify two or three population-based and health-related interventions at your institution or in your community. Determine whether the approach has been successful in changing outcomes and/or reducing health-related costs. Identify the aggregate population and what parameters were used in this intervention. Identify any changes in policy associated with these interventions.

EXERCISE 1.4 This chapter includes a description of the health effects of alcohol. Design an educational program for teens that addresses the negative health effects of alcohol. First, research the health effects of alcohol and select three to five health effects to address. Identify your target population and design an educational intervention for your target population. What outcomes will you look at to determine whether your intervention works? What approach will you use to engage your target population? How does your state regulate the purchase of alcohol? What more could your state do?

TABLE 1.2 Example Population Parameters

POPULATION	FRAMING DEFINITIONS	PARAMETERS
Patients who have been diagnosed with CHF and who live in the community	Adult (18 years of age and older) patients discharged from an urban medical center with a primary diagnosis of CHF	P1 = diagnosis P2 = age P3 = location/service area
Population of New Jersey	All permanent residents of New Jersey	P1 = geographical location P2 = permanent residency

CHF, congestive heart failure.

EXERCISE 1.5 The relationship between obesity and cancer is described and discussed in this chapter. Conduct a search to answer the following questions. The incidence rates for six cancers associated with obesity are increasing in young Americans. Identify them. What is the prevalence rate of obesity in people younger than 18 in your state? Which children are at highest risk for obesity in your state? Are there any prevention programs in your state that address this issue? Are they effective? Has your state passed and enacted any laws designed to decrease obesity? Are they effective? If they are not effective, explain why you believe they are not working.

> A robust set of instructor resources designed to supplement this text is located at http://connect.springerpub.com/content/book/978-0-8261-4377-8. Qualifying instructors may request access by emailing textbook@springerpub.com.

REFERENCES

Abdelaal, M., le Roux, C. W., & Docherty, N. G. (2017). Morbidity and mortality associated with obesity. *Annals of Translational Medicine, 5*(7), 161. https://doi.org/10.21037/atm.2017.03.107

American Association of Colleges of Nursing. (2021). *The essentials: Core competencies for professional nursing education.* Author. Retrieved from https://www.aacnnursing.org/Essentials

American Heart Association. (2011). *Most Americans don't understand health effects of wine and sea salt, survey finds.* Author. Retrieved from https://www.prnewswire.com/news-releases/most-americans-dont-understand-health-effects-of-wine-and-sea-salt-survey-finds-120595304.html

American Institute for Cancer Research. (2019). *2019 AICR cancer risk awareness survey*. Retrieved from https://www.aicr.org/assets/can-prevent/docs/2019-Survey.pdf

American Nurses Association. (2023). *What is evidence-based practice in nursing?* Retrieved from https://www.nursingworld.org/practice-policy/nursing-excellence/evidence-based-practice-in-nursing/

Antoniou, G., Lambourg, E., Steele, J. D., & Colvin, L. A. (2023). The effect of adverse childhood experiences on chronic pain and major depression in adulthood: A systematic review and meta-analysis. *British Journal of Anaesthesia, 130*(6), 729–746. https://doi.org/10.1016/j.bja.2023.03.008

Betz, M. E., Wintersteen, M., Boudreaux, E. D., Brown, G., Capoccia, L., Currier, G., Goldstein, J., King, C., Manton, A., Stanley, B., Moutier, C., & Harkavy-Friedman, J. (2016). Reducing suicide risk: Challenges and opportunities in the emergency department. *Annals of Emergency Medicine, 68*(6), 758–765. https://doi.org/10.1016/j.annemergmed.2016.05.030

Cawley, J., Biener, A., Meyerhoefer, C., Ding, Y., Zvenyach, T., Smolarz, B. G., & Ramasamy, A. (2021). Direct medical costs of obesity in the United States and the most populous states. *Journal of Managed Care & Specialty Pharmacy, 27*(3), 354–366. https://doi.org/10.18553/jmcp.2021.20410

Centers for Disease Control and Prevention. (2021). *Adverse childhood experiences (ACE)*. Retrieved from https://www.cdc.gov/violenceprevention/aces/index.html

Centers for Disease Control and Prevention. (2022a). *Deaths from excessive alcohol use in the United States*. Retrieved from https://www.cdc.gov/alcohol/features/excessive-alcohol-deaths.html

Centers for Disease Control and Prevention. (2022b). *Overweight and obesity*. Retrieved from Why It Matters | Overweight & Obesity | CDC

Centers for Disease Control and Prevention. (2023a). *Leading causes of death*. Retrieved from https://www.cdc.gov/nchs/fastats/leading-causes-of-death.htm

Centers for Disease Control and Prevention. (2023b). *Diabetes*. Retrieved from https://www.cdc.gov/diabetes/library/spotlights/diabetes-facts-stats.html#:~:text=37.3%20million%20Americans%E2%80%94about%201,t%20know%20they%20have%20it

Centers for Disease Control. (2023c). *Suicide and self-harm*. Retrieved from https://www.cdc.gov/nchs/fastats/suicide.htm

Centers for Disease Control. (2023d). *Facts about suicide*. Retrieved from https://www.cdc.gov/suicide/facts/index.html

Centers for Disease Control. (2023e). *NCCDPHD.* Retrieved from https://www.cdc.gov/chronicdisease/index.htm

Centers for Disease Control and Prevention. (2023f). *NCCDPHD: About the center.* Retrieved from https://www.cdc.gov/chronicdisease/center/index.htm

Centers for Disease Control and Prevention. (2023g). *Sodium intake and health.* Retrieved from https://www.cdc.gov/salt/index.htm

Centers for Medicare & Medicaid Services. (2023). *NHE fact sheet.* Retrieved from https://www.cms.gov/research-statistics-data-and-systems/statistics-trends-and-reports/nationalhealthexpenddata/nhe-fact-sheet

Collins, S., Doty, M., Robertson, R., & Garber, T. (2011). *How the recession has left millions of workers without health insurance, and how health reform will bring relief: Findings from the Commonwealth Fund Biennial Health Insurance Survey of 2010.* Retrieved from https://www.commonwealthfund.org/publications/fund-reports/2011/mar/help-horizon-how-recession-has-left-millions-workers-without

Constantin, J., & Wehby, G. L. (2023). Effects of recent medicaid expansions on infant mortality by race and ethnicity. *American Journal of Preventive Medicine, 64*(3), 377–384. https://doi.org/10.1016/j.amepre.2022.09.026

Conway, D., & Mykyta. L. (2022, September 15). *Decline in share of people without health insurance driven by increase in public coverage in 36 states.* U.S. Census Bureau. Retrieved from Uninsured Rate Declined in 28 States 2019-2021 (census.gov)

Dhungana, S., Koirala, R., Ojha, S. P., & Thapa, S. B. (2022). Association of childhood trauma, and resilience, with quality of life in patients seeking treatment at a psychiatry outpatient: A cross-sectional study from Nepal. *PLoS One, 17*(10), e0275637. https://doi.org/10.1371/journal.pone.0275637

Dossey, B. (2000). *Florence Nightingale: Mystic, visionary, healer.* Springhouse Corporation.

Dubois, L., Feng, C., Bédard, B., Yu, Y., Luo, Z.-C., Marc, I., & Fraser, W. D. (2022). Breast-feeding, rapid growth in the first year of life and excess weight at the age of 2 years: The 3D cohort study. *Public Health Nutrition, 25*(12), 1–11. https://doi.org/10.1017/S1368980022000015

Dunlap, L. J., Orme, S., Zarkin, G. A., Arias, S. A., Miller, I. W., Camargo, C. A., Jr, Sullivan, A. F., Allen, M. H., Goldstein, A. B., Manton, A. P., Clark, R., & Boudreaux, E. D. (2019). Screening and intervention for suicide prevention: A cost-effectiveness analysis of the ED-SAFE interventions. *Psychiatric Services 70*(12), 1082–1087. https://doi.org/10.1176/appi.ps.201800445

Evans, G. D. (2003). Clara Barton: Teacher, nurse, Civil War heroine, founder of the American Red Cross. *International History of Nursing Journal, 7*(3), 75–82.

Felitti, V., Anda, R., Nordenberg, D., Williamson, D., Spitz, A., Edwards, V., . . . Marks, J. (1998). Relationship of childhood abuse and household dysfunction to many of the leading causes of death in adults: The adverse childhood experiences (ACE) study. *American Journal of Preventative Medicine, 14,* 245–258. https://doi.org/10.1016/s0749-3797(98)00017-8

Finkelstein, E., Trogdon, J., Cohen, J., & Dietz, W. (2009). Annual medical spending attributable to obesity: Payer-and service-specific estimates. *Health Affairs, 28*(5), w822–w831. https://doi.org/10.1377/hlthaff.28.5.w822

Goding Sauer, A., Fedewa, S. A., Bandi, P., Minihan, A. K., Stoklosa, M., Drope, J., Gapstur, S. M., Jemal, A., & Islami, F. (2021). Proportion of cancer cases and deaths attributable to alcohol consumption by US state, 2013–2016. *Cancer Epidemiology, 71*(Pt A), 101893. https://doi.org/10.1016/j.canep.2021.101893

Guth, M., & Ammula, M. (2021, May). *Building on the evidence base: Studies on the effects of Medicaid expansion, February 2020 to March 2021.* Retrieved from the KFF website: https://www.kff.org/medicaid/report/building-on-the-evidence-base-studies-on-the-effects-of-medicaid-expansion-february-2020-to-march-2021/

Hyland, M. E., Alkhalaf, A. M., & Whalley, B. (2012). Beating and insulting children as a risk for adult cancer, cardiac disease and asthma. *Journal of Behavioral Medicine, 36*(6), 632–640. https://doi.org/10.1007/s10865-012-9457-6

Institute of Medicine. (2011). *Initiative on the future of nursing.* Retrieved from http://www.thefutureofnursing.org/recommendations

Jin, Y., Xu, S., Wang, Y., Li, H., Wang, X., Sun, X., & Wang, Y. (2022). Associations between PTSD symptoms and other psychiatric symptoms among college students exposed to childhood sexual abuse: A network analysis. *European Journal of Psychotraumatology, 13*(2), 2141508. https://doi.org/10.1080/20008066.2022.2141508

Kaiser Family Foundation. (2022). *2022 Employer health benefits survey*. Retrieved from https://www.kff.org/health-costs/report/2022-employer-health-benefits-survey/

Kaiser Family Foundation. (2023). *KFF health tracking poll: The public's view on the ACA*. Retrieved from https://www.kff.org/interactive/kff-health-tracking-poll-The-publics-views-on-the-aca/#?response=Favorable--Unfavorable&aRange=twoYear

Khatana, S. A., Bhatla, A., Nathan, A. S., Giri, J., Shen, C., Kazi, D. S., & Groeneveld, P. W. (2019, April). *3—Association of Medicaid expansion with cardiovascular mortality—A quasi-experimental analysis*. Paper presented at American Heart Association, Quality of Care & Outcomes Research, Arlington, VA

Levitt, L., Cox, C., Dawson, L., Pestaina, K., Salganicoff, A., & Sobel, L. (2023, April). *Q&A: Implications of the ruling on the ACA's preventive services requirement*. Retrieved from KFF website: https://www.kff.org/policy-watch/qa-implications-of-the-ruling-on-the-acas-preventive-services-requirement/

Lipsey, S. (1993, July/August). Mathematical education in the life of Florence Nightingale. *Newsletter of the Association for Women in Mathematics, 23*(4), 11–12.

Martin, M. (2023). Explore KY history. *Frontier Nursing Service*. Retrieved from https://explorekyhistory.ky.gov/items/show/583

Mazurenko, O., Balio, C. P., Agarwal, R., Carroll, A. E., & Menachemi, N. (2018). The effects of Medicaid expansion under the ACA: A systematic review. *Health Affairs (Project Hope), 37*(6), 944–950. https://doi.org/10.1377/hlthaff.2017.1491

McKelvey, L. M., Saccente, J. E., & Swindle, T. M. (2019). Adverse childhood experiences in infancy and toddlerhood predict obesity and health outcomes in middle childhood. *Childhood Obesity, 15*(3), 206–215. https://doi.org/10.1089/chi.2018.0225

NCSBN. (2023). *Nurse licensure compact*. Retrieved from https://nursecompact.com/

Obama, B. (2009, August 16). Why we need healthcare reform. *The New York Times*, WK9.

Organisation for Economic Co-operation and Development. (2022, September). *Understanding differences in health expenditure between the United States and OECD countries*. Retrieved from https://www.oecd.org/health/Health-expenditure-differences-USA-OECD-countries-Brief-July-2022.pdf

Population. (2019). *Merriam Webster dictionary*. Houghton Mifflin. Retrieved from https://www.merriam-webster.com/dictionary/population

SAVE. (2023). *Suicide statistics*. Retrieved from https://save.org/about-suicide/suicide-statistics/

Seon, J., Cho, H., Choi, G.-Y., Son, E., Allen, J., Nelson, A., & Kwon, I. (2021). Adverse childhood experiences, intimate partner violence victimization, and self-perceived health and depression among college students. *Journal of Family Violence, 37*(4), 691–706. https://doi.org/10.1007/s10896-021-00286-1

The Commonwealth Fund. (2023). *U.S. health care from a global perspective, 2022: Accelerating spending, worsening outcomes*. Retrieved from https://www.commonwealthfund.org/publications/issue-briefs/2023/jan/us-health-care-global-perspective-2022

U.S. Department of Health and Human Services. (2023). *Healthy People 2023*. Retrieved from Reduce the proportion of children and adolescents with obesity — NWS-04 - Healthy People 2030 | health.gov

van Zyl, T.-L., O'Neill, T., & Rushe, T. (2023). Distinct Psychological Profiles Linking Childhood Adversity and Substance Misuse in High-Risk Young Adults. *Journal of Family Violence, 38*(4), 633–645. https://doi.org/10.1007/s10896-022-00397-3

Webber-Ritchey, K. J., Habtezgi, D., Wu, X., & Samek, A. (2023). Examining the association between parental factors and childhood obesity. *Journal of Community Health Nursing, 40*(2), 94–105. https://doi.org/10.1080/07370016.2022.2125809

Wiseman, K. P., Seidenberg, A. B., & Klein, W. M. P. (2022). Clinician role in patient awareness regarding carcinogenic nature of alcohol consumption in the US: a nationally representative survey. *Journal of General Internal Medicine, 37*(8), 2116–2119. https://doi.org/10.1007/s11606-021-07113-9

World Health Organization. (2023a). *Alcohol*. Retrieved from https://www.who.int/health-topics/alcohol#tab=tab_1

World Health Organization. (2023b). *Noncommunicable diseases*. Retrieved from https://www.who.int/news-room/fact-sheets/detail/noncommunicable-diseases#:~:text=Noncommunicable%20diseases%20(NCDs)%20kill%2041,%2D%20and%20middle%2Dincome%20countries

CHAPTER 2

PRINCIPLES OF PUBLIC AND COMMUNITY HEALTH

KAREN T. D'ALONZO

INTRODUCTION

The terms "public health" and "community health" are inseparably linked. Both disciplines are dedicated to preventing disease, prolonging life, and promoting healthy behaviors. Rather than focusing on individual patients, advanced practice registered nurses (APRNs) who work in these settings seek to improve the health of entire populations by studying risk factors, comorbidities, and other trends that impact overall health and healthcare delivery. Although the terms public health and community health are sometimes used interchangeably, they are, in fact, two distinctly different approaches to population health.

Charles-Edward A. Winslow's definition of *public health*, written in 1920, is still the standard today: "...the science and art of preventing disease, prolonging life, and promoting health through the organized efforts and informed choices of society, organizations, public and private communities, and individuals" (Winslow, 1920). Overall, public health is concerned with the scientific processes underlying the protection of the health of populations, ranging in size from a small neighborhood to a hemisphere. Modern-day public health activities for APRNs may include designing health education programs to lower the risk of cardiovascular disease, promoting interventions that prevent the spread of communicable diseases such as coronavirus disease 2019 (COVID-19), assisting communities during natural disasters, and developing policies to improve the quality of health in at-risk neighborhoods.

APRNs who practice in the field of public health are referred to as *public health nurses*, a term reportedly first coined by Lillian Wald in 1893 (Buhler-Wilkerson, 1993). The American Public Health Association (APHA) defines *public health nursing* as "the practice of promoting and protecting the health of populations using knowledge from nursing, social, and public health sciences" (APHA, 2013). For public health nurses, the community is the client and the nurse is the guardian of the public's health. Public health nurses comprise the largest segment of the public health workforce (Kub et al., 2017) and serve in many different critical roles.

The term "community health" became popularized in the mid-20th century (Abrams, 2004) and is generally seen as a subset of public health. Both terms have a similar focus on populations, but community health primarily concerns itself with addressing those factors that contribute to socioeconomic challenges and disparities that, in turn, result in excess morbidity and mortality. Examples of contemporary community health activities for APRNs may include addressing food insecurity/ensuring access to healthy food, improving availability of after-school and childcare programs, and providing safe spaces for physical activity. Community health efforts usually involve a defined geographical area and collaboration among community members, school systems, local government, and the healthcare provider system.

APRNs working in community health often find themselves responsible for implementing broader public health measures to optimize the health of members of a community. In doing so, they often begin with a community assessment, in order to identify the community's healthcare needs and priorities. The initial component of such an assessment is often a windshield or "drive-through" survey (see Chapter 11, "Building Relationships and Engaging Communities Through Collaboration"). A thorough community assessment includes gathering information from stakeholders, key informants, and community coalitions to include varied viewpoints.

This chapter introduces the reader to the basic principles of public health and community health nursing. In accordance with the American Association of Colleges of Nursing (AACN) 2021 *The Essentials: Core Competencies for Professional Nursing Education* (AACN, 2021), this chapter will begin with a discussion of the many definitions of community from a population-focused perspective. The various levels of public and community health practice will be identified. The concept of the "social determinants of health" will be analyzed along with the various factors that influence the health of the community. Finally, the chapter will conclude by explaining the overall purpose of public health interventions, the ethical principles underlying such interventions, and lastly, the various methods that APRNs can use to improve public health.

BACKGROUND

"If access to health care is considered a human right, who is considered human enough to have that right?"

—Paul Farmer

The prevention of disease and disability for all people is a goal of nursing practice. In the field of public health, APRNs do this primarily by addressing the conditions in which people can be healthy (Porche, 2004). One commonality to both public health and community health nursing is the emphasis on population-based practice. *Population-based practice* is defined as "community and/or clinical populations that consider the environmental, occupational, cultural, socio-economic, and other dimensions of health and derives evidence from population-level data and statistics" (Starfield et al., 2008). In order to impact the health of an entire community, the APRN targets specific groups and designs interventions at multiple levels (individual, aggregate or group, family, and community). The level that the APRN targets largely depends upon whether the population of interest needs aggregate- or community-based care.

As explained in Chapter 1, "Introduction to Population-Based Nursing," an aggregate is a subgroup of a population, often designated as having similar characteristics (e.g., the elderly) or a similar geographical location (e.g., residents living in a particular housing complex). A high-risk aggregate is a subgroup or subpopulation of the community that has a high-risk commonality among its members, such as risky lifestyle behaviors (e.g., intravenous drug users) or high-risk health conditions (e.g., patients with chronic kidney disease). Although some researchers include racial/ethnic groups as examples of aggregates, others argue aggregation of such subgroups may mask important differences in health and health risks (Gordon et al., 2019). For example, Hispanic subgroups have different degrees of health risk which are frequently obscured when they are lumped together. For example, overall smoking rates among Hispanic people (14%) are lower than among White people (24%) but are substantially higher among Puerto Rican males (26%) and Cuban males (22%) (Kaplan et al., 2014).

The aggregate concept is used in public health practice to design interventions that target a specific subpopulation(s) within a geographical or geopolitical community. Alternatively, the community-based approach is appropriate when the APRN wants to focus an intervention on the entire community, using population-based data (e.g., initiating learn-to-swim classes in a community where few individuals can swim). An individual within a given population can be a member of several different communities at the same time, depending on the defining characteristics of the community.

Population-based APRNs are responsible for the following (AACN, 2021):

1. managing population health;
2. engaging in effective partnerships;
3. considering the socioeconomic impact of the delivery of healthcare;
4. advancing equitable population health policy;
5. demonstrating advocacy strategies; and
6. advancing preparedness to protect population health during disasters and public health emergencies.

An APRN in a population-focused practice intervenes with communities, the systems that impact communities, and/or the individuals and families that comprise communities. For example, in the event of a natural disaster such as a hurricane, the APRN might work with the geographical community itself to determine the degree of damage and ensure adequate access to roadways and resources. The APRN would also work with the political system to assess the need for funds to repair storm-related damage and to provide police protection to prevent looting. Lastly, the APRN might work with individuals and families to address access to food, medications, and healthcare. Community-focused practice changes community norms, attitudes, awareness, practices, and behaviors. One example would be an APRN who maintains a master list of individuals who are available to assist homeowners to shovel their sidewalks promptly after a snowfall to prevent falls. Systems-focused practice changes organizations, policies, laws, and power structures of the systems that affect health. For example, an APRN might lobby a town to install crosswalks or speed bumps in high-traffic areas to avoid pedestrian accidents. Individual/family-focused practice changes knowledge, attitudes, beliefs, values, practices, and behaviors of individuals (identified as belonging to a population), alone or as part of a family, class, or group. For example, an APRN might teach a patient and family members how to safely dispose of insulin syringes used at home. Interventions at each level of practice contribute to the overall goal of improving population health.

SOCIAL DETERMINANTS OF HEALTH

There are many examples of extra-personal factors that can have a major impact on people's health, well-being, and quality of life. These factors are collectively referred to as *social determinants of health* (SDOH). Because they are established conditions related to economic, social, and physical environments that occur outside the healthcare system and are unrelated to healthcare delivery, they are referred to as "upstream" factors (Distelhorst et al., 2021). SDOH are defined as the conditions in the environments where people are born, live, learn, work, play, worship, and age that affect a wide range of health, functioning, and quality-of-life outcomes and risks (National Center for Health Statistics, 2016). SDOH can be grouped into five categories (Figure 2.1).

Specific examples of SDOH include housing, transportation, and neighborhoods; racism, discrimination, and violence; education, job opportunities, and income; access to nutritious foods and physical activity opportunities; air and water quality; and language and literacy skills. SDOH contribute to wide health disparities and inequities that cannot be eliminated or mitigated by individuals making healthier choices. Instead, public health organizations and their partners in sectors like education, transportation, and housing need to take action to improve the conditions in people's environments.

One example is an APRN works in a community that has been hard-hit by COVID-19. Many of the inhabitants are "essential workers"—individuals employed in the service industry who work outside the home, despite the fear and/or likelihood of contracting COVID-19 and spreading it to family members. Many of these workers live in cramped quarters and have difficulty isolating themselves. The role of the APRN might involve working with community members to limit the spread of the disease by encouraging vaccinations and masking.

Exposure to air, water, and land pollution in the environment are other examples of SDOH that can impact health. A recent example was the Flint water crisis which began in 2014, when tens of thousands of Michigan residents—42 percent of whom live in poverty and 54 percent of whom are Black—were exposed to lead-contaminated water for 20 months. While it will take time to know the long-term consequences, past research

FIGURE 2.1

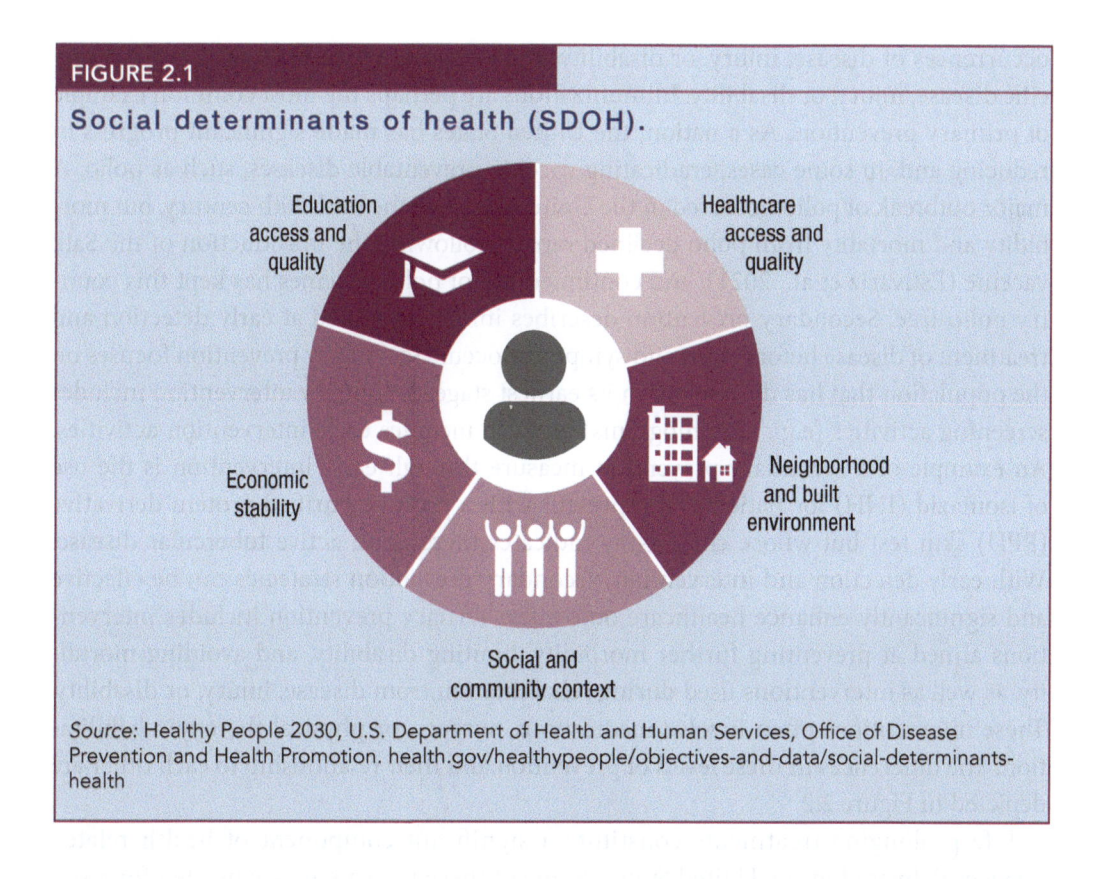

Social determinants of health (SDOH).

- Education access and quality
- Healthcare access and quality
- Economic stability
- Neighborhood and built environment
- Social and community context

Source: Healthy People 2030, U.S. Department of Health and Human Services, Office of Disease Prevention and Health Promotion. health.gov/healthypeople/objectives-and-data/social-determinants-health

has shown that lead is a neurotoxin linked to hypertension, kidney damage, decreased bone and muscle growth, behavioral disturbances, and loss of intellectual function, especially in children (Campbell et al., 2016; Sanders et al., 2009). Through support of programs such as the Clean Water Act, public health policies that address SDOH, and effective SDOH interventions, APRNs can improve the environments in which people live (AACN, 2021). In turn, these actions have the capacity to reduce health disparities and advance the health and well-being of all people.

OBJECTIVES OF PUBLIC HEALTH

The objectives of public health can be succinctly summarized as (WHO, 2021):

- preventing disease,
- prolonging life, and
- promoting health.

Prevention is considered the keystone of public health and is the focus of many public health interventions across the lifespan. There are three levels of prevention: primary, secondary, and tertiary (Leavell & Clark, 1965).

As we will learn in Chapter 4, "Epidemiological Methods and Measurements in Population-Based Nursing Practice: Part I," primary prevention activities aim to prevent occurrences of disease, injury, or disability in a population that does not have the specific disease, injury, or disability. Immunizations are perhaps the most common example of primary prevention. As a nation, the United States has made significant progress in reducing and, in some cases, eradicating vaccine-preventable diseases, such as polio. A major outbreak of polio occurred in the United States in the mid-20th century, but morbidity and mortality from polio declined rapidly following the introduction of the Salk vaccine (Estivariz et al., 2021), and continued use of polio vaccines has kept this country polio-free. Secondary prevention describes initiatives aimed at early detection and treatment of disease before signs and symptoms occur. Secondary prevention focuses on the population that has disease but in its earliest stage. Secondary intervention includes screening activities (e.g., mammograms) but also includes early intervention activities. An example of a secondary prevention measure through early intervention is the use of isoniazid (INH) for patients who present with a positive purified protein derivative (PPD) skin test but whose chest x-ray indicates there is no active tubercular disease. With early detection and intervention, secondary prevention strategies can be effective and significantly enhance healthcare outcomes. Tertiary prevention includes interventions aimed at preventing further morbidity, limiting disability, and avoiding mortality, as well as interventions used during rehabilitation from disease, injury, or disability. These interventions often involve medications, surgery, or physical therapy/rehabilitation. The differences in these levels of prevention and their relationship to each other are depicted in Figure 2.2.

Life-prolonging treatments constitute a significant component of health-related services delivered in the United States. Some of these treatments are needed for a relatively short period of time, while others may be needed for the rest of an individual's life. Examples of life-prolonging treatments include medications (e.g., insulin and antibiotics), intravenous treatments, tube feeding, dialysis treatments, and ventilator use. The decision to consent to life-prolonging treatments is a complex one that may be affected by factors such as age, likelihood that the illness can be cured or managed, and potential side effects of treatment. Public health programs have contributed to the prolongation of life expectancy of U.S. residents from 47 years in 1900 to 76 years in 2022 (Arias et al., 2022). Much of the improvement in life expectancy in the United States during this time period can be attributed to measures instituted to prevent

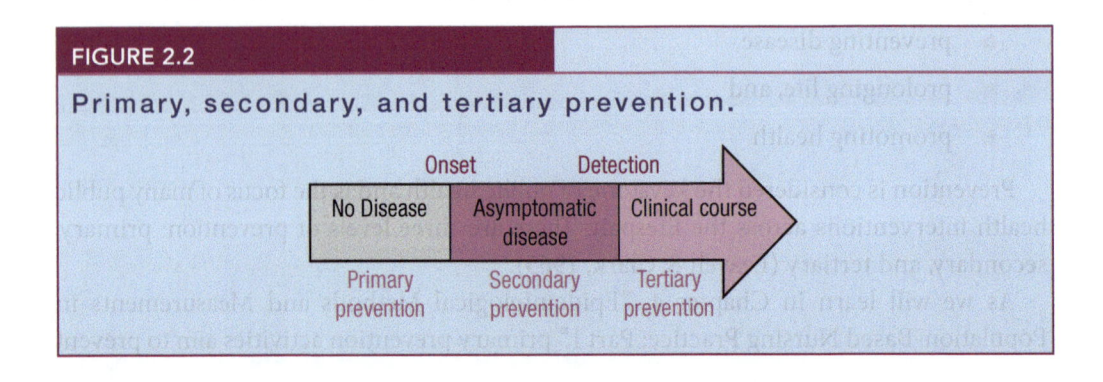

FIGURE 2.2

Primary, secondary, and tertiary prevention.

No Disease	Onset	Asymptomatic disease	Detection	Clinical course
Primary prevention		Secondary prevention		Tertiary prevention

infectious diseases (such as tuberculosis, HIV/AIDS, and rabies) and decreases in infant mortality (Morbidity and Mortality Weekly Report, 2011). Improvements in sanitation, milk purification, and institutional structures to monitor and reduce infant mortality played a crucial role in the decline in infant mortality in the early 1900s (Bhatia et al., 2019).

Unfortunately, for some groups of individuals, increased life expectancy includes at least some periods of diminished health and function, often referred to as a decrease in health-related quality of life (HRQOL). HRQOL surveillance supports the basic functions of public health—assessment, policy development, and assurance. HRQOL surveillance is used to identify unmet population health needs including recognizing trends, disparities, and determinants of health in the population (assessment). HRQOL surveillance data can be used to inform and support decision-making and program development (policy development). Finally, HRQOL surveillance data can be used for program evaluation to assure that the population is benefiting from public health programs (assurance). For example, a community has a free and reduced-price lunch program for elementary school students that runs during the school year. After some parent groups complained that their children did not have access to the same lunch services during the summer (when the parents were at work), the community developed a program where the lunches would be delivered to the children's homes during the summer using an off-duty school bus. In this case, parental and student HRQOL could be measured before and after the institution of the innovative summer school lunch program.

HRQOL data is important to help practitioners understand the burden of physical and mental illness and disability and to provide a focus for comprehensive community health programs. The Centers for Disease Control and Prevention (CDC) has developed a HRQOL tool that measures population health-related quality of life called the "Healthy Days Measures" (CDC, 2000). In recent years, several organizations have found these Healthy Days Measures useful at the national level for (1) identifying health disparities and (2) tracking population trends (Dumas et al., 2020; Slabaugh, 2017). Lastly, Healthy Days Measures provide support for the development of a measure of population health consistent with the WHO definition of *health* as "a state of complete physical, mental and social well-being and not merely the absence of disease or infirmity" (WHO, 2020).

To help policymakers and other stakeholders identify opportunities to improve health equity in their states, the State Health Access Data Assistance Center (SHADAC) has ranked HRQOL for the 50 states and the District of Columbia. Data from 2021 indicated that the District of Columbia reported the lowest average number of physically unhealthy days per month, at 3.0 days, while West Virginia reported the highest average number, at 5.5 days. South Dakota reported the lowest average number of mentally unhealthy days per month, at 3.3 days, while West Virginia again reported the highest, at 5.7 days (SHADAC, 2021). An APRN who works in a state with a high number of mentally unhealthy days could conduct a small qualitative study in their community to identify those factors that appear to impact mental health and then promote strategies to ameliorate them.

COST-SAVING OR COST-EFFECTIVE?

A fundamental assumption of public health is that providing enhanced preventive healthcare services can cut spending on unnecessary healthcare utilization. In public health, *prevention strategies* refer to activities targeted at a community that are designed to prevent problems before they occur. Community-based prevention is not focused on changing individual risks but rather on promoting strategies that target populations at risk. Community-based prevention programs and policies can be implemented in a variety of settings, including workplaces, schools, families, and communities (Poland et al., 2000). Identification of population-specific social health determinants and community health factors is an important step toward improving population health and designing interventions to prevent the excessive and unnecessary use of healthcare resources such as ambulatory services and emergency department resources.

In theory, community-based preventive interventions are a good idea, and there is evidence that some community-based preventive healthcare programs are effective. One frequently cited example is the North Karelia study in Finland (Puska & Uutela, 2000, pp. 73–96) that was designed to reduce the community's high rates of death from coronary heart disease. Impressive decreases in smoking rates (among men), as well as decreases in serum cholesterol, and mean blood pressure were attributed to the implementation of strategies introduced through this program.

Other examples of effective community-level interventions include substance abuse prevention programs; these have been shown to lessen the economic burden caused by addiction across many sectors of society (Ridenour et al., 2022). There are also several examples of tobacco control policies that have been highly successful (Best et al., 2007; Carson et al., 2011) as well as interventions to promote bicycle helmet use among youth (Owen et al., 2011). A good source for a list of efficacious community-level interventions is the Community Guide to Preventive Services (also known as The Community Guide [www.thecommunityguide.org]). Similar to the Cochrane Library, The Community Guide uses systematic and objective methods to evaluate evidence for the effectiveness of community-level preventive interventions. Where possible, The Community Guide also reviews evidence of the economic efficiency of the intervention (Briss et al., 2004).

There is currently insufficient evidence to support the notion that community-based preventive strategies as a whole are economically advantageous. Some preventive programs are cost-saving (they yield more in returns than they cost), while others have been found to be cost-effective (they provide adequate improvements in health and well-being for their cost, though they do not save money overall) (Owen et al., 2012). Examples of cost-effective interventions include smoking cessation programs, alcohol prevention strategies, and measures taken to prevent sexually transmitted diseases. The term *cost-effective analysis (CEA)* is used to evaluate a community public health prevention program when the program costs money but also generates health benefits. CEA provides information on the health benefits and cost impacts of an intervention compared to an alternative intervention (status quo or "usual care"). If the intervention is cost-saving, the results are presented as net cost savings. An example of such is an analysis of a workplace influenza immunization program that computes the number of cases of influenza

FIGURE 2.3

Calculation of incremental cost-effectiveness ratio (ICER).

$$\text{ICER} = \frac{\text{cost of healthy menu} - \text{cost of old lunch menu}}{\text{\# of obese children healthy menu} - \text{\# obese children old menu}}$$

prevented. If the intervention is effective but more costly, the results are presented as a cost-effectiveness ratio. A *cost-effectiveness ratio* is the net cost divided by changes in health outcomes. A good example is the introduction of a healthy lunch menu in the schools in a specific district where the health outcome measure is the number of obese students. The amount of money needed to prevent one case of childhood obesity can be calculated. This calculation, using the incremental cost-effectiveness ratio (ICER), is illustrated in Figure 2.3.

There are no specific guidelines regarding interpretation of the ICER; one community may decide the investment is money well spent, while another community may feel the funds should be allocated for another cause.

Perhaps the most compelling reason to engage in preventive care is an ethical one—as it pertains to serious illnesses, preventive care avoids unnecessary suffering and premature death. Ethics play a significant role in public health decision-making.

PUBLIC HEALTH ETHICS

Public health ethics are used to understand and clarify principles and values which guide public health actions. Principles and values provide a framework for decision-making and a means of justifying decisions. From a practical perspective, public health ethics is the application of relevant principles and values to public health decision-making. Several public health ethics frameworks that have been introduced since the late 1990s are discussed in the following pages. Although there is no one widely accepted ethical framework in the field of public health, they each share many of the same bioethical underpinnings and values. These four principles—autonomy, beneficence, nonmaleficence, and justice—were first outlined by Thomas Beauchamp and James Childress in the 1970s (Beauchamp & Childress, 2013):

a. **Autonomy:** It can be argued that in the United States, autonomy is the most fundamental principle in bioethics. In public health, autonomy is often contrasted with coercion, as demonstrated in the need to balance the desire to improve health outcomes by changing individual behaviors with respect for individual freedom. A more contemporary interpretation implies that autonomy is about creating an environment where "each person is free to choose life options, including healthy behaviors, out of a sense of authentic self-reflection"

(Zimmerman, 2017). Public health education (such as when an APRN presents a community workshop on the human papillomavirus [HPV] vaccine) allows individuals to make informed decisions and hence exercise their right to autonomy.

b. **Beneficence:** The ethical principle of beneficence requires that potential benefits to individuals and to society be maximized and that potential harms be minimized. Beneficence implies a moral obligation to help other persons, to protect individual welfare, and to promote the common welfare. An example of beneficence is laws that require proof of vaccination against childhood illnesses as a requirement for admission to a public school. The effectiveness and efficiency of public health programs are closely related to the idea of beneficence (Coughlin, 2008).

c. **Nonmaleficence:** The principle of nonmaleficence requires that harmful acts be avoided. This principle recognizes that intentionally or negligently causing harm is a fundamental moral wrong. However, the principle of nonmaleficence does not rule out balancing potential harms against potential benefits. For example, the risks and potential harms of public health interventions (e.g., the discomfort and inconvenience of masking and/or quarantine) must be weighed against the benefits to the public in general and especially those at high risk.

d. **Justice:** From a public health perspective, each person should share equally in the distribution of the potential benefits of public services. Some theorists would argue that society has an obligation to correct inequalities in the distribution of resources and that those who are least well-off should benefit most from available resources. Such an approach to defining justice in public health would support maximizing benefits to underserved people and to protecting vulnerable groups (Powers & Fadden, 2006).

There are several suggested frameworks for public health ethics. They are generally divided into one of two types: practice-based and theory-based frameworks. Practice-based frameworks summarize foundational values and provide operating principles that direct a course of action for practitioners faced with ethical quandaries in the public health sphere. An example of a practice-based public health ethicist is Nancy Kass (Kass, 2001). Kass espoused the importance of ensuring the minimal level of interference to improve population health, preserving the rights of citizens, while not greatly reducing program effectiveness, reducing social inequities and health disparities, and providing evidence of program benefits (Lee, 2012). In contrast, theory-based frameworks outline the fundamental unifying principles from which all ethical decisions can be derived. For example, in the 1990s, Jonathan Mann proposed a human rights framework for dealing with modern public health challenges (Mann, 1996). Mann believed that human rights are critical determinants of health and that governments should respect the human rights of all persons in order to ensure health. Proponents of theory-based frameworks believe that public health practitioners must commit to linking human rights with public health. A summary of the various public health ethics frameworks is presented in Table 2.1.

TABLE 2.1 Public Health Ethics Frameworks

AUTHOR, CITATION	PHILOSOPHICAL UNDERPINNING	FOUNDATIONAL VALUE(S)	OPERATING PRINCIPLE(S)
Practice-based frameworks			
N. E. Kass, "An Ethics Framework for Public Health," *American Journal of Public Health* 91, no. 11 (2001): 1776–1782.	Empirical • Bioethics • Research ethics	• Negative right to noninterference • Positive right or obligation to improve the public's health • Social justice	• Minimal interference for improvements of population health • Obligation to reduce inequalities • Reducing harms and burdens
J. R. Childress, R. R. Faden, R. D. Gaare, L. O. Gostin, J. Kahn, R. J. Bonnie, N. E. Kass, A. C. Mastroianni, J. D. Moreno, and P. Nieburg, "Public Health Ethics: Mapping the Terrain," *Journal of Law, Medicine, and Ethics* 30, no. 2 (2002): 170–178.	Empirical • Human rights • Works with several philosophical approaches	• Producing benefits • Preventing, removing harms • Producing maximal balance of benefits to harms • Distributing burdens and benefits • Ensuring participation • Respecting autonomy • Protecting confidentiality • Keeping commitments • Disclosing information truthfully • Building and maintaining trust	• Effectiveness • Proportionality: benefits must outweigh the infringement • Necessity: ensuring that any infringement is necessary • Least infringement: only the least possible infringement on autonomy is justified • Public justification: transparency and accountability require public explanation of infringement
R. E. G. Upshur, "Principles for the Justification of Public Health Intervention," *Canadian Journal of Public Health* 93, no. 2 (2002): 101–103.	Empirical • Heuristic • Applicable to diversity of public health decisions	Intimated: • Individual liberty • Nondiscrimination • Social duty • Honesty and truthfulness	• Harm principle • Least restrictive or coercive means • Reciprocity principle • Transparency principle
A. K. Thompson, K. Faith, J. L. Gibson, and R. E. G. Upshur, "Pandemic Influenza Preparedness: An Ethical Framework to Guide Decision-Making," *BMC Medical Ethics* 7 (2006): E12.	Empirical • Applicable to public health emergency situations	• Duty to provide care • Equity • Individual liberty • Privacy • Proportionality • Protection from harm • Reciprocity • Solidarity • Stewardship • Trust	• Inclusiveness • Openness and transparency • Reasonableness • Responsiveness

(continued)

TABLE 2.1 Public Health Ethics Frameworks *(continued)*

AUTHOR, CITATION	PHILOSOPHICAL UNDERPINNING	FOUNDATIONAL VALUE(S)	OPERATING PRINCIPLE(S)
N. M. Baum, S. E. Gollust, S. D. Goold, and P. D. Jacobson, "Looking Ahead: Addressing Ethical Challenges in Public Health Practice," *Journal of Law, Medicine, and Ethics* 35, no. 4 (2007): 657–667.	Empirical	• Population-level utility • Evidence • Justice/fairness • Accountability • Costs/efficiencies • Political feasibility • Beneficence • Nonmaleficence • Autonomy	• Unmask normative assumptions and ethical trade-offs explicitly • Add ethical value to economic analyses • Illuminate and clarify ethical considerations connected to policies or program decisions • Clarify limits of public health mission
G. R. Swain, K. A. Burns, and P. Etkind, "Preparedness: Medical Ethics Versus Public Health Ethics," *Journal of Public Health Management Practice* 14, no. 4 (2008): 354–357.	Empirical	• Interdependence • Community trust • Fundamentality • Justice	*From Kass's model (5):* • Minimal interference for improvement of population health • Obligation to reduce inequities • Reducing harms and burdens • Providing evidence of benefits *Plus:* • Focus on fundamental causes of disease • Community participation, collaboration, communication, and consent
H. W. Jaffe and T. Hope, "Treating for the Common Good: A Proposed Ethical Framework," *Public Health Ethics* 3, no. 3 (2010): 193–198.	Empirical	• Respect for persons/autonomy • Beneficence • Nonmaleficence • Justice	• Valid consent procedure • Risk of harm to recipients is low or negligible • Public health benefit cannot be produced by alternative means • Public health benefit justifies risk to harm to individuals • Data on harm collected to increase accuracy of risk and harm estimates • Intervention is scrutinized by independent body

(continued)

Theory-based frameworks

J. M. Mann, "Health and Human Rights," *BMJ* 312, no. 7036 (1996): 924–925.	Human rights	• Human rights are critical determinants of health • Basic minimum that governments should ensure for all persons in order to ensure health	• Health is contextual and more than medicine • Public health practitioners must commit to linking human rights with public health
M. J. Roberts and M. R. Reich, "Ethical Analysis in Public Health," *The Lancet* 359, no. 9311 (2002): 1055–1059.	Ethics-of-care Feminism Consequentialism	• Caring relationships are not impartial, impersonal, or equal • Relationships fundamentally unequal • One cannot and should not care for all humans equally	• Caring roles are important part of life plan • Support for the caring role is important for both the caregiver and society

B. Jennings, "Public Health and Civic Republicanism: Toward an Alternative Framework for Public Health Ethics," in A. Dawson and M. Verweij, eds., *Ethics, Prevention, and Public Health* (New York: Oxford University Press, 2007).	Civic republicanism
	Political philosophy
		• Freedom
		  ○ Life in the absence of arbitrary power
		  ○ Relationships of mutuality and reciprocity
		• Respect diversity
		• Civic virtue
		• Concept of the "public"
			• Tap into latent civic virtue
			• Education

C. Petrini and S. Gainotti, "A Personalist Approach to Public-Health Ethics," *Bull World Health Organization* 86, no. 8 (2008): 624–629.	Personalism Utilitarianism Kantian theories Communitarianism	• Autonomy • Confidentiality • Equity • Equal opportunity for health resources • Solidarity and sociality	• Respect for individual rights • Individual good is basis for common good • Cases exist where freedom must be sacrificed for the common good • Precaution principle (making temporary decisions based on available evidence, modifying with new evidence

(continued)

TABLE 2.1 Public Health Ethics Frameworks (*continued*)

AUTHOR, CITATION	PHILOSOPHICAL UNDERPINNING	FOUNDATIONAL VALUE(S)	OPERATING PRINCIPLE(S)
Nuffield Council on Bioethics, *Public Health: Ethical Issues*, London: Nuffield Council on Bioethics, 2007, available at www.nuffieldbioethics.org/go/ourwork/publichealth/introduction (last visited January 4, 2012).	<ul><li>Political liberalism</li><li>John Stuart Mill's classic harm principle</li><li>Colletivism/community</li><li>Paternalism/libertarian paternalism</li></ul>	<ul><li>Equality between citizens</li><li>Protection of individual freedom limits state authority</li><li>Social contract that state power may be used to advance welfare</li><li>Autonomy as self-governance</li><li>Health is important for a good life</li><li>Health is defined by individuals</li><li>Limiting liberty is acceptable only when purpose is to prevent harm to others</li><li>Third-party participation in public health delivery</li></ul>	<ul><li>Reduce risks persons impose on each other</li><li>Use regulation to ensure environmental conditions that sustain good health</li><li>Attend to health of children and vulnerable persons</li><li>Provide programs that help make it easy for people to lead healthy lives</li><li>Ensure access to appropriate medical services</li><li>Reduce unfair health inequalities</li><li>Do not coerce adults</li><li>Minimize interventions that are introduced without some form of consent, individual, community, or democratic decision-making</li><li>Minimize interventions that are perceived as intrusive or in conflict with important personal values</li></ul>
N. P. Kenny, S. B. Sherwin, and F. E. Baylis, "Re-visioning Public Health Ethics: A Relational Perspective," *Canadian Journal of Public Health* 101, no. 3 (2010): 9–11.	Relational ethics	<ul><li>Relational autonomy: persons are socially, politically, and economically situated</li><li>Relational social justice: fair access to social goods (rights, opportunities, power, self-respect)</li><li>Relational solidarity: attending to needs of all, especially vulnerable and systematically disadvantaged</li></ul>	<ul><li>Transparency</li><li>Fairness</li><li>Inclusivity</li><li>Interconnectedness</li><li>Responsive to systemic inequalities</li></ul>

Source: Adapted from Lee, L. (2012). Public health ethics theory: Review and path to convergence. *Journal of Law, Medicine & Ethics, 40*(1), 85–98. doi:10.1111/j.1748-720X.2012.00648.x

Public health practitioners are often faced with ethical dilemmas when there are conflicts between these practice-based and theory-based ethical frameworks. In individualistic societies such as the United States, citizens prize their ability to make decisions about their health with minimal interference from public health officials. This emphasis on autonomy became an issue during the COVID-19 pandemic, where large numbers of individuals were either wary of being vaccinated ("vaccine skeptics") or simply refused to be vaccinated. Although autonomy is a salient consideration, herd immunity can only be achieved through widespread vaccination—that is, when the majority of a population is immune to a disease or virus. Herd immunity is relevant to the ethical doctrine of utilitarianism—that is, that actions are justified or right when they benefit the majority and protect the most vulnerable. APRNs can support the public's right to autonomy and at the same time help to protect the health of the majority through the provision of accurate and up-to-date public health education and their support of evidence-based policies.

PUBLIC HEALTH METHODS

Public health approaches to preventing disease, prolonging life, and promoting health generally involve one or more of the following activities:

- Defining and measuring the problem;
- Determining the cause or risk factors for the problem;
- Determining how to prevent or ameliorate the problem; and
- Implementing effective strategies on a larger scale and evaluating the impact.

As a result, APRNs who work in public health settings may find themselves engaged in a number of different roles. These roles can include collecting data to identify health risks (e.g., using tools to screen for social determinants of health in a primary care setting and integrating the results into electronic health record [EHR] systems), monitoring the incidence and prevalence of disease (e.g., required reporting of communicable diseases to the State Department of Health), educating the public (e.g., how to quit smoking), and designing/promoting policies to improve public health (e.g., running for public office or serving on a local board of health).

Public health APRNs often work for government agencies, nonprofit groups, community health centers, and other organizations that aim to improve health at the community level. They may work alone or on multidisciplinary teams, and they often supervise other healthcare and lay personnel. In addition to working with communities, they work behind the scenes, planning activities, managing budgets, and evaluating the effectiveness of public health programs.

SUMMARY

APRNs play an important role in improving population health in many settings (AACN, 2021). Whether they are defined as public health nurses or community health nurses, the common denominator is the focus on community as client. APRNs have ample opportunities to access and use available data to contribute to the current body of knowledge that forms the basis for evidence-based practice in various levels of practice: systems, social, virtual, and individual perspectives. In particular, social determinants of health and disparities data are areas that APRNs can use to develop community-focused, socioculturally appropriate, cost-effective interventions. It is important to promote the common good while preserving an individual's right to autonomy. By engaging in these activities, APRNs carry on the noble tradition of public health nursing begun by Lillian Wald over 100 years ago.

END-OF-CHAPTER RESOURCES

EXERCISES AND DISCUSSION QUESTIONS

EXERCISE 2.1 An APRN is working in a regional perinatal center, coordinating nursing care provided to high-risk obstetric patients. The APRN knows there are racial and ethnic disparities in maternal mortality.

- Where could the APRN go to find information on maternal mortality disparities?
- What SDOH are associated with maternal mortality?
- How might an APRN participate in local efforts to reduce maternal mortality rates at the population level?
- Which principle of ethics would guide the APRN's attempts to support maximizing benefits to the underserved maternal population and to protect such vulnerable groups? Why?

EXERCISE 2.2 An APRN who is interested in reducing opiate-related overdoses in high schools develops an online training program to teach all school employees to administer Narcan (naloxone).

- What are the Leading Health Indicators (LHIs) found in *Healthy People 2030?*
- In examining The Community Guide topics, which ones are most relevant to this scenario?
- What outcomes might the APRN monitor for effectiveness of the program?
- What other population-level strategies could the APRN implement to address the issue?

EXERCISE 2.3 Type 2 diabetes mellitus (T2DM) affects a growing number of Americans. An APRN works in a local hospital that is part of a collaborative of community agencies strategically addressing T2DM from a community perspective.

- What SDOH should the community look at in relation to risk or incidence of disease?
- What resources could the APRN use to identify different outcomes related to T2DM?
- What outcomes related to T2DM are of most interest to community members?
- Using the Agency for Healthcare Research and Qulaity's (AHRQ) Healthcare Quality and Disparities Report Data Query (nhqrnet.ahrq.inhqrdr/data/submit), what national- and statelevel data are available to the APRN?

A robust set of instructor resources designed to supplement this text is located at http://connect.springerpub.com/content/book/978-0-8261-4377-8. Qualifying instructors may request access by emailing textbook@springerpub.com.

REFERENCES

Abrams, S. E. (2004). From function to competency in public health nursing, 1931 to 2003. *Public Health Nursing, 21*(5), 507–510. http://doi.org//10.1111/j.0737-1209.2004.021514.x

American Association of Colleges of Nursing. (2021). *The essentials: Core competencies for professional nursing education*. Available online: https://www.aacnnursing.org/Essentials

American Public Health Association Public Health Nursing Section. (2013). *The definition and practice of public health nursing: A statement of the public health nursing section*. American Public Health Association.

Arias, E., Tejada-Vera, B., Kochanek, K. D., & Ahmad, F. B. (2022). *Provisional life expectancy estimates for 2021. Vital statistics rapid release* (Vol. 23). National Center for Health Statistics. http://doi.org//10.15620/cdc:118999

Beauchamp, T. L., & Childress, J. F. (2013). *Principles of biomedical ethics* (7th ed.). Oxford University Press.

Best, A., Clark, P. I., Leischow, S. J., & Trochim, W. (2007). *Greater than the sum: Systems thinking in tobacco control*. National Institutes of Health.

Bhatia, A., Krieger, N., & Subramanian, S. V. (2019). Learning from history about reducing infant mortality: Contrasting the centrality of structural interventions to early 20th-century successes in the United States to their neglect in current global initiatives. *The Milbank quarterly, 97*(1), 285–345. https://doi.org/10.1111/1468-0009.12376

Briss, P., Rimer, B., Reilley, B., Coates, R. C., Lee, N. C., Mullen, P., Corso, P., Hutchinson, A. B., Hiatt, R., Kerner, J., George, P., White, C., Gandhi, N., Saraiya, M., Breslow, R., Isham, G., Teutsch, S. M., Hinman, A. R., & Lawrence R. (2004). Promoting informed decisions about cancer screening in communities and healthcare systems. *American Journal of Preventive Medicine, 26*(1), 67–80. https://doi.org//10.1016/j.amepre.2003.09.012

Buhler-Wilkerson, K. (1993). Bringing care to the people: Lillian Wald legacy to public health nursing. *American Journal of Public Health, 83*(12), 1778–1786. https://doi.org//10.2105/ajph.83.12.1778

Campbell, C., Greenberg, R., Mankikar, D., & Ross, R. D. (2016). A case study of environmental injustice: The failure in flint. *International Journal of Environmental Research and Public Health, 13*(10), 951. https://doi.org/10.3390/ijerph13100951

Carson, K. V., Brinn, M. P., Labiszewski, N. A., Esterman, A. J., Chang, A. B., & Smith B. J. (2011). Community interventions for preventing smoking in young people. *Cochrane Database of Systematic Reviews, 7*, CD001291. http://doi.org//10.1002/14651858.CD001291.pub2

Center for Disease Control and Prevention. (2000). *Measuring healthy days*. CDC.

Coughlin, S. S. (2008). How Many principles for public health ethics? *The Open Public Health Journal, 1*, 8–16. https://doi.org/10.2174/1874944500801010008

Distelhorst, K. S., Graor, C. H., & Hansen, D. M. (2021). Upstream factors in population health: A concept analysis to advance nursing theory. *ANS. Advances in Nursing Science, 44*(3), 210–223. https://doi.org/10.1097/ANS.0000000000000362

Dumas, S. E., Dongchung, T. Y., Sanderson, M. L., Bartley, K., & Levanon Seligson, A. (2020). A comparison of the four healthy days measures (HRQOL-4) with a single measure of self-rated general health in a population-based health survey in New York City. *Health and Quality of Life Outcomes, 18*(1), 315. https://doi.org/10.1186/s12955-020-01560-4

Estivariz, C.F., Link-Gelles, R., & Shimabukuro, T. (2021). Chapter 18: Poliomyelitis. In E. Hall, A. Wodi, J. Hamborsky, V. Morelli, & S. Schillie (Eds.), *Epidemiology and prevention of vaccine-preventable diseases* (The Pink Book) (14th ed.). Centers for Disease Control and Prevention (CDC).

Gordon, N. P., Lin, T. Y., Rau, J., & Lo, J. C. (2019). Aggregation of Asian-American subgroups masks meaningful differences in health and health risks among Asian ethnicities: An electronic health record-based cohort study. *BMC Public Health, 19*(1), 1551. https://doi.org/10.1186/s12889-019-7683-3

Kaplan, R. C., Bangdiwala, S. I., Barnhart, J. M., Castañeda, S. F., Gellman, M. D., Lee, D. J., Pérez-Stable, E. J., Talavera, G. A., Youngblood, M. E., & Giachello, A. L. (2014). Smoking among U.S. Hispanic/Latino adults: The Hispanic community health study/study of Latinos. *American Journal of Preventive Medicine, 46*(5), 496–506. https://doi.org/10.1016/j.amepre.2014.01.014

Kass, N. E. (2001). An ethics framework for public health. *American Journal of Public Health, 91*(11), 1776–1782. https://doi.org/10.2105/ajph.91.11.1776

Kub, J. E., Kulbok, P. A., Miner, S., & Merrill, J. A. (2017). Increasing the capacity of public health nursing to strengthen the public health infrastructure and to promote and protect the health of communities and populations. *Nursing Outlook, 65*(5), 661–664. https://doi.org/10.1016/j.outlook.2017.08.009

Leavell, H. R., & Clark, E. G. (1965). *Preventive medicine for the doctor in his community* (3rd ed.). McGraw-Hill.

Lee L. M. (2012). Public health ethics theory: Review and path to convergence. *The Journal of Law, Medicine & Ethics: A Journal of the American Society of Law, Medicine & Ethics, 40*(1), 85–98. https://doi.org/10.1111/j.1748-720X.2012.00648.x

Mann, J. M. (1996). Health and human rights. *BMJ, 312*(7036), 924–925. https://doi.org//10.1136/bmj.312.7036.924

Morbidity and Mortality Weekly Report. (2011, May 20). Ten great public health achievements — United States, 2001–2010. *MMWR, 60*(19), 619–623.

National Center for Health Statistics. (2016). Chapter 39: *Social determinants of health*. Healthy People 2020 Midcourse Review.

Owen, R., Kendrick, D., Mulvaney, C., Coleman, T., & Royal, S. (2011). Non-legislative interventions for the promotion of cycle helmet wearing by children. *Cochrane Library, 2*, CD003985. https://doi.org//10.1002/14651858.CD003985.pub3

Owen, L., Morgan, A., Fischer, A., Ellis, S., Hoy, A., & Kelly, M. P. (2012). The cost-effectiveness of public health interventions. *Journal of Public Health (Oxford, England), 34*(1), 37–45. https://doi.org/10.1093/pubmed/fdr075

Poland, J. C., Green, L. W., & Rootman, I. (2000). *Settings in health promotion: Linking theory and practice*. SAGE Publications.

Porche, D. J. (2004). *Public health policy and politics*. SAGE Publications. https://doi.org/10.4135/9781483328669

Powers, M., & Faden, R. (2006) *Social justice: The moral foundations of public health and health policy*. Oxford University Press.

Puska, P., & Uutela, A. (2000). Community intervention in cardiovascular health promotion: North Karelia, 1972–1999. In N. Schneiderman, M. A. Speers, J. M. Silva, H. Tomes, & J. H. Gentry (Eds.), *Integrating behavioral and social sciences with public health*. American Psychological Association. https://doi.org/10.1037/10388-004

Ridenour, T. A., Murray, D. W., Hinde, J., Glasheen, C., Wilkinson, A., Rackers, H., & Coyne-Beasley, T. (2022). Addressing barriers to primary care screening and referral to prevention for youth risky health behaviors: Evidence regarding potential cost-savings and provider concerns. *Prevention Science: The Official Journal of the Society for Prevention Research, 23*(2), 212–223. https://doi.org/10.1007/s11121-021-01321-9

Sanders, T., Liu, Y., Buchner, V., & Tchounwou, P. B. (2009). Neurotoxic effects and biomarkers of lead exposure: A review. *Reviews on Environmental health, 24*(1), 15–45. https://doi.org/10.1515/reveh.2009.24.1.15

Slabaugh, S. L., Shah, M., Zack, M., Happe, L., Cordier, T., Havens, E., Davidson, E., Miao, M., Prewitt, T., & Jia, H. (2017). Leveraging health-related quality of life in population health management: The case for healthy days. *Population Health Management, 20*(1), 13–22. https://doi.org/10.1089/pop.2015.0162

Starfield, B., Hyde, J., Gérvas, J., & Heath, I. (2008). The concept of prevention: A good idea gone astray? *Journal of Epidemiology and Community Health, 62*(7), 580–583. https://doi.org/10.1136/jech.2007.071027

State Health Access Data Assistance Center. (2021). *State Health Compare*. Available online: https://statehealthcompare.shadac.org/

U.S. Department of Health and Human Services, Office of Disease Prevention and Health Promotion. *Social Determinants of Health, Healthy People 2030*. Available online: https://health.gov/healthypeople/objectives-and-data/social-determinants-health

Winslow, C. E. A. (1920). The untilled field of public health. *Modern Medicine, 2*(1306), 183–191. http://doi.org/10.1126/science.51.1306.23

World Health Organization. (2020). Constitution of the World Health Organization. In *World Health Organization: Basic documents* (49th ed.). World Health Organization.

World Health Organization. (2021). *Health promotion glossary of terms*. Available online: https://www.who.int/publications/i/item/9789240038349

Zimmerman, F. J. (2017). Public health and autonomy: A critical reappraisal. *Hastings Center Report, 47*(6), 38–45. https://doi.org/10.1002/hast.784

CHAPTER 3

IDENTIFYING OUTCOMES IN POPULATION-BASED NURSING

ALYSSA E. ERIKSON

INTRODUCTION

Nurses have a long and rich history of wanting to do the most good for the most people. It is imperative that advanced practice registered nurses (APRNs) continue that tradition by delivering care that improves the health of populations. By assessing community, aggregate, family, and individual factors and conditions that have a strong influence on health, APRNs are equipped to deliver effective and evidence-based care. Identifying population-level healthcare needs and healthcare disparities can improve equity in health outcomes at all levels.

The American Association of Colleges of Nursing's (AACN) updated *Essentials* (2021) provides a reimagined model for nursing education with 10 domains and associated competencies for two levels of professional nursing education: entry and advanced. This chapter addresses the competencies for advanced-level education that fall within Domain 3: Population Health and Domain 5: Quality and Safety.

Regardless of whether APRNs practice with a focus on clinical prevention or population health, the ability to define, identify, and analyze outcomes is imperative for improving the health status of individuals and populations (AACN, 2022; Office of Disease Prevention and Health Promotion [ODPHP], 2022).

The purpose of this chapter is to explore how APRNs can identify determinants of health and define population outcomes. Specific examples from various settings are given, such as acute care, primary care, long-term care, and the community, as well as outcomes related to health disparities and national health objectives. The identification of factors that lead to certain outcomes or key health indicators is an essential first step in planning effective interventions and is used later in the evaluation process. By comparing outcomes, APRNs can advocate for needed resources and changes in policies at local, regional, state, and/or national levels by identifying areas for improvement in practice, comparing evidence needed for effective practice, and better understanding health disparities.

Health disparities are not fair or socially just. They are preventable. They reflect an uneven distribution of social determinants and environmental, economic, and political factors. *Health disparities* can be defined as "a particular type of health difference that is closely linked with social, economic, and/or environmental disadvantage" (ODPHP, 2022, p. 31). *Health equity* is both a process and an outcome that is defined as "the state in which everyone has a fair and just opportunity to attain their highest level of health" (Braveman et al., 2017; Centers for Disease Control and Prevention [CDC], 2022c). The National Academies of Sciences, Engineering, and Medicine's (2021) report *The Future of Nursing 2020–2030: Charting a Path to Achieve Health Equity* details how nurses at all levels can be change agents to achieve the goal of health equity. Along with professionals from other disciplines and community members, APRNs play an important collaborative role in the work required to improve health outcomes for all.

IDENTIFYING AND DEFINING POPULATION OUTCOMES

BACKGROUND

One of the earliest records of observed outcomes by nurses dates back to 1854, during the Crimean War at the Scutari Hospital in Turkey under Florence Nightingale's leadership and pioneering work. Nightingale, credited as the founder of modern nursing, documented a decrease in mortality among the British soldiers after providing more nutritious food, cleaning up the environment, and improving the sewage system (Fee & Garofalo, 2010). Despite these exemplary nursing outcomes in the 1850s, variation and challenges with outcome documentation persisted as the nursing profession matured. By the mid-1990s, documentation of nursing outcomes started to improve (Griffiths, 1995; Hill, 1999; Lang & Marek, 1991; van Maanen, 1979). Early work in nursing outcomes focused on costs, and it was clear that a more comprehensive model that included other types of outcomes was needed to advance healthcare and reflect the various outcomes that result from nursing interventions (Jones, 2016). Today, nursing interventions are based on evidence using models of practice that include standards and synchronization with other systems to deliver quality of care, patient safety, and optimal population health outcomes (National Academies of Sciences, Engineering, and Medicine, 2021; Oner et al., 2021; Siaki et al., 2023; Xiao et al., 2017). Health reform efforts to improve quality and access to care and to reduce costs spurred more work to examine outcomes while also examining their relationship to indicators of structure and process (see Chapter 9, "Evaluation of Practice at the Population Level"). The Patient-Centered Outcomes Research Institute (PCORI), for example, developed out of the Patient Protection and Affordable Care Act (ACA) of 2010 and uniquely engages patients and the healthcare community on research projects (Newhouse et al., 2015), such as the **Preemptive Pharmacogenomic Testing for Preventing Adverse Drug Reactions** (PREPARE) study which improved outcomes for African American/Black and Hispanic/Latinx adults with moderate to severe asthma (Israel et al., 2022).

DEFINING, CATEGORIZING, AND IDENTIFYING OUTCOMES

Health outcomes are usually defined as an end result that follows some kind of healthcare provision, treatment, or intervention and may describe a patient's condition or health status (Agency for Healthcare Research and Quality [AHRQ], n.d.; Jones, 2016; Kleinpell & Gawlinski, 2005). Using a population perspective, a health outcome can be measured using public health metrics, such as mortality and life expectancies, that are used to demonstrate the contribution of certain diseases to population mortality. New trends also emphasize the inclusion of qualitative metrics that are based on subjective data, such as self-perceived health status, psychological state, or ability to function, that can illustrate collective social well-being (Wolff et al., 2018).

Evaluating population-based outcomes and their impact on population health involves looking at what to assess and how to assess it. Establishing the impact takes time and requires using an evaluation that links interventions to long-term outcomes such as reducing disease morbidity and mortality at the population level. APRNs can best determine the effectiveness of an intervention and long-term impact by focusing on an accurate assessment and interpretation of data that are generated or collected using individual, population, and community health indicators (Anderson & McFarlane, 2018).

Classifying and categorizing outcomes can be done in several ways. Outcomes may be classified into categories by describing "who" is measured, such as individuals, aggregates, communities, populations, or organizations; by identifying the "what" or the type of outcome, such as care, patient, or performance-related outcomes (Kapu et al., 2021, pp. 1–18; Kleinpell & Gawlinski, 2005); and by determining the "when" or the time it takes to achieve an outcome, such as short-term, intermediate, or long-term outcomes (Rich, 2021, pp. 519–532). Table 3.1 provides examples of various outcomes using these different classification systems. Each outcome type is listed by beneficiary and has a related example of the type of measurement, the potential outcome, and the potential impact of that outcome. Many of them also include a time frame for the outcome.

The Donabedian (1980) framework is frequently used in nursing and healthcare to evaluate quality of care and relies on the examination of three components: *structure, process,* and *outcome. Structure* refers to healthcare resources, such as the number and type of health and social service agencies, and can also include utilization indicators. *Process* describes how the healthcare is delivered. *Outcome* refers to the change in health status related to the intervention provided (Donabedian, 1980). This framework is particularly useful in describing the health of a community. It is based on the concept of community as client and focuses on the health of the collective or population instead of the individual (Gibson & Thatcher, 2019, pp. 396–421).

Using Donabedian's framework, a community's health can be described in terms of its *structure* by the number and type of health and social agencies present, number of public health nurses, health services utilization indicators, and the community's educational and socioeconomic levels in relation to demographic measures of ethnicity, gender, and

3 IDENTIFYING OUTCOMES IN POPULATION-BASED NURSING 43

TABLE 3.1 Examples of Outcomes, Measures, and Impact by Beneficiary, Type, and Time Frame

BENEFICIARY (WHO?)	MEASURE	POTENTIAL OUTCOME	IMPACT
Individual outcomes	BP measurement	Decreased BP	The degree to which perceived health status is improved by BP management
Aggregate outcomes	Weekly weights of participants in an exercise class	Reduced mean weight for exercise class members each week	Sustained weight maintenance using BMI parameters
Community outcomes	A town's seat belt usage per 100 drivers ≥18 years of age computed yearly	Increased yearly rate of a town's seat belt usage per 100 drivers ≥18 years of age	Decrease in the town's percentage of automobile accident injuries/fatalities in drivers ≥18 years of age
Population outcomes	Reported number of infant deaths within 1 year of birth per 1,000 infants	Decreased infant mortality rate compared to previous year	5-year decrease in infant mortality rate
TYPE (WHAT?)	**MEASURE**	**POTENTIAL OUTCOME**	**IMPACT**
Care-related outcomes	Annual rate of hospital-acquired infections determined from hospital infectious disease reports	Decreased hospital-acquired infections rate from previous year	Decreased length of stay and decreased mortality in patients with hospital-acquired infections
Patient-related outcomes	Observation of insulin injection administration technique	Correct demonstration by patient of safe insulin administration technique	Decreased hemoglobin A1C and decreased incidence of microvascular complications
Performance-related outcomes	Chart review for completed checklist of asthma best-practices protocol	Nursing staff adherence to asthma best-practices protocol	Decreased emergency department visits due to asthma
TIME FRAME (WHEN?)	**MEASURE**	**POTENTIAL OUTCOME**	**IMPACT**
Short-term outcomes	Self-report of nipple discomfort among first-time breastfeeding mothers in a postpartum unit	Absence of nipple discomfort among first-time breastfeeding mothers 1 week after hospital discharge from a postpartum unit	Improved breastfeeding rates among women discharged from a postpartum unit

(continued)

TABLE 3.1 Examples of Outcomes, Measures, and Impact by Beneficiary, Type, and Time Frame (*continued*)

TIME FRAME (WHEN?)	MEASURE	POTENTIAL OUTCOME	IMPACT
Intermediate outcomes	Self-report of tobacco usage by first-time outpatient clinic users during the calendar year	An increase in smoking-cessation rates among outpatient clinic users during the calendar year	Decrease in smoking-related illnesses among outpatient clinic users during the calendar year
Long-term outcomes	COVID-19 annual vaccination rates per state	Annual reduction of COVID-19 infection rates per state	Annual reduction of mortality related to COVID-19 per state

BMI, body mass index; BP, blood pressure; COVID-19, coronavirus disease 2019.

age. A community's health *process* can be measured by its healthcare delivery methods and how well community members work together to build capacity and solve their problems, which reflects the ability to share power and resources and to respond to needs and changes (Minkler et al., 2021, pp. 35–52). Most publicly reported measures on healthcare quality are related to process (AHRQ, 2015). Community health outcomes can include measures associated with vital statistics (e.g., births, deaths, marriages, divorces, fetal deaths, and induced termination of pregnancies); morbidity or illness data and trends; social determinants of health (SDOH), such as housing, unemployment, and poverty rates; and health risk profiles of aggregates by specific areas, including neighborhood safety, access to fresh fruits and vegetables, as well as availability of physical activity venues such as parks, playgrounds, and neighborhood sports fields (Anderson & McFarlane, 2018). Other indicators of a community's health status may include the number of premature deaths, quality of life, disabilities, risk factors, and injuries. Community health outcomes models are used to assess the interaction between the physical and the social environments (including the built environment) and the impact on health at the individual, population, and community levels (Chatelan & Khalatbari-Soltani, 2022; DeGuzman & Kulbok, 2012). The *built environment* refers to the physical structures where people live, work, are educated, and recreate (CDC, 2021a). Guided by these models of practice and research, APRNs can work in partnership with community members to assess the community's health status through structure, process, and outcome measures; identify and monitor relevant health outcomes; and develop appropriate interventions to improve those outcomes (Bigbee & Issel, 2012; Emery et al., 2023; Payán et al., 2017).

VITAL STATISTICS

Vital statistics provide important outcome measures that APRNs can monitor and compare over time and analyze by demographic variables to detect issues such as health disparities. In the United States, the National Center for Health Statistics (NCHS) located within the CDC collects information from a variety of sources, such as birth and death certificates, health records, surveys, physical exams, and laboratory testing (CDC, 2022b). Personnel from local health departments review the data from death certificates, including demographic data, looking at the immediate cause of death and any contributing factors of death and recording multiple causes of death. Local data are sent to a state office for collation and then sent to the NCHS, which provides this information to the public on its website (www.cdc.gov/nchs). State and national provisional data is available on its Vital Statistics Rapid Release page (www.cdc.gov/nchs/nvss/vsrr/provisional-tables.htm). APRNs can access national and global health statistics from multiple agency sources, including government agencies, to identify health trends and patterns. However, due to the lack of agencies and/or resources in certain populations or regions, health information might not be available or might be limited in scope.

United States Census Bureau

The U.S. Census Bureau (www.census.gov), part of the U.S. Department of Commerce, is an excellent source of information of population-level demographics and other statistics. Its mission is "to serve as the nation's leading provider of quality data about its people and economy" (U.S. Census Bureau, 2022). The Census Bureau collects data through regular surveys on the nation's people, geography, and economy. It is best known for conducting the Decennial Census of Population and Housing survey. The information collected through this census is used to allocate the number of representatives each state can elect and send to the U.S. Congress. It is also used to determine the level of funding for critical programs, such as Medicare. The Census Bureau administers and analyzes the National Sample Survey of Registered Nurses (NSSRN) for the Health Resources and Services Administration (HRSA). Its website provides access to robust search tools, maps, and tables. APRNs can use data from the Census Bureau to better understand the communities they work with, especially in the area of SDOH.

BEHAVIORAL RISK FACTOR SURVEILLANCE SYSTEM

In the early 1980s, personal health behaviors became a key source of information that paved the way in understanding risk behavior and its impact on morbidity and mortality. The Behavioral Risk Factor Surveillance System (BRFSS; www.cdc.gov/brfss) was established to collect state-level data, such as perceived health status and primary source of health insurance, via a telephone survey. The survey allows states to estimate the prevalence of disease (e.g., hypertension, high cholesterol, or asthma) for regions that can be compared across states (CDC, 2018). The annual BRFSS questionnaires can be accessed on the CDC's website (www.cdc.gov/brfss/questionnaires/index.htm). The data generated by this surveillance system have been pivotal in assessing and addressing urgent or emerging health issues. The ability to reach cell phone users has expanded BRFSS's accessibility to populations that were not accessible by prior data collection methods. This has increased representation and produced a higher quality of information than when the survey was solely conducted through landline phones.

It is the world's largest continuously conducted health survey system and serves as model for other countries. In 2009, almost all states added questions concerning adverse childhood experiences (ACEs) to the annual BRFSS. APRNs can search for city, county, and state data on health-related risk behaviors, chronic health conditions, and use of preventive services using various tools available on the BRFSS website (www.cdc.gov/brfss).

SOCIAL DETERMINANTS OF HEALTH

SDOH and disparities data can be used by APRNs to inform and guide their practice to develop culturally appropriate interventions. SDOH are recognized situations related to where people are born, grow up, work, and live and the systems of care available to them to deal with illness and disease (Braveman & Gottlieb, 2014; CDC, 2022e; Hacker et al., 2022; ODPHP, 2022). Examples of SDOH associated with disparities include poverty, educational level, racism, income, and housing. Health inequalities can lead to poor quality of life, poor self-rated health, multiple morbidities, limited access to resources, unnecessary risks and vulnerabilities, and premature death. The AHRQ's 2022 *National Healthcare Quality and Disparities Report* (NHQDR) noted that SDOH had a greater effect on population health and well-being than programs or services. This finding illustrates why it is so important for APRNs to work with interprofessional teams to address SDOH. One good resource is the *Compendium of Federal Datasets Addressing Health Disparities* (2019), which APRNs can use to find data, especially on SDOH, from a collection of federally funded agencies.

APRNs may encounter a lack of available data and status for immigrant, refugee, and/or migrant populations. They may be able to access health information for these populations through partnerships with other sectors outside of health, such as housing, labor, education, and community-based or faith-based organization, that offer services to immigrant communities. A national resource is the U.S. Department of Labor's annual survey on agricultural workers, specifically migrant farmworkers, that collects data related to birthplace, work authorization, demographics, household structure, language, education, housing, employment, and health (www.dol.gov/agencies/eta/national-agricultural-workers-survey/research).

MORBIDITY AND MORTALITY DATA

APRNs are often responsible for reviewing morbidity and mortality trends and can use this information to advocate for improved health policy and additional resources or to develop and implement innovative interventions. Provisional weekly updates of reportable diseases can be accessed electronically through the *Morbidity and Mortality Weekly Report* (MMWR), published by the CDC. Morbidity data are less standardized in general than mortality data because state legislatures and local agencies decide what illnesses must be reported to the CDC. Reporting cases of infectious diseases and related conditions is an important step in controlling and preventing the spread of communicable disease. The list of reportable or notifiable diseases can change as some diseases may become eradicated and other, new diseases and conditions are discovered such as the COVID-19 and mpox viruses. The accuracy of morbidity data is diminished if healthcare providers fail to report a disease or illness for fear of violating an individual's privacy or because they may not be aware of reporting requirements or because the healthcare provider misdiagnosed the illness (Porche, 2023). It is imperative that APRNs educate themselves on the reporting requirements in their state. Certain diseases with easy and/or rapid transmission are more likely to harm a population's health. Infectious or communicable diseases, such as certain sexually transmitted infections (STIs) or other diseases, such as COVID-19, rabies, rubella, plague, measles, tetanus, and foodborne illnesses, can lead to significant morbidity and mortality if not reported promptly (Friis & Sellers, 2020).

Another way to evaluate morbidity is derived from population surveys that are conducted to determine the frequency of acute and chronic illnesses and disability as well as other population characteristics. The U.S. National Health Interview Survey (NHIS) is an example of a morbidity survey that was first authorized by Congress in 1956 for the purpose of informing the U.S. population about various health measures and indicators. To obtain a representative national sample, the NHIS continuously surveys households throughout the year on a variety of health topics, such as physical and mental health status, chronic conditions, and access to and use of healthcare services. One finding from the 2021 data indicated a disparity in telemedicine use, with Hispanic, non-Hispanic Black, and non-Hispanic Asian persons less likely to use telemedicine than non-Hispanic White and non-Hispanic American Indian or Native Alaskan persons (Lucas & Villarroel, 2022). The NHIS debuted a redesign in 2019 to improve its content and structure. The redesign emphasizes content with a strong link to public health, such as intermediate health outcomes for leading causes of morbidity/mortality. It also targets major federal health promotion initiatives and healthcare access and utilization (CDC, 2022a).

The NHIS is one sector of the data collection program at the NCHS, housed within the CDC. The NCHS works with public and private partners to collect data that provide reliable and valid evidence on a population's health status, influences on health, and health outcomes (CDC, 2023). APRNs can review these data to identify health disparities among subgroups based on ethnicity and/or socioeconomic status, monitor trends with health status and with healthcare delivery systems, support research endeavors, identify health problems, evaluate health policies, and access important information that can be used to improve policies and health services. The NHIS data can be accessed at www.cdc.gov/nchs/nhis.

In addition to population surveys such as the NHIS, the NCHS collects data using other surveys with each method yielding information that is readily available on the Internet for use by healthcare providers, researchers, and educators. First, the *National Vital Statistics System* provides information about state and local vital statistics, including teen birth rates, prenatal care, birth weights, risk factors related to poor pregnancy outcomes, infant mortality rates, life expectancy, and leading causes of death (www.cdc.gov/nchs/nvss). Second, the *National Health and Nutrition Examination*

Survey (NHANES) is conducted through mobile examination centers held at randomly selected sites throughout the United States. Data are obtained from interviews (e.g., environmental exposures, risk factors), and additional data are collected from physical examinations, diagnostic procedures, laboratory tests, and indicators of growth and development, including weight, diet, and nutrition (www.cdc.gov/nchs/nhanes.htm). Third, the *National Healthcare Surveys* obtain data using a collection of surveys targeted toward various healthcare providers and healthcare settings (www.cdc.gov/nchs/dhcs). A variety of data is collected, including information on patient safety and safety indicators, clinical management of specific health conditions, disparities in healthcare utilization and health quality, and information about the use of healthcare innovations. All these survey data are collated and made available for policymakers, practitioners, and researchers and all provide useful outcome information for APRNs. Additional surveys can be found on the NCHS website, but the aforementioned surveys are most useful for analyzing outcomes data.

IDENTIFYING OUTCOMES

How do APRNs decide what outcomes to study? There are a variety of outcomes that exist in relation to cost, clinical and functional data, social conditions, and community and environmental indicators. Often, outcomes will reflect the desired or anticipated effects of the intervention that are related to the problem or population of interest. Another way to select outcomes is by reviewing available epidemiological and social epidemiological data for outcomes that may be of interest or relevance to an APRN's intervention or study (Galea & Link, 2013; Minkler et al., 2021, pp. 35–52; Porche, 2023). Using the following case study example of designing an intervention to reduce teenage motor vehicle collisions (MVCs), an APRN could seek out epidemiological data from the *National Highway Traffic Safety Administration's* (NHTSA) *Fatality Analysis Reporting System* and review annual data and trends for fatalities in drivers ages 15 to 19 (crashstats.nhtsa.dot.gov). Outcomes can also be identified using County Health Rankings and Roadmaps (CHR&R), a user-friendly online data source. It allows an APRN to compare similarly sized counties on various measures, such as premature death, low birthweight, or drug overdose deaths (www.countyhealthrankings.org). Paul et al. (2021) used data from the CHR&R, Bureau of Labor, and U.S. Department of Agriculture to identify the impact of county-level SDOH on COVID-19 mortality rates. Their analysis revealed that urban and rural counties with a high percentage of Black residents, and/or high HIV, and/or high diabetes experienced higher COVID-19 mortality rate than those counties with lower percentages of these three variables. Additionally, education was found to have an inverse association with COVID-19 mortality rates; higher levels of education correlated with lower rates. Understanding how such factors impact the health of a community can help APRNs to target appropriate community level outcomes for improvement.

There is no shortage of usable resources for identifying outcomes. The Community Preventive Services Task Force (CPSTF), established by the Department of Health and Human Services (DHHS) in 1996, updates and publishes *The Community Guide,* a helpful online resource for community-focused health promotion and disease prevention interventions (available at www.thecommunityguide.org). It provides evidence-based recommendations for public health interventions, analyses from systematic reviews to determine program and policy effectiveness, information on whether an intervention might work in one's community, and information about the intervention's costs and benefits. In 2022, the task force added seven key goal areas that focus on advancing health equity and addressing the SDOH (i.e., the what) especially for historically disadvantaged racial and ethnic populations and those affected by marked income disparities (i.e., the who). APRNs can review topics or areas of focus and strategies that work for various outcomes. For example, systematic reviews are available on adolescent health. By spending a few minutes exploring the website, one can find numerous outcomes such as number of self-reported risk behaviors, including engagement in any sexual activity, frequency of sexual activity, number of partners, frequency of unprotected sexual activity, use of protection to prevent STIs, use of protection to prevent pregnancy, and self-reported or clinically documented STIs. Other community guide topics are listed in Table 3.2 with example outcomes adapted from the website (United States DHHS, 2023).

CASE STUDY

An APRN who is employed by a large school district identifies an increase in asthma exacerbation episodes in adolescents from one year to the next. Before designing an intervention, the APRN first reviewed morbidity and mortality trends for the community. Then, they reviewed other sources of relevant data, such as asthma-related emergency department and hospitalization rates, asthma diagnoses, student medication records, school absences, indoor and outdoor air quality, average household incomes, and ethnic and racial disparities. The APRN decides to develop a plan of care to target risk factors associated with asthma in adolescents. They approach other school nurses, health professionals, community stakeholders, and education administrators to collaborate on an evidence-based, school-based asthma education program. The team reviews recommendations from CPSTF (2019) on *School-Based Self-Management Interventions for Children and Adolescents with Asthma*. They decide to implement various interventions targeted at increasing asthma education in the schools, such as ensuring every student has a personalized asthma plan, running group sessions on using rescue medications, and educating students on potential triggers at school and home.

1. What health outcomes should the team use to evaluate the success of the program?

2. When should the team conduct evaluations?

3. What is the value of collaborating with community stakeholders such as pediatric primary care providers?

4. What are some policy additions and/or changes that the team might suggest?

TABLE 3.2 Community Guide Topics and Outcome Examples

TOPICS	OUTCOME EXAMPLES
Adolescent health	Alcohol, tobacco, and drug usage; injury, violence, and suicide rates; BMI, physical activity, and educational attainment
Asthma	Symptom-free days, quality-of-life scores, school or work absenteeism, environmental mold remediation, medication usage, hospital admissions
Cancer	Cigarette smoking, physical activity, nutrition, screening test results
Diabetes	Hemoglobin A1C, incidence of skin infections, obesity, peripheral neuropathy, renal insufficiency
Excessive alcohol consumption	Alcohol-related injuries or death, motor vehicle accidents, liver disease rates, alcohol poisoning rates
Health communication and HIT	Use of reliable digital and mobile technology for HIT or appointment reminders, health literacy level, communication by provider of understandable HIT, difficulty using HIT
Heart disease and stroke prevention	Blood pressure, physical activity, cholesterol levels, BMI
HIV, STIs, and teen pregnancy	Abstinence, condom use, incidence of STIs or pregnancy
Mental health	Depression scale scores, hospital admissions, attendance at school or work, suicidal ideation or attempts
Motor vehicle injury	Use of child safety seats, use of seat belts, driver blood alcohol concentration, distracted driving rates, moving violations
Nutrition	Daily intake of fruits and vegetables, BMI; sugary drinks intake, fat intake, fiber intake, access to free school lunch
Obesity	Daily physical activity, screen time, weight loss, BMI
Oral health	Dental caries; incidence of oral or throat cancer; use of helmets, face masks, and mouth guards in contact sports; reduced or discontinued use of chewing tobacco; dental insurance coverage
Physical activity	Muscle strength and endurance activities, moderate- or vigorous-intensity aerobic physical activity
Pregnancy health	Gestational hypertension, gestational diabetes, folic acid intake, maternal mortality, infant mortality
Preparedness and response	Infectious disease rates, healthcare workforce, mortality rate
SDOH	Income disparities, racial and ethnic disparities, number of tenant-based housing voucher programs, number of school-based health centers
Tobacco	Out-of-pocket costs for cessation therapies, creation of smoke-free policies, retail tobacco sales to youth

(continued)

TABLE 3.2 Community Guide Topics and Outcome Examples (*continued*)

TOPICS	OUTCOME EXAMPLES
Vaccination	Number of infectious cases, hospitalizations, deaths from vaccine-preventable disease, immunization rates, immunization failures
Violence	Number of violence-related hospitalizations and deaths, participation in therapeutic foster care, school-based violence prevention programs, reduction of nonaccidental trauma in infants and toddlers
Worksite health	Stair usage by employees, gym membership by employees, use of weight management counseling by employees

BMI, body mass index; HIT, health information technology; SDOH, social determinants of health.
Source: Adapted from U.S. Department of Health and Human Services, Community Preventive Services Task Force. (2023). *The community guide.* Retrieved from www.thecommunityguide.org

Trust for America's Health (TFAH) is another resource to inform APRNs' outcome identification (www.tfah.org). TFAH's work is centered on causes of poor health and prevention. Its vision is of a nation that values health and well-being for all. It is a resource for issues such as public health funding; obesity; the drug, alcohol, and suicide crisis in America; emergency preparedness; and health disparities. It also allows an APRN to examine state-level data and rankings on key health indicators (e.g., percentage of the population who received the seasonal flu vaccination, percent of adults who have obesity, and drug- and alcohol-related deaths).

OUTCOME MONITORING

After identifying outcomes, monitoring of measures to assess effectiveness of interventions is increasingly important and, in many cases, is a necessity to justify program implementation or program funding. For example, outcome monitoring is used to assess quality of healthcare by examining the association between the level of improved health services and the desired health outcomes of individuals and populations (Blumenthal et al., 2015). This is best done by having a quality improvement (QI) plan that systematically and consistently implements improvement strategies to address areas that are deficient and not meeting benchmarks. The Institute for Healthcare Improvement (IHI) is a useful resource for determining a QI plan and provides a QI Essentials Toolkit with 10 tools (e.g., Plan-Do-Study-Act [PDSA] worksheet) to guide QI projects (www.ihi.org/resources/Pages/Tools/Quality-Improvement-Essentials-Toolkit.aspx).

Outcomes are an expected part of what APRNs must collect when their focus is on populations. When combined with an evidence-based practice approach, outcomes can help provide standards or parameters for developing innovative interventions, instituting approaches more likely to impact the problem, and/or developing new practice guidelines or protocols. Through working with populations, APRNs contribute to meeting the IHI (2022) Triple Aim: (1) improve the health of the population, (2) enhance the experience of the patient, and (3) reduce the per capita cost of health. For example, an APRN working in a community-based clinic with a Hispanic population may gather information on factors related to an increased rate of type 2 diabetes mellitus, such as hypertension, obesity, or language barriers. An assessment can be made to determine if differences in health outcomes exist based on social support, family structures, barriers to obtaining medications or durable medical equipment, or other variables of interest. Once these outcomes are assessed, actions can be taken to address the issues that may contribute to poor health outcomes or increased incidence, such as implementing a cost-effective intervention, such as hiring community health workers (CHWs) (Chang et al., 2018). A reassessment of outcomes is necessary after an intervention to determine if a change has occurred. Nundy et al. (2022) advocate for adding the goal of advancing health equity to the Triple Aim framework. According to these authors, "quality improvement without equity is a hollow victory" (p. 521).

Outcomes can also be used to measure quality of care in an outpatient setting. For example, APRNs in a maternity care practice set a goal to increase the percentage of publicly insured women who attend their standard postpartum visit (Kuster et al., 2022). They added an additional postpartum visit between birth and the 6-week follow-up appointment. After 5 months, they achieved an increase in the percentage of women who attend their postpartum visits.

NURSE-SENSITIVE QUALITY INDICATORS

As documented evidence of patient safety concerns grew in the United States and at a time when healthcare costs were increasing and healthcare quality was being questioned, various nursing organizations started to focus on establishing a coordinated system for evaluating patient safety. In 1994, the American Nurses Association (ANA) developed Nursing's Safety and Quality Initiative, which started studies of patient safety with the goal of advocating healthy change. It was clear that nurse managers and administrators needed sound data for comparing their hospital units with similar units across the nation as a means of improving quality by developing and refining quality improvement initiatives and monitoring progress. The indicators needed to be specific or sensitive to nursing care rather than ones that reflected medical care or institutional care. The indicators would have to be highly correlated with nursing quality and be measurable with a high degree of reliability and validity. Furthermore, the indicator must not pose undue hardships on personnel tasked with collecting the data. Donabedian's (1982) framework of focusing on structure, process, and patient-centered outcomes was used for identifying and honing the indicators. *Structure* indicators included staff mix and nursing care hours per patient day; *process* indicators included maintenance of skin integrity and nurse satisfaction; and patient-focused *outcomes* included nosocomial infections, patient fall rates, patient satisfaction with pain management, patient education, nursing care, and overall care (Ayanian & Markel, 2016).

The National Database of Nursing Quality Indicators® (NDNQI®) was created in 1998 by the ANA as part of the initiative to make changes to improve safety and quality of care, to help educate nurses about measurement, and to invest in research studies that examined safe and high-quality patient care. The NDNQI® helped standardize information that was submitted by hospital units throughout the United States on indicators related to nursing structure (staffing level, educational level), process measures, and outcome measures. Hospitals use these results to compare their performance with those of other hospitals with similar demographic makeup and patient population. NDNQI®

was purchased by Press Ganey Associates in 2014. Technical assistance and continuing education are provided by liaisons to ensure that reliable and valid data collection methods are used by hospital personnel. This database provides a wealth of information on a quarterly and annual basis of more than 2,000 facilities in the United States (Press Ganey Associates, n.d.). In addition to hospital indicators, nurse-sensitive indicators for community-based healthcare settings also exist. The ability to collect and compare data on nurse-sensitive indicators and the ability to develop new indicators over time enhance the NDNQI® initiative and provide APRNs with important information to help measure, compare, and improve the health and safety of populations.

STANDARDIZED LANGUAGE IN NURSING

The use of standardized language is important in any field to ensure a level of communication that is both consistent and effective in ensuring quality outcomes. Specifically, in nursing and other health professions, standardized language is critical for patient safety and quality of care. By establishing a uniform nursing language in electronic health records, research, and the development of evidence-based practice, APRNs have a stronger foundation to communicate and improve patient outcomes and standards of care. The North American Nursing Diagnosis Association (NANDA) was developed in the 1970s to classify and standardize nursing diagnoses. Now referred to as NANDA International, Inc. or NANDA-I, the nursing diagnoses include a name or label, signs and symptoms or defining characteristics, and risk factors associated with the diagnosis. The 12th edition of *Nursing Diagnoses: Definitions and Classifications 2021–2023* reflects new trends in nursing healthcare (www.nanda.org). Members of NANDA-I worked with nursing researchers at the University of Iowa to develop the Nursing Interventions Classification (NIC) and the Nursing Outcomes Classification (NOC). The Center for Nursing Classification and Clinical Effectiveness (CNC, n.d.) continually researches and develops NICs and NOCs and their connectedness to NANDA-I to reflect a standardized way of communicating with defined terms within and across various national and international settings. As APRNs contribute to the body of evidence-based practice and collaborate with others to generate more evidence of effective practice, their work may benefit from reviewing and using the NIC, NOC, and NANDA-I language for diagnoses, nursing interventions, and patient outcomes (Butcher et al., 2018; Herdman et al., 2021; Moorhead et al., 2018). It is imperative that APRNs use standardized language in their research and in their practice so that outcomes can be compared in similar ways with larger databases for evaluation and research purposes.

NATIONAL HEALTHCARE OBJECTIVES

THE AGENCY FOR HEALTHCARE RESEARCH AND QUALITY'S NATIONAL HEALTHCARE QUALITY AND DISPARITIES REPORT

Since 2003, the AHRQ has partnered with members of the DHHS to report on healthcare quality improvement by publishing the NHQDR. The intent of this report is to respond to the status of healthcare quality in the United States, identify where improvement is most needed, and describe how the quality of healthcare that is given to Americans changes over time. This report includes more than 250 measures of quality and disparities and uses the Three Aims for Improving Healthcare as its framework. Its six priority quality domains are person-centered care, patient safety, healthy living, effective treatment, care coordination, and care affordability (AHRQ, 2022). The four *Special Emphasis Topics* in the 2022 report are maternal health, child and adolescent mental health, substance use disorders, and oral health. A key finding related to the four *Special Emphasis Topics* is that maternal mortality rates in the United States are increasing and are higher than the maternal mortality rates in other industrialized countries (AHRQ, 2022). In another key finding, the rate of opioid overdose deaths in the United States increased by 36.8% from 2019 to 2020.

The AHRQ offers robust NHQDR data tools (datatools.ahrq.gov/nhqdr) that APRNs can use to retrieve data linked to their geographical location and populations of interest. Additionally, the AHRQ's website has useful information for APRNs that they can use to identify and monitor outcomes (www.qualityindicators.ahrq.gov). Other tools, referred to as indicators, can be used by APRNs to identify outcomes or measures of the quality of healthcare. The inpatient quality indicators are designed to help hospitals identify issues and problems in need of quality improvement. Hospital administrative data is used to calculate morbidity and mortality rates for specific conditions and procedures, hospital- and area-level procedure utilization rates, and number of procedures (for select procedures). In addition to the inpatient quality indicators, other sets of quality indicators are available, including preventive quality indicators, patient safety indicators, and pediatric quality indicators.

Healthy People 2030

Healthy People 2030, released by the United States' ODPHP in August 2020, serves as a blueprint or road map to improve the health of all Americans. The *Healthy People* initiative started in 1979 when the surgeon general released a report that focused on promoting health and preventing disease for all Americans and released *Healthy People 1990*. Every 10 years, with leadership provided by the DHHS, an appointed advisory committee and numerous public and private groups, local and state policymakers and officials, and numerous organizations (voluntary, advocacy, faith based, and for-profit businesses) use information that is solicited regionally, statewide, and nationally to help craft the vision, mission, and overarching goals. These groups and organizations also develop strategies to improve health and prevent disease with the ultimate goal of helping Americans live longer and healthier lives. The resulting objectives, whether on the county, state, or national level, are intended for use by broad audiences and stakeholders to help motivate, guide, and focus action for a healthier nation.

The *Healthy People 2030*'s three priority areas are health equity, health literacy, and SDOH. Its mission is to "promote, strengthen, and evaluate the nation's efforts to improve the health and well-being of all people" (United States DHHS, n.d.). It moves beyond an individual-level approach to interventions and guides the creation of policies to promote the social and physical environments that are conducive to health. Changes to the 2030 version include a reduced number of core objectives, comprehensive data standards, a more user-friendly online interface, addition of emerging topics like e-cigarettes and substance use disorders, and a compendium of evidence-based strategies. *Healthy People 2030* has eight overall health and well-being measures (OHMs), which are broad, global outcomes, to assess progress toward its overarching vision for "a society in which all people can achieve their full potential for health and well-being across the lifespan." The eight OHMs are categorized into three tiers: well-being, healthy life expectancy, and summary mortality and health. The OHMs include three types of objectives: core objectives (measurable targets associated with evidence-based interventions), developmental objectives (public health issues with evidence-based interventions but unreliable data), and research objectives (public health issues with evolving evidence-based interventions). Some of the objectives were retained from *Healthy People 2020* because they were not met, some objectives were modified, and some are entirely new to *Healthy People 2030*. The SDOH framework continues to guide work in identifying and addressing factors that can widen health disparities. One notable change to *Healthy People 2030*'s SDOH objectives is explicit 10-year targets, compared to *Healthy People 2020* which had only informational objectives related to SDOH. The Leading Health Indicators (LHIs) are 23 high-priority core objectives that require urgent action to improve prevalent diseases and conditions affecting the U.S. population across the lifespan. The LHIs are listed in Table 3.3.

APRNs and other users can tailor information available from *Healthy People 2030* for their specific use and needs. The online tools can be used to identify needs and priority populations, set targets specific to a work setting, find practical tools and learn about successful initiatives, monitor national progress, and set benchmarks. The *Healthy People* website is continually improved to facilitate easy access of the data and to make sense of the findings. Information about *Healthy People 2030* can be found at www.healthypeople.gov. See Table 3.3 for a summary of the *Healthy People 2030* initiatives with its vision, mission, goals, foundational principles, overarching goals, LHIs, and objective topic areas. Each topic area has a list of objectives with data sources, baseline, and target measures to achieve.

Health Disparities

With each successive version, *Healthy People* has sharpened its focus on health equity. This focus is exemplified in *Healthy People 2030*'s overarching goal to "Eliminate health disparities, achieve health equity, and attain health literacy to improve the health and well-being of all." *Healthy People 2030* is tracking metrics related to health disparities to assess progress toward achieving health equity, such as the number of asthma deaths by race/ethnicity, age, and geographical location. *Healthy People 2030* utilizes the following definitions for health equity and health disparity:

> **Health equity**: The attainment of the highest level of health for all people. Achieving health equity requires valuing everyone equally with focused and ongoing societal efforts to address avoidable inequalities, historical and contemporary injustices, and the elimination of health and healthcare disparities (CDC, 2022d).

TABLE 3.3 Vision, Mission, Goals, Foundational Principles, Overarching Goals, Leading Health Indicators, and Objective Topic Areas of *Healthy People 2030*

Vision	A society in which all people can achieve their full potential for health and well-being across the lifespan
Mission	• To promote, strengthen, and evaluate the nation's efforts to improve the health and well-being of all people
Foundational principles	The following foundational principles guide decisions about *Healthy People 2030*: • The health and well-being of all people and communities is essential to a thriving, equitable society. • Promoting health and well-being and preventing disease are linked efforts that encompass physical, mental, and social health dimensions. • Investing to achieve the full potential for health and well-being for all provides valuable benefits to society. • Achieving health and well-being requires eliminating health disparities, achieving health equity, and attaining health literacy. • Healthy physical, social, and economic environments strengthen the potential to achieve health and well-being. • Promoting and achieving health and well-being nationwide is a shared responsibility that is distributed across the national, state, tribal, and community levels, including the public, private, and not-for-profit sectors. Working to attain the full potential for health and well-being of the population is a component of decision-making and policy formulation across all sectors.
Overarching goals	• Attain healthy, thriving lives and well-being free of preventable disease, disability, injury, and premature death • Eliminate health disparities, achieve health equity, and attain health literacy to improve the health and well-being of all • Create social, physical, and economic environments that promote attaining the full potential for health and well-being for all • Promote healthy development, healthy behaviors, and well-being across all life stages • Engage leadership, key constituents, and the public across multiple sectors to take action and design policies that improve the health and well-being of all
Leading Health Indicators	
All ages	• Children, adolescents, and adults who use the oral health care system (2+ years) • Consumption of calories from added sugars by persons aged 2 years and over (2+ years) • Drug overdose deaths • Exposure to unhealthy air • Homicides • Household food insecurity and hunger • Persons who are vaccinated annually against seasonal influenza • Persons who know their HIV status (13+ years) • Persons with medical insurance (<65 years) • Suicides
Infants	• Infant deaths

(continued)

TABLE 3.3 Vision, Mission, Goals, Foundational Principles, Overarching Goals, Leading Health Indicators, and Objective Topic Areas of *Healthy People 2030* (*continued*)

Children and adolescents	• Fourth-grade students whose reading skills are at or above the proficient achievement level for their grade • Adolescents with major depressive episodes who receive treatment • Children and adolescents with obesity • Current use of any tobacco products among adolescents
Adults and older adults	• Adults engaging in binge drinking of alcoholic beverages during the past 30 days • Adults who meet current minimum guidelines for aerobic physical activity and muscle strengthening activity • Adults who receive a colorectal cancer screening based on the most recent guidelines • Adults with hypertension whose blood pressure is under control • Cigarette smoking in adults • Employment among the working age population • Maternal deaths • New cases of diagnosed diabetes in the population
Healthy People 2030 **Topic Areas**	
Health conditions	Addiction Arthritis Blood disorders Cancer Chronic kidney disease Chronic pain Dementias Diabetes Foodborne illness Healthcare-associated infections Heart disease and stroke Infectious disease Mental health and mental disorders Oral conditions Osteoporosis Overweight and obesity Pregnancy and childbirth Respiratory disease Sensory or communication disorders STIs
Health behaviors	Child and adolescent development Drug and alcohol use Emergency preparedness Family planning Health communication Injury prevention Nutrition and healthy eating Physical activity Preventive care Safe food handling Sleep Tobacco use Vaccination Violence prevention

(*continued*)

TABLE 3.3 Vision, Mission, Goals, Foundational Principles, Overarching Goals, Leading Health Indicators, and Objective Topic Areas of *Healthy People 2030* (*continued*)

Populations	Adolescents Children Infants LGBTQ+ Men Older adults Parents or caregivers People with disabilities Women Workforce
Settings and systems	Community Environmental health Global health Health care Health insurance HIT Health policy Hospital and emergency services Housing and homes Public health infrastructure Schools Transportation Workplace
SDOH	Economic stability Education access and quality Healthcare access and quality Neighborhood and built environment Social and community context

Source: Adapted from the U.S. Department of Health and Human Services. (n.d.). *Healthy People 2030*. Retrieved from health.gov/healthypeople; health.gov/healthypeople/about/healthy-people-2030-framework; health.gov/healthypeople/objectives-and-data/leading-health-indicators

> **Health disparity**: A particular type of health difference that is closely linked with social, economic, and/or environmental disadvantage. Health disparities adversely affect groups of people who have systematically experienced greater obstacles to health based on their racial or ethnic group; religion; socioeconomic status; gender; age; mental health; cognitive, sensory, or physical disability; sexual orientation or gender identity; geographical location; or other characteristics historically linked to discrimination or exclusion (CDC, 2022e).

By monitoring differences among groups, health professionals can identify why and where population disparities occur. This in turn facilitates the implementation of evidence-based strategies to reduce health disparities and improve equity in health and the delivery of healthcare.

There are numerous dimensions of disparities or differences related to health that can adversely affect groups of people because of specific characteristics or obstacles. It is widely recognized now that the SDOH, such as housing, education, access to public transportation, access to safe water, access to fresh food, and the built environment, are all related to a population's health (AHRQ, 2022). In addition to ethnicity, other characteristics also contribute to the presence of disparities or the achievement of good health such as gender; sexual orientation; geographical location; working environment; cognitive, sensory, or physical disability; and socioeconomic status. *Healthy People 2030* aims to improve health disparities in populations by tracking morbidity and mortality outcomes in relation to factors found to be associated with disparities.

ONLINE RESOURCES

APRNs have numerous online resources they can access to improve the quality of and timely access to healthcare and to decrease health disparities. Several of these are mentioned earlier in this chapter. Kleinpell and Kapu (2017) identify 13 resources for quality measures that are relevant to APRN practice. One is the *Nurse Practitioner Outcomes Toolkit* available through the American Association of Nurse Practitioners (AANP). Think Cultural Health (thinkculturalhealth.hhs.gov) is an initiative from the Office of Minority Health and Health Equity (OMHHE) that offers a variety of information, training, and resources to implement culturally and linguistically appropriate services (CLAS) across healthcare settings. Established in 1988, the OMHHE is housed within the DHHS. Healthcare disparities are complex to address as they go beyond differences in biological characteristics and health behaviors (microlevel properties). Racist and discriminatory behaviors and policies, cultural barriers, lack of access to care, and interaction with the environment (macrolevel properties) play a major role in creating the problem (see Chapter 12, "Challenges in Program Implementation").

National Quality Partners™ (www.qualityforum.org/National_Quality_Partners.aspx) includes key private and public stakeholders who have agreed to work on major health priorities of patients and families, palliative and end-of-life care, care coordination, patient safety, and population health. Another excellent resource is the Association of American Medical Colleges' (AAMC) Center for Health Justice (www.aamchealthjustice.org). AAMC Center for Health Justice is a collaborative effort to improve the health of communities and dismantle injustices that contribute to disparities (AAMC, n.d.). The website includes resources for building trust with communities, community engagement toolkits, and developing a systems approach to community health and equity.

Established in 2000 and housed within the National Institute of Health (NIH) is the National Institute on Minority Health and Health Disparities (NIMHD). It supports researchers who address issues of health inequity. Its website highlights successful initiatives and programs (www.nimhd.nih.gov/programs/edu-training), such as the Transdisciplinary Collaborative Centers (TCCs) for Health Disparities Research Program, which funds regional coalitions. APRNs can contact the principal investigators or other research staff to obtain information, to explore collaborative endeavors with researchers, to participate with community-based participatory research, to assist with translational research studies, and to share expertise with the aim of decreasing health disparities among vulnerable populations.

Also, within the NIH, is the National Cancer Institute's Division of Cancer Control and Population Sciences (DCCPS), which has a variety of resources available, including funding opportunities, reports and health surveys, datasets, tool kits for research projects, and cost-cutting areas such as health disparities, patient-centered communication, and care coordination (cancercontrol.cancer.gov). There is also a health disparities calculator (HD*Calc). HD*Calc is statistical software that can be downloaded and used to generate and calculate a range of disparity measurements (seer.cancer.gov/hdcalc).

EXAMPLES OF HEALTH DISPARITIES

Even a cursory review of reports and studies available through government agencies and various other organizations as well as peer-reviewed journals reveals numerous examples of healthcare disparities in the United States. The following are just a few examples.

Despite advances in diabetes prevention and treatment, American Indian/Alaska Natives (AI/AN) have a higher age-adjusted percentage of people with diabetes mellitus (as compared to White people), followed by non-Hispanic Black people and Hispanic people (CDC, 2022c), as well as a disparity in disease-related complications, like nephropathy (Haw et al., 2021). AI/AN groups, as well as Black and Hispanic people, are disproportionately affected by COVID-19 infection rates, hospitalizations, and death (Hill & Artiga, 2022). African American/Black persons continue to have a higher death rate than White persons for all-cause mortality (Benjamins et al., 2021). Most striking is that the maternal mortality rate is three times higher for Black women than non-Hispanic White women and the overall rate has increased in recent years (Hoyert, 2023). Further, even though the infant mortality rate in the United States has declined in recent years, when controlling for socioeconomic factors, the Black infant mortality rate is more than double (2.4x) that of rates for non-Hispanic White people (Ely & Driscoll, 2022). Researchers in the area of health literacy have found disparities based on the literacy level of the client and the ability of the provider to facilitate patient understanding of treatment and management of a disease. Studies on the impact of health literacy on outcomes have found that there is poor access to care, lower health-related quality of life, and lower health knowledge among people with low health literacy which should inform interventions that target multiple levels of care (Cajita et al., 2016; Hälleberg et al., 2018; Levy & Janke, 2016).

Evidence-based interventions can be successful in addressing such disparities, especially when they aim to change systems and structures (AHRQ, 2022; Brown et al., 2019). One research team successfully integrated a diabetes education program within a faith-based framework for use in Black churches to support health behavior changes (Whitney et al., 2017). To address the higher prevalence of diabetes in Hispanic/Latinx populations, researchers in the Diabetes Among Latinos Best Practices Trial (DIALBEST) randomly assigned a group of Latinx with type 2 diabetes to CHWs. They received CLAS through education sessions on nutrition, blood glucose monitoring, medication adherence, and other topics. The researchers found that subjects in the CHWs group had improved HbA1C at 3, 6, 12, and 18 months post-intervention, but there was no change in serum lipid levels, hypertension, or weight (Pérez-Escamilla et al., 2015). Similar findings were found across 53 studies in a scoping review on CHWs' role in diabetes management (Egbujie et al., 2018). In studies investigating underserved older adults, a systematic review by Marsh et al. (2021) found that self-management education delivered through telemedicine and CHWs lowered A1C levels. Policies are being written and adopted at all levels of government to address healthcare disparities. Some of these policies can be reviewed on the National Conference of State Legislatures' (NCSL) website at www.ncsl.org/research/health/population-groups/health-disparities.aspx.

APRNs also need to address health disparities that exist in LGBTQ+ populations. These disparities can begin during adolescence. The *Healthy People 2030* objectives for the LGBTQ+ population reflect these disparities. These objectives address the need to increase cervical cancer screening, reduce the proportion of LGBTQ+ high school students who abuse drugs, reduce suicidal thoughts in LGBTQ+ students, reduce the incidence of HIV diagnoses, and reduce the syphilis rate in gay men (ODPHP, n.d.). The LGBTQ+ population encounters stigma, discrimination, bullying, and violence which exacerbate the disparities and access to care (Dawson et al., 2021). To address these issues, APRNs must design interventions that use inclusive language and are gender-affirming (Goldhammer et al., 2021).

In summary, health disparities are preventable, and effective strategies to reverse these disparities and achieve health equity are urgently needed. Although much research has been done to better understand healthcare disparities, researchers suggest that a multi-dimensional approach is needed to reverse problems associated with a long history of systemic, structural, and institutional racism that is embedded in every social system (Braveman et al., 2022; Hardeman et al., 2018). In fact, the CDC (CDC, 2021b) declared racism as a serious threat to public health, which highlights the call to action and advocacy for APRNs. For the purpose of eliminating health disparities and effectuating racial equity, the National Collaborative for Health Equity (NCHE) is a resource for research, collaboration, and leadership. Only through radically changing structures and systems through policy and advocacy will health equity be possible (Braveman et al., 2017; NCHE, n.d.; Zambrano & Williams, 2022).

It is critical that APRNs advocate for the elimination of health disparities to achieve health equity, as this work is of vital importance and urgently needed. From an ethical standpoint, working to eliminate health disparities is the right thing to do. Strategies may include advocating for health insurance coverage for low-income populations; incorporating SDOH into a broader framework of care delivery; assessing the interaction among social environments, genetics, and population health; recruiting diverse participation in research studies with community-based participatory research and specifically with practice-based research networks; using culturally and linguistically appropriate communication and written handouts; promoting and facilitating community partnerships; and implementing strategies to diversify the nursing workforce to better reflect the populations served (Green, 2020; Hill-Briggs et al., 2021; Quinones et al., 2015; Sentell et al., 2014; Williams & Purdie-Vaughns, 2016).

APRNs have successfully tested interventions to decrease health disparities, and by careful and thorough review of the current literature and resources available, they have the tools to develop additional effective and culturally sensitive interventions and to identify outcomes in order to achieve better and more equitable health outcomes.

SUMMARY

APRNs have a critical role in improving population health by intervening at every level from the individual to the community. Before an effective intervention can take place, it is imperative that realistic and measurable outcomes are first identified and defined so that they can be measured and analyzed. Outcomes may be classified by the beneficiary of the health intervention, by type (e.g., care, patient, or performance related), and by time frame of achievement. Outcomes may also be categorized by clinical or disease-specific outcomes, function, cost-effectiveness, self-perception health status, and satisfaction outcomes. A commonly used framework to classify outcomes is Donabedian's framework of structure, process, and outcomes. This framework has been used for describing a community's health as well as for classifying nurse-sensitive indicators. Outcomes are an important part of the standardized language that nursing leaders and researchers continue to refine and operationalize as a means of improving healthcare.

The national healthcare objectives in *Healthy People 2030* provide a blueprint of health promotion and disease prevention objectives that are designed to improve the health of all people in the United States. Building on the goal of *Healthy People*, APRNs can use these web-based resources to identify outcomes and compare them with national and state data that can be further analyzed by stratifying for a population's ethnicity, race, income, education, and/or gender. Federal agencies, such as the AHRQ, the CDC, OMHHE, and the NIH's NIMHD, provide ready access to a plethora of information and resources that can be used to identify and define outcomes.

APRNs have a tremendous opportunity to access and use available data to contribute to the current body of knowledge that forms the basis for evidence-based practice. By selecting and using well-defined indicators and comparing those to national norms, APRNs can provide important information on trends or patterns of quality of care. This information has the potential to stimulate the development of creative and innovative programs or interventions to improve health outcomes. Evidence of improved outcomes will help APRNs to justify and advocate for change through policy, practice, and research, with the ultimate goal of providing quality, equitable care for all.

END-OF-CHAPTER RESOURCES

EXERCISES AND DISCUSSION QUESTIONS

EXERCISE 3.1 An APRN is working in a community clinic, providing postnatal care to a diverse population of families. The APRN knows there are disparities that occur for maternal and infant mortality related to ethnicity.

1. Where could the APRN go to find information on maternal and infant mortality disparities?
2. What is the ethnic disparity in maternal and infant mortality?
3. What SDOH are associated with maternal and infant mortality?
4. How might an APRN participate in local efforts to reduce maternal and infant mortality rates on a population level?

EXERCISE 3.2 An APRN who is interested in reducing opiate-related overdoses in high schools develops an online training program to teach all school employees to administer Narcan® (naloxone).

1. What are related LHIs found in *Healthy People 2030*?
2. In examining *The Community Guide* topics, which ones are most relevant to this scenario?
3. What outcomes might the APRN monitor for effectiveness of the program?
4. What other population-level strategies could the APRN implement to address the issue?

EXERCISE 3.3 APRNs should not only recognize health disparities, they should also make it part of their practice to develop strategies to reduce or eliminate them. Review information from *Healthy People 2030* and the CDC's Office of Minority Health and Health Disparities websites.

1. What health disparities can you find that are relevant to a geographical area?
2. What CLAS interventions could an APRN implement in their specific practice that are consistent with the National CLAS Standards?
3. What outcomes could an APRN monitor related to an identified health disparity in their geographical area?
4. Which objectives in *Healthy People 2030* could help this effort?

EXERCISE 3.4 Diabetes affects a growing number of Americans. An APRN working in a local hospital is part of a collaborative of community agencies strategically addressing diabetes from a community perspective.

1. What SDOH should the community look at in relation to risk or incidence of diabetes?
2. What resources could the APRN use to identify different outcomes related to diabetes?
3. What outcomes related to diabetes are of most interest to community members?
4. Using the AHRQ's NHQDR Data Query (datatools.ahrq.gov/nhqdr), what related national- and state-level data are available to the APRN?

A robust set of instructor resources designed to supplement this text is located at http://connect.springerpub.com/content/book/978-0-8261-4377-8. Qualifying instructors may request access by emailing textbook@springerpub.com.

REFERENCES

Agency for Healthcare Research and Quality. (2022, October). *National healthcare quality and disparities report*. AHRQ Pub. No. 22(23)-0030. Rockville, MD. Agency for Healthcare Research and Quality.

Agency for Healthcare Research and Quality. (n.d.). *Topic: Outcomes*. https://www.ahrq.gov/topics/outcomes.html

Agency for Healthcare Research and Quality. (2015, July). *Types of health care quality measures*. https://www.ahrq.gov/talkingquality/measures/types.html

American Association of Colleges of Nursing. (2021). *The essentials: Core competencies for professional nursing education*. https://www.aacnnursing.org/Portals/42/AcademicNursing/pdf/Essentials-2021.pdf

American Association of Colleges of Nursing. (2022). *The state of doctor of nursing practice education in 2022*. https://www.aacnnursing.org/Portals/42/News/Surveys-Data/State-of-the-DNP-Summary-Report-June-2022.pdf

Anderson, E. T., & McFarlane, J. (2018). *Community as partner: Theory and practice in nursing* (8th ed.). Lippincott Williams & Wilkins.

Association of American Medical Colleges Center for Health Justice. (n.d.). *Who we are and what we do*. Retrieved from https://www.aamchealthjustice.org/who-we-are-and-what-we-do

Ayanian, J. Z., & Markel, H. (2016). Donabedian's Lasting Framework for Health Care Quality. *The New England Journal of Medicine, 375*(3), 205–207. https://doi.org/10.1056/NEJMp1605101

Benjamins, M. R., Silva, A., Saiyed, N. S., & De Maio, F. G. (2021). Comparison of all-cause mortality rates and inequities between black and white populations across the 30 most populous US cities. *JAMA Network Open, 4*(1), e2032086. https://doi.org/10.1001/jamanetworkopen.2020.32086

Bigbee, J. L., & Issel, L. M. (2012). Conceptual models for population-focused public health nursing interventions and outcomes: The state of the art. *Public Health Nursing, 29*(4), 370–379. https://doi.org/10.1111/j.1525-1446.2011.01006.x

Blumenthal, D., Malphrus, E., McGinnis, J. M., Committee on Core Metrics for Better Health at Lower Cost, & Institute of Medicine (Eds.). (2015). *Vital signs: Core metrics for health and health care progress*. National Academies Press.

Braveman, P., Arkin, E., Orleans, T., Proctor, D., & Plough, A. (2017). *What is health equity? And what difference does a definition make?* Robert Wood Johnson Foundation. Retrieved from https://resources.equityinitiative.org/handle/ei/418

Braveman, P. A., Arkin, E., Proctor, D., Kauh, T., & Holm, N. (2022). Systemic and structural racism: Definitions, examples, health damages, and approaches to dismantling. *Health Affairs, 41*(2), 171–178. https://doi.org/10.1377/hlthaff.2021.01394

Braveman, P., & Gottlieb, L. (2014). The social determinants of health: It's time to consider the causes of the causes. *Public Health Reports, 129*(Suppl. 2), 19–31. https://doi.org/10.1177/00333549141291S206

Brown, A. F., Ma, G. X., Miranda, J., Eng, E., Castille, D., Brockie, T., Jones, P., Airhihenbuwa, C. O., Farhat, T., Zhu, L., & Trinh-Shevrin, C. (2019). Structural interventions to reduce and eliminate health disparities. *American Journal of Public Health, 109*(S1), S72–S78. https://doi.org/10.2105/AJPH.2018.304844

Butcher, H. K., Bulechek, G. M., Dochterman, J. M., & Wagner, C. M. (Eds.). (2018). *Nursing interventions classification (NIC)* (7th ed.). Elsevier.

Cajita, M. I., Cajita, T. R., & Hae-Ra, H. (2016). Health literacy and heart failure. *Journal of Cardiovascular Nursing, 31*(2), 121–130. https://doi.org/10.1097/JCN.0000000000000229

Centers for Disease Control and Prevention. (2018). *BRFSS Frequently Asked Questions (FAQs)*. https://www.cdc.gov/brfss/about/brfss_faq.htm

Centers for Disease Control and Prevention. (2021a). *Built environment assessment tool manual*. https://www.cdc.gov/physicalactivity/resources/built-environment-assessment/index.htm

Centers for Disease Control and Prevention. (2021b, April 8). *Media statement from CDC director Rochelle P. Walensky, MD, MPH, on racism and health*. CDC Newsroom. https://www.cdc.gov/media/releases/2021/s0408-racism-health.html

Centers for Disease Control and Prevention. (2022a, March 22). *2019 questionnaire redesign*. Retrieved from https://www.cdc.gov/nchs/nhis/2019_quest_redesign.htm

Centers for Disease Control and Prevention. (2022b, July 15). *About the national center for health statistics*. https://www.cdc.gov/nchs/about/index.htm

Centers for Disease Control and Prevention. (2022c). *National Diabetes Statistics Report*. https://www.cdc.gov/diabetes/data/statistics-report/index.html

Centers for Disease Control and Prevention. (2022d, July 1). *What is health equity?* https://www.cdc.gov/healthequity/whatis/index.html

Centers for Disease Control and Prevention. (2022e, December 8). *Social determinants of health at CDC*. https://www.cdc.gov/about/sdoh/index.html

Centers for Disease Control and Prevention. (2023, February 3). *National health care surveys*. Retrieved from https://www.cdc.gov/nchs/dhcs/index.htm

Center for Nursing Classification and Clinical Effectiveness (CNC). (n.d.). *Center for Nursing Classification and Clinical Effectiveness (CNC)*. https://nursing.uiowa.edu/center-for-nursing-classification-and-clinical-effectiveness#:~:text=The%20Center%20for%20Nursing%20Classification,Nursing%20Outcomes%20Classification%20(NOC).

Chang, A., Patberg, E., Cueto, V., Hua, L., Singh, B., Kenya, S., Alonzo, Y, & Carrasquillo, O. (2018). Community health workers, access to care, and service utilization among Florida Latinos: A randomized controlled trial. *American Journal of Public Health, 108*(9), 1249–1251. https://doi.org/10.2105/AJPH.2018.304542

Chatelan, A., & Khalatbari-Soltani, S. (2022). Evaluating and rethinking public health for the 21st century: Toward vulnerable population interventions. *Frontiers in Public Health, 10*, 1033270. https://doi.org/10.3389/fpubh.2022.1033270

Community Preventative Services Task Force. (2019, July). *Asthma: School-based self-management inteventions for children and adolescents with asthma*. Finding and Rational Statement. https://www.thecommunityguide.org/media/pdf/asthma-school-based-self-management.pdf

Dawson, L., Frederiksen, B., Long, M., Ranji, U., & Kates, J. (2021). *LGBT+ people's health and experiences accessing care*. Kaiser Family Foundation. https://www.kff.org/report-section/lgbt-peoples-health-and-experiences-accessing-care-report/

DeGuzman, P. B., & Kulbok, P. A. (2012). Changing health outcomes of vulnerable populations through nursing's influence on neighborhood built environment: A framework for nursing research. *Journal of Nursing Scholarship, 44*(4), 341–348. https://doi.org/10.1111/j.1547-5069.2012.01470.x

Donabedian, A. (1980). *Explorations in quality assessment and monitoring*. Health Administration Press.

Donabedian, A. (1982). *The criteria and standards of quality*. Health Administration Press.

Egbujie, B. A., Delobell, P. A., Levitt, N., Puone, T., Sanders, D., & van Wyk, B. (2018). Role of community health workers in type 2 diabetes mellitus self-management: A scoping review. *PLoS One, 13*(6), e0198424. https://doi.org/10.1371/journal.pone.0198424

Ely, D. M., & Driscoll, A. K. (2022). Infant mortality in the United States, 2020: Data from the period linked birth/infant death file. *National Vital Statistics Reports; 71*(5). Hyattsville, MD: National Center for Health Statistics. doi: https://dx.doi.org/10.15620/cdc:120700

Fee, E., & Garofalo, M. E. (2010). Florence Nightingale and the Crimean war. *American Journal of Public Health, 100*(9), 1591. https://doi.org/10.2105/AJPH.2009.188607

Friis, R. H., & Sellers, T. A. (2020). *Epidemiology for public health practice* (6th ed.). Jones & Bartlett.

Galea, S., & Link, B. G. (2013). Six paths for the future of social epidemiology. *American Journal of Epidemiology, 178*(6), 843–849. https://doi.org/10.1093/aje/kwt148

Green, C. (2020). Equity and diversity in nursing education. *Teaching and Learning in Nursing, 15*(4), 280–283. https://doi.org/10.1016/j.teln.2020.07.004

Gibson, M. E., & Thatcher, E. J. (2019). Community as client: Assessment and analysis. In M. Stanhope & J. Lancaster (Eds.), *Public health nursing: Population-centered health care in the community* (10th ed.). Mosby.

Goldhammer, H., Smart, A. C., Kissock, L. A., & Keuroghlian, A. S. (2021). Organizational strategies and inclusive language to build culturally responsive health care environments for lesbian, gay, bisexual, transgender, and queer people. *Journal of Health Care for the Poor and Underserved, 32*(1), 18–29. https://doi.org/10.1353/hpu.2021.0004

Griffiths, P. (1995). Progress in measuring nursing outcomes. *Journal of Advanced Nursing, 21*(6), 1092–1100. https://doi.org/10.1046/j.1365-2648.1995.21061092.x

Hacker, K., Auerbach, J., Ikeda, R., Philip, C., Houry, D., & SDOH Task Force. (2022). Social determinants of health—An approach taken at CDC. *Journal of Public Health Management and Practice, 28*(6), 589–594. https://doi.org/10.1097/PHH.0000000000001626

Hälleberg, N. M., Nilsson, U., Dahlberg, K., & Jaensson, M. (2018). Association between functional health literacy and postoperative recovery, health care contacts, and health-related quality of life among patients undergoing day surgery: Secondary analysis of a randomized clinical trial. *JAMA Surgery, 153*(8), 738–745. https://doi.org/10.1001/jamasurg.2018.0672

Hardeman, R. R., Murphy, K. A., Karbeah, J., & Kozhimannil, K. B. (2018). Naming institutionalized racism in the public health literature: A systematic literature review. *Public Health Reports, 133*(3), 240–249. https://doi.org/10.1177/0033354918760574

Haw, J. S., Shah, M., Turbow, S., Egeolu, M., & Umpierrez, G. (2021). Diabetes complications in racial and ethnic minority populations in the USA. *Current Diabetes Reports, 21*(1), 2. https://doi.org/10.1007/s11892-020-01369-x

Herdman, T. H., Kamitsuri, S., & Lopes, C. (Eds). (2021). *NANDA international nursing diagnoses: Definitions & classifications, 2021–2023* (12th ed.). Thieme.

Hill, M. (1999). Outcomes measurement requires nursing to shift to outcome-based practice. *Nursing Administration Quarterly, 24*(1), 1–16. https://doi.org/10.1097/00006216-199910000-00003

Hill-Briggs, F., Adler, N. E., Berkowitz, S. A., Chin, M. H., Gary-Webb, T. L., Navas-Acien, A., Thornton, P. L., & Haire-Joshu, D. (2021). Social determinants of health and diabetes: A scientific review. *Diabetes Care, 44*(1), 258–279. https://doi.org/10.2337/dci20-0053

Hoyert, D. L. (2023). *Maternal mortality rates in the United States, 2021.* NCHS Health E-Stats. https://dx.doi.org/10.15620/cdc:113967

Institute for Healthcare Improvement. (2022). *Triple aim for populations.* Retrieved from http://www.ihi.org/Topics/TripleAim/Pages/default.aspx

Jones, T. (2016). Outcome measurement in nursing: Imperatives, ideals, history, and challenges. *Online Journal of Issues in Nursing, 21*(2), 1. https://dx.doi.org/10.3912/OJIN.Vol21No02Man01

Kapu, A. N., Sicoutris, C., Broyhill, B. S., & Kleinpell, R. M. (2021). Measuring outcomes in advanced practice nursing: Practice-specific quality metrics. In R. Kleinpell (Ed.), *Outcome assessment in advanced practice nursing* (5th ed.). Springer Publishing Company.

Kleinpell, R., & Gawlinski, A. (2005). Assessing outcomes in advanced practice nursing practice: The use of quality indicators and evidence-based practice. *AACN Clinical Issues, 16*(1), 43–57. https://dx.doi.org/10.1097/00044067-200501000-00006

Kleinpell, R., & Kapu, A. N. (2017). Quality measures for nurse practitioner practice evaluation. *Journal of the American Association of Nurse Practitioners, 29*(8), 446–451. https://dx.doi.org/10.1002/2327-6924.12474

Lang, N. M., & Marek, K. D. (1991). The policy and politics of patient outcomes. *Journal of Nursing Quality Assurance, 5*(2), 7–12.

Levy, H., & Janke, A. (2016). Health literacy and access to care. *Journal of Health Communication, 21*(Suppl. 1), 43–50. https://dx.doi.org/10.1080/10810730.2015.1131776

Lucas, J. W. & Villarroel, M. A. (2022, October). *Telemedicine use among adults: United States, 2021*. NCHS Data Brief No. 445. https://www.cdc.gov/nchs/products/databriefs/db445.htm

Marsh, Z., Nguyen, Y., Teegala, Y., & Cotter, V. T. (2021). Diabetes management among underserved older adults through telemedicine and community health workers. *Journal of the American Association of Nurse Practitioners, 34*(1), 26–31. https://doi.org/10.1097/JXX.0000000000000595

Minkler, M., Wallerstein, I., & Hyde, C. A. (2021). Chapter 3: Improving health through community organization and community building: Perspectives from health education and social work. In M. Minkler & Wakimoto, P. (Eds.), *Community organizing and community building for health and welfare* (4th ed.). Rutgers University Press.

Moorhead, S., Swanson, E., Johnson, M., & Maas, M. L. (Eds.). (2018). *Nursing outcomes classification (NOC): Measurement of health outcomes* (6th ed.). Elsevier.

National Academies of Sciences, Engineering, and Medicine. (2021). *The future of nursing 2020–2030: Charting a path to achieve health equity*. The National Academies Press. https://doi.org/10.17226/25982

National Collaborative for Health Equity. (n.d.). Health through policy creating pathways to racial justice. https://www.nationalcollaborative.org/healing-through-policy/

Newhouse, R., Barksdale, D. J., & Miller, J. A. (2015). The patient-centered outcomes research institute: Research done differently. *Nursing Research, 64*(1), 72–77. https://doi.org/10.1097/NNR.0000000000000070

Nundy, S., Cooper, L. A., & Mate, K. S. (2022). The quintuple aim for health care improvement: A new imperative to advance health equity. *JAMA, 327*(6), 521–522. https://doi.org/10.1001/jama.2021.25181

Office of Disease Prevention and Health Promotion. (2022, March). *Health equity and health disparities environmental scan*. U.S. Department of Health and Human Services. https://health.gov/sites/default/files/2022-04/HP2030-HealthEquityEnvironmentalScan.pdf

Office of Disease Prevention and Health Promotion. (n.d.). *LGBT. Healthy People 2030*. U.S. Department of Health and Human Services. https://health.gov/healthypeople/objectives-and-data/browse-objectives/lgbt

Oner, B., Zengul, F. D., Oner, N., Ivankova, N. V., Karadag, A., & Patrician, P. A. (2021). Nursing-sensitive indicators for nursing care: A systematic review (1997–2017). *NursingOpen, 8*(3), 1005–1022. https://doi.org/10.1002/nop2.654

Paul, R., Arif, A., Pokhrel, K., & Ghosh, S. (2021). The association of social determinants of health with COVID-19 mortality in rural and urban counties. *The Journal of Rural Health, 37*(2), 278–286. https://doi.org/10.1111/jrh.12557

Payán, D. D., Sloane, D. C., Illum, J., Vargas, R. B., Lee, D., Galloway-Gilliam, L., & Lewis, L. B. (2017). Catalyzing implementation of evidence-based interventions in safety net settings: A clinical–community partnership in south Los Angeles. *Health Promotion Practice, 18*(4), 586–597. https://doi.org/10.1177/1524839917705418

Pérez-Escamilla, R., Damio, G., Chhabra, J., Fernandez, M. L., Segura-Pérez, S., Vega-López, S., Kollannor-Samuel, G., Calle, M., Shebl, F. M., & D'Agostino, D. (2015). Impact of a community health workers-led structured program on blood glucose control among Latinos with type 2 diabetes: The DIALBEST trial. *Diabetes Care, 38*(2), 197–205. https://doi.org/10.2337/dc14-0327

Porche, D. J. (2023). *Epidemiology for the advanced practice nurse: A population health approach*. Springer Publishing, LLC.

Press Ganey Associates. (n.d.). *National Database of Nursing Quality Indicators® (NDNQI®)*. Retrieved from https://www.pressganey.com/platform/ndnqi/

Quinones, A. R., Talavera, G. A., Castaneda, S. F., & Saha, S. (2015). Interventions that reach into communities – promising directions for reducing racial and ethnic disparities in healthcare. *Journal of Racial and Ethnic Health Disparities, 2*(3), 336–340. https://doi.org/10.1007/s40615-014-0078-3

Rich, K. A. (2021). Chapter 18: Evaluating outcomes of innovations. In N. A. Schmidt & J. M. Brown (Eds.), *Evidence-based practice: Appraisal and application of research* (5th ed.). Jones & Bartlett.

Sentell, T., Zhang, W., Davis, J., Baker, K. K., & Braun, K. L. (2014). The influence of community and individual health literacy on self-reported health status. *Journal of General Internal Medicine, 29*(2), 298–304. https://doi.org/10.1007/s11606-013-2638-3

Siaki, L., Patrician, P., Loan, L., Matlock, A., Start, R., Gardner, C., & McCarthy, M. (2023). Ambulatory care nurse-sensitive indicators: A scoping review of the literature 2006–2021. *Journal of Nursing Care Quality, 38*(1), 76–81. https://doi.org/10.1097/NCQ.0000000000000660

United States Census Bureau. (2022, August 3). *What we do*. https://www.census.gov/about/what.html

United States Department of Health and Human Services. (n.d.). *Healthy People 2030: Building a healthy future for all*. https://health.gov/healthypeople

United States Department of Health and Human Services. (n.d.). *Healthy People 2030 framework*. https://health.gov/healthypeople/about/healthy-people-2030-framework

U.S. Department of Health and Human Services, Community Preventive Services Task Force. (2023). *The community guide*. Retrieved from https://www.thecommunityguide.org

van Maanen, H. M. T. (1979). Perspectives and problems on quality of nursing care: An overview of contributions from North America and recent developments in Europe. *Journal of Advanced Nursing, 4*(4), 377–389. https://doi.org/10.1111/j.1365-2648.1979.tb00872.x

Williams, D. R., & Purdie-Vaughns, V. (2016). Needed interventions to reduce racial/ethnic disparities in health. *Journal of Health Politics, Policy and Law, 41*(4), 627–651. https://doi.org/10.1215/03616878-3620857

Whitney, E., Kindred, E., Pratt, A., O'Neal, Y., Harrison, R. C. P., & Peek, M. E. (2017). Culturally tailoring a patient empowerment and diabetes education curriculum for the African-American church. *The Diabetes Educator, 43*(5), 441–448. https://doi.org/10.1177/0145721717725280

Wolff, B., Mahoney, F., Lohiniva, A. L., & Corkum, M. (2018). Collecting and analyzing qualitative data. *The CDC field epidemiology manual*. https://www.cdc.gov/eis/field-epi-manual/chapters/Qualitative-Data.html

Xiao, S., Widger, K., Tourangeau, A., & Berta, W. (2017). Nursing process health care indicators. *Journal of Nursing Care Quality, 32*(1), 32–39. https://doi.org/10.1097/ncq.0000000000000207

Zambrano, R. E. & Williams, D. R. (2022). The intellectual roots of current knowledge on racism and health: Relevance to policy and the national equity discourse. *Health Affairs, 41*(2), 163–170. https://doi.org/10.1377/hlthaff.2021.01439

INTERNET RESOURCES

Agency for Healthcare Research and Quality (AHRQ): www.qualityindicators.ahrq.gov

Association of American Medical Colleges (AAMC) Center for Health Justice: https://www.aamchealthjustice.org/

CMS, "Hospital Compare": https://www.medicare.gov/hospitalcompare/search.html

County Health Rankings and Roadmaps: http://www.countyhealthrankings.org

Healthy People 2030: https://health.gov/healthypeople

Institute for Healthcare Improvement/Quality Improvement Essentials Toolkit: http://www.ihi.org/resources/Pages/Tools/Quality-Improvement-Essentials-Toolkit.aspx

NANDA International: www.NANDA.org

National Cancer Institute, Division of Cancer Control & Population Sciences: http://cancercontrol.cancer.gov

National Cancer Institute, Health Disparities Calculator: http://seer.cancer.gov/hdcalc

National Center for Health Statistics (NCHS): http://www.cdc.gov/nchs

National Center for Health Statistics / National Vital Statistics Program: www.cdc.gov/nchs/nvss

National Conference of State Legislature (NCSL): http://www.ncsl.org/research/health/population-groups/health-disparities.aspx

National Health and Nutrition Examination Survey (NHNES): www.cdc.gov/nchs/nhanes.htm

National Quality Partners': https://www.qualityforum.org/National_Quality_Partners.aspx

NIH, National Institute on Minority Health and Health Disparities: https://www.nimhd.nih.gov/programs/edu-training

The Behavioral Risk Factor Surveillance System (BRFSS): http://www.cdc.gov/brfss

The Community Guide: www.thecommunityguide.org

The National Healthcare Surveys: www.cdc.gov/nchs/dhcs

Trust for America's Health: https://www.tfah.org

CHAPTER 4

EPIDEMIOLOGICAL METHODS AND MEASUREMENTS IN POPULATION-BASED NURSING PRACTICE: PART I

ANN L. CUPP CURLEY

INTRODUCTION

Evidence-based practice as it relates to population-based nursing combines clinical practice and public health through the use of population health sciences in clinical practice (Heller & Page, 2002). *Epidemiology* is the science of public health. It is concerned with the study of the factors determining and influencing the frequency and distribution of disease, injury, and other health-related events and their causes and the use of this knowledge to control health problems (Celentano & Szklo, 2018). In addition to epidemiology, an understanding of other scientific disciplines, such as biology and biostatistics, is also important for identifying associations and determining causation when looking at exposures and outcomes as they relate to population health.

Population-based care focuses on populations at risk, analysis of aggregate data, evaluation of demographic factors, and recognition of health disparities. It is concerned with the patterns of delivery of care and outcome measurements at the population or subpopulation level. The purpose of this chapter is to provide readers with an understanding of the natural history of disease and the approaches that are integral for the prevention of disease. It addresses the advanced-level nursing core competencies specified in Domain *3: Population* (American Association of Colleges of Nursing [AACN], 2021). Basic concepts are introduced that are necessary to understand how to measure disease outcomes and select study designs that are best suited for population-based research. Emphasis is placed on measuring disease occurrence with a fundamental discussion of how to calculate incidence, prevalence, and mortality rates. Successful advanced practice nursing in population health depends upon the ability to recognize the difference between the individual and population approaches to the collection and use of data and the ability to assess needs and evaluate outcomes at the population level. Concepts surrounding survival data are also discussed along with strategies to guide advanced practice registered nurses (APRNs) on how to calculate and interpret survival data.

THE NATURAL HISTORY OF DISEASE

The *natural history of disease* refers to the progression of a disease from its *preclinical state* (prior to symptoms) to its *clinical state* (from onset of symptoms to cure, control, disability, or death). Disease is not something that occurs suddenly, but rather it is a multifactorial process that is dynamic and occurs over time. It evolves and changes and is sometimes initiated by events that take place years, even decades, before symptoms first appear. Many diseases have a natural life history that can extend over a very long period of time. The natural history of disease is described in stages. Understanding the different stages allows for a better understanding of the approach to the prevention and control of disease.

STAGE OF SUSCEPTIBILITY

The *stage of susceptibility* refers to the time prior to disease development. In the presence of certain risk factors, genetics, or environment, disease may develop and the severity can vary among individuals. Risk factors are those factors that are associated with an increased likelihood of disease developing over time. The idea that individuals could modify "risk factors" tied to heart disease, stroke, and other diseases is one of the key findings of the Framingham Heart Study (Framingham Heart Study, 2022). Started in 1948 and still in operation, this study is one of the most important population studies ever carried out in the United States. Before Framingham, for example, most healthcare providers believed that atherosclerosis was an inevitable part of the aging process. Although not all risk factors are amenable to change (e.g., genetic factors) and some risk factors are largely beyond the control of any one individual (e.g., environmental factors), the identification of risk factors is important and fundamental to disease prevention.

PRECLINICAL STAGE OF DISEASE

During the preclinical phase, the disease process has begun but there are no obvious symptoms. Although there is no clear manifestation of disease, because of the interaction of biological factors, changes have started to occur. During this stage, however, the changes are not always detectable. Screening technologies have been developed to detect the presence of some diseases before clinical symptoms appear. The Papanicolaou (Pap) smear is an example of an effective screening method for detecting cancer in a premalignant state to improve mortality related to cervical cancer. The use of the Pap smear as a screening tool facilitates early detection and treatment of premalignant changes of the cervix prior to development of malignancy.

CLINICAL STAGE OF DISEASE

In the clinical stage of disease, sufficient physiologic and/or functional changes occur, leading to the development of recognizable symptoms of disease. It might also be accurately referred to as the treatment stage. For some people, the disease may completely resolve (either spontaneously or with medical intervention), whereas for some it will lead to disability and/or death. It is for this reason that the clinical stage of disease is sometimes subdivided for better medical management. Staging systems used in malignancies to better define the extent of disease involvement are an example of a system that can help guide the type of treatment modality selected based on the stage. In many cases, staging can provide an estimate of prognosis. Another example is the identification of disability as a specific subcategory of the treatment stage. Disability occurs when a clinical disease leaves a person either temporarily or permanently disabled. When people become disabled, the goal of the treatment is to mitigate the effects of disease and to help these individuals to function to their optimal abilities. This is very different from the goal for someone who can be treated and restored to the level of functioning that they enjoyed prior to the illness.

THE NONCLINICAL DISEASE STAGE

This nonclinical or unapparent disease stage can be broken into four subparts. The first subpart is the *preclinical stage*, which, as mentioned earlier, is the acquisition of disease prior to development of symptoms and is destined to become disease. The second subpart is the *subclinical stage* that occurs when someone has the disease but it is not destined to develop clinically. The third subpart is the *chronic or persistent stage of disease*, which is disease that persists over time. And finally, there is the fourth subpart or *latent stage* in which one has disease with no active multiplication of the biological agent (Celentano & Szklo, 2018).

THE ICEBERG PHENOMENON

For most health problems, the number of identified cases is exceeded by the number of unidentified cases. This occurrence, referred to as the "iceberg phenomenon," makes it difficult to assess the true burden of disease. Many diseases do not have obvious symptoms, as stated earlier, and may go unrecognized for many years. Unrecognized diseases, such as diabetes, hypertension, and mental illness, create a significant problem with identifying populations at risk and estimating service needs. Complications also arise when patients are not recognized or treated during an early stage of a disease when interventions are most effective. Additionally, patients who do not have symptoms or do not recognize their symptoms may not seek medical care and, in many cases, even if they do have a diagnosis, do not take their medications as they perceive that they are healthy when they are asymptomatic.

CASE STUDY

You are an APRN working as a primary care provider (PCP) in a large medical practice. The practice is located in a county where the median age of residents is 58. The median age in the United States is 38. You note that several of your patients have Parkinson's disease (PD). Each of these patients is followed by a neurologist. As you sift through the professional literature, you learn that more than 1,040,000 people in the United States live with PD and approximately 90,000 new cases are diagnosed every year. The midyear population of the United States is 331,002,650. There is no current treatment that halts the progression of the disease and management evolves as the disease progresses. You want to learn more about the disease in order to provide relevant and up-to-date care for this patient population as well as to be able to collaborate effectively with both the patients and their neurologists.

1. *What is the natural history of PD?*

   Answer: PD is a neurological disease characterized by a breakdown of neurons in the brain that produce dopamine. The decrease in dopamine levels leads to impaired movement and the other symptoms of PD.

   There are five stages in PD.

   Stage 1: Mildest form of PD. There may be either no outward symptoms or symptoms that are so mild that they go unnoticed. If they are present, they do not interfere with daily tasks. Symptoms that do occur (such as tremor) are one-sided at this stage.

   Medications can be effective in minimizing symptoms at this stage.

   Stage 2: Moderate form of PD. Stiffness, tremors, and trembling may be more noticeable, and changes in facial expressions can occur. No impairment of balance at this stage. Difficulties walking may develop or increase, and the person's posture may start to change. Symptoms may occur bilaterally.

   People at this stage can generally live alone but it may take longer for them to complete tasks.

   Stage 3: This is the middle stage. Although symptoms may be similar to stage 2, balance and reflexes become markedly worse. Movement slows.

   This is the stage at which falls become more common.

   Stage 4: It becomes significantly harder for people at this stage to complete daily tasks. People at this stage might need to use an assistive device to walk.

   It may be dangerous for people to live alone at this stage.

   Stage 5: Most advanced stage of PD. People require wheelchairs and are unable to stand alone.

   At this last stage, people require 24-hour assistance.

   There is no way to predict how much time it will take for someone to move from one stage to another. (Parkinson's Foundation, 2023)

(continued)

2. *Why is it important to understand the natural history of a disease such as PD?*

   Answer: Understanding the progression of the disease helps the person with PD to plan for future needs. It helps the healthcare provider to provide appropriate patient education, treatment, and care and to monitor progression of the disease.

3. *Using the data that is provided, calculate the incidence and prevalence per 100,000 for PD in the United States.*

   Answer:
   U.S. incidence: 90,000/331,002,650 × 100,000 = 27.2 per 100,000
   U.S. prevalence: 1,040,000/331,002,650 × 100,000 = 314.2 per 100,000

4. *Would you expect the incidence and prevalence rates of PD in your practice to be the same, higher, or lower than the U.S. rates?*

   Answer: You might expect them to be higher, given the median age in your county versus the median age in the United States.

PREVENTION

Understanding the natural history of disease is as important as understanding the causal factors of disease because it provides the APRN with the knowledge that is required to design programs or interventions that target populations at risk. Understanding how disease develops is fundamental to the concept of prevention and provides a framework for disease prevention and control. The primary goal of prevention is to prevent disease before it occurs. The concept of prevention has evolved to include measures taken to interrupt or slow the progression of disease or to lessen its impact. There are three levels of prevention.

PRIMARY PREVENTION

Primary prevention refers to the process of altering susceptibility or reducing exposure to susceptible individuals and includes general health promotion and specific measures designed to prevent disease prior to a person getting the disease. Interventions designed for primary prevention are carried out during the stage of susceptibility and can include things such as providing immunizations to change a person's susceptibility. Actions taken to prevent tobacco usage are another example of primary prevention. Tobacco use is one of the health behaviors targeted by *Healthy People 2030* to improve health. It is estimated that cigarette smoking is responsible for one out of every five deaths in the United States, making it the leading cause of preventable mortality in the country (Centers for Disease Control and Prevention [CDC], 2022a). Prevention or cessation of smoking can reduce the development of many smoking-related diseases. Taxes on cigarettes, education programs, and support groups to help people stop smoking and the creation of smoke-free zones are all examples of primary prevention measures. The CDC linked a series of tobacco control efforts by Minnesota to a decrease in adult smoking prevalence rates. From 1999 to 2010, Minnesota implemented a series of anti-smoking initiatives, including a statewide smoke-free law, cigarette tax increases, media campaigns, and statewide cessation efforts. Adult smoking prevalence decreased from 22.1% in 1999 to 16.1% in 2010 (CDC, 2011). In 2013, Minnesota increased the tax on a pack of cigarettes an additional $1.60. Following this increase, smoking decreased by 33% among Minnesota's 11th graders and by 10% among adult residents. Smokers reported that the tax increase did influence their smoking behaviors (Minnesota Department of Health, 2018). This is an excellent example of a successful statewide primary prevention effort to reduce smoking prevalence through a variety of initiatives.

In 2019, U.S. Tobacco 21 (T21) was passed by Congress and signed into law by President Donald Trump. It raised the minimum age to buy tobacco products in the United States to 21. This measure received wide bipartisan support following the dramatic success of a similar measure in California that was enacted in 2016 (Kim et al., 2021). Subsequent studies of the impact of this legislation have so far revealed mixed results. One study found that the perception that it was easy to buy tobacco among sixth to 12th graders dropped from 67.2% before legislation to 58.9% after but that the law was more protective of non-Hispanic Whites than others (Agaku et al., 2022). The authors of a second study concluded from their analyses that existing T21 state policies are not sufficient to reduce youth tobacco use and intentions to use (Patel et al., 2022). Both sets of researchers cited the need for more consistent enforcement of T21 policies across states. Although access laws can be an effective tool in reducing risky behaviors, as demonstrated by the results in Minnesota, they are most effective when combined with other evidence-based interventions.

SECONDARY PREVENTION

The early detection and prompt treatment of a disease at the earliest possible stage are referred to as *secondary prevention*. The goals of secondary prevention are to either identify and cure a disease at a very early stage or slow its progression to prevent complications and limit disability. Secondary prevention measures are carried out during the preclinical or presymptomatic stage of disease. Screening programs are designed to detect specific diseases in their early stages while they are curable and to prevent or reduce morbidity and mortality related to a later diagnosis of disease. Examples of secondary prevention include the Pap smear mentioned earlier, annual testing of cholesterol levels, mammography, and rapid HIV testing of asymptomatic individuals.

TERTIARY PREVENTION

Tertiary prevention strategies are implemented during the middle or late stages of clinical disease and refer to measures taken to alleviate disability and restore effective functioning. Attempts are made to slow the progression or to cure the disease. In cases in which permanent changes have taken place, interventions are planned and designed to help people lead a productive and satisfying life by maximizing the use of remaining capabilities (rehabilitation). Cardiac rehabilitation programs that provide physical and occupational therapies to postoperative cardiac patients are an example of tertiary prevention.

CAUSATION

THE EPIDEMIOLOGICAL TRIANGLE

The relationship between risk factors and disease is complex. Research studies may describe a relationship between a risk factor and disease, but how do we know that this relationship is causal? An understanding of causation is important if APRNs want to effectively impact the health of populations. The *epidemiological triangle* is a model that has historically been used to explain causation. The model consists of three interactive factors: the causative agent (those factors for which presence or absence cause disease—biological, chemical, physical, nutritional), a susceptible host (things such as age, gender, race, immune status, genetics), and the environment (including diverse elements such as water, food, neighborhood, pollution). A change in the agent, host, and environmental balance can lead to disease (Harkness, 1995). The underlying assumptions of this model are that causative factors can be both intrinsic and extrinsic to the host and that the cause of disease is related to interaction among these three factors. This model was developed initially to explain the transmission of infectious diseases and is particularly useful when the focus of epidemiology is on acute diseases. It is less helpful for understanding and explaining the processes associated with chronic disease. With the rise of chronic diseases as the primary cause of morbidity and mortality in the 21st century, a model that recognizes multiple causative factors was needed to better understand this complex interaction.

THE WEB OF CAUSATION

The dynamic nature of chronic diseases calls for a more sophisticated model for explaining causation than the epidemiological triangle. Introduction of the *web of causation* concept first appeared in the 1960s when chronic diseases overtook infectious diseases as the leading cause of morbidity and mortality in the United States. The foundation of this concept is that disease develops as the result of many antecedent factors and not as a result of a single, isolated cause. Each factor is itself the result of a complex pattern of events that can be best perceived as interrelated in the complex configuration of a web. The use of a web is helpful for visualizing how difficult it is to untangle the many events that can precede the onset of a chronic illness.

Critics have argued that this model places too much emphasis on epidemiological methods and too little on theories of disease causation. As theories evolved about the relationship between smoking and cancer, the U.S. Surgeon General appointed a committee to review the evidence. This committee developed a set of guidelines for judging whether an observed association is causal. These guidelines include temporal relationship, strength of the association, dose–response relationship, replication of the findings, biological plausibility, consideration of alternative explanation, cessation of exposure, consistency with other knowledge, and specificity of the association (Celentano & Szklo, 2018). For a more detailed discussion on this model, see Chapter 5, "Epidemiological Methods and Measurements in Population-Based Nursing Practice: Part II."

METHODS OF ANALYSIS

Successful population-based approaches depend on the ability to recognize the difference between the collection and use of data from individuals and populations and the ability to assess needs and evaluate outcomes at the population level. Several of the more recent theories of causation can be helpful in determining whether an exposure is causally related to the development of disease. In particular, calculating the strength of association using statistics is one of several criteria that can be used to determine causality. However, statistics must be used with caution. Health is a multidimensional variable; factors that affect health and that interact to affect health are numerous. Many relationships are possible. There are problems inherent in the use of statistics to explain differences among groups. Although statistics can describe disparities, they cannot explain them. It is left to the researchers to explain the differences. In addition to statistics, one must also be aware of the validity and reliability of the data. There are problems associated with the categorizing and gathering of statistics that can have an effect on how the data should be interpreted. In order to be successful in research, one must do more than just collect data: One must look at the theoretical issues associated with explaining the relationship among the variables. Additionally, even if a relationship is found to be statistically significant, that does not ensure that it is clinically significant. Recognizing limitations in research and in practice is the most important step prior to making conclusions in any setting. Therefore, it is important that APRNs have a commitment to higher standards with an emphasis placed on adherence to careful and thorough procedural and ethical practice.

Methods derived from epidemiology can be useful in identifying the etiology or the cause of a disease. Among the important steps in this process are identifying risk factors and their impact on a population, determining the extent of a disease and/or adverse events found in a population, and evaluating both existing and new preventive and therapeutic measures and modes of healthcare delivery. Applying strong epidemiological methods with a sound application and interpretation of statistics is the foundation for evidence-based practice. The integration of evidence can lead to the creation of good public policy and regulatory decisions.

DESCRIPTIVE EPIDEMIOLOGY

Rates

Knowledge of how illness and injury are distributed within a population can provide valuable information on disease etiology and can lay the foundation for the introduction of new prevention programs. It is important to know how to measure disease in populations, and rates are a useful method for measuring attributes over time, such as disease and injury in any population. Rates can also be used to identify trends and evaluate outcomes and can allow for comparisons within and between groups. The *Morbidity and Mortality Weekly Report* (*MMWR*; located at www.cdc.gov/mmwr/index.html) is a publication of the CDC and contains updated information on incidence and prevalence of many diseases and conditions. These rates provide healthcare providers with up-to-date information on the risks and burdens of various diseases and conditions as well as recommendations (CDC, 2022b). The information obtained from the *MMWR* can be used to identify trends and provide policymakers with information for designating resources. The following is an example of such information*:

> During 2020, death rates for drug overdose causes were higher in urban areas than in rural areas for those aged 15–24 years (17.2 compared with 13.3), 45–64 years (43.4 compared with 33.5), and ≥65 years (10.0 compared with 6.2). Among adults aged 25–44, drug overdose death rates were not significantly different between urban and rural areas (50.3 compared with 51.6). Drug overdose death rates were lower for adults aged ≥65 years compared with other age groups in both urban and rural areas. (CDC, 2022c)

By publishing incidence rates and comparing those rates among groups, it highlights the disparity between different demographic profiles related to death rates for drug overdose causes. Information such as this can be useful to both clinicians and policymakers who make decisions about interventions and services.

When calculating rates, the numerator is the number of events that occur during a specified period of time and is divided by the denominator, which is the average population at risk during that specified time period. This number is multiplied by a constant—either 100; 1,000; 10,000; or 100,000—and is expressed per that number. The purpose of expressing rates per 100,000, for example, is to have a constant denominator, and it allows investigators to compare rates among groups with different population sizes. To put it simply, the rate is calculated as follows:

$$\text{Rate} = \text{Numerator/Denominator} \times \text{Constant multiplier}$$

In order to calculate rates, the APRN must first have a clear and explicit definition of the patient population and of the event. An important consideration when calculating rates is that anyone represented in the denominator must have the potential to enter the group in the numerator and all persons represented in the numerator must come from the denominator.

Rates can be either crude or specific. Crude rates apply to an entire population without any reference to any characteristics of the individuals within it. For example, to calculate the crude mortality rate, the numerator is the total number of deaths during a specific period of time divided by the denominator, which is the average number of

---

In this example, incidence rates are calculated per 100,000 population. Included together in the calculation are death by suicide, accidental overdose, and undetermined cause.

people in the population during that specified period of time (including those who have died). Typically, the population value for a 1-year period is determined using the midyear population.

Specific rates can also be calculated for a population that has been categorized into groups. Suppose that an APRN wants to calculate the number of new mothers who initiate breastfeeding in a specific hospital in 2023. The formula would be as follows:

$$\frac{\text{Total number of breastfeeding infants in community hospital in 2023}}{\text{Total number of live births in the same community hospital in 2023}} \times \text{Constant multiplier}$$

In order to compare rates in two or more groups, the events in the numerator must be defined in the same way, the time intervals must be the same, and the constant multiplier must be the same. Rates can be used to compare two different groups or one group during two different time periods. Returning to the example about breastfeeding, the breastfeeding rates could be compared in the same hospital but at two different times, before and after implementation of a planned intervention to increase breastfeeding rates.

Formulae for the rates discussed in this chapter can be found in Exhibit 4.1 (Fulton, Goudreau, & Swartzell, 2021).

EXHIBIT 4.1

LIST OF USEFUL FORMULAE

Calculating Rates

Incidence rate describes the occurrence of *new* disease cases in a community over a period of time relative to the size of the population at risk.

$$\text{Incidence rate} = \frac{\text{Number of new cases during a specified period}}{\text{Population at risk during the same specified period}} \times \text{Constant multiplier}$$

Prevalence rate is the number of *all* existing cases of a specific disease in a population *at a given point in time* relative to the population at risk.

$$\text{Prevalence rate} = \frac{\text{Number of existing cases at a specified period}}{\text{Population at risk at the same specified period}} \times \text{Constant multiplier}$$

(continued)

EXHIBIT 4.1

Crude rates summarize the occurrence of births (crude birth rate) or deaths (crude death rate). The numerator is the number of events and the denominator is the average population size (usually estimated as a midyear population).

$$\text{Crude death rate} = \frac{\text{Number of deaths in a population during a specified period}}{\text{Population estimate during same specified period}} \times \text{Constant multiplier}$$

Specific rates are used to overcome some of the biases seen with crude rates. They are used to control for variables such as age, race, gender, and disease.

$$\text{Age-specific death rate} = \frac{\text{Number of deaths for a specified age group during a specified time}}{\text{Population estimate for the specified age group during same specified time}} \times \text{Constant multiplier}$$

Case fatality rate is used to measure the percentage of people who die from a certain disease. This rate tells you how fatal or severe a disease is compared to other diseases.

$$\text{Case fatality rate} = \frac{\text{Number of individuals dying after disease onset or diagnosis}}{\text{Number of individuals with the specified disease}} \times 100$$

Proportionate mortality ratio is useful for determining the leading causes of death.

$$\text{Proportionate mortality ratio} = \frac{\text{Number of deaths from a specified cause during specified time period}}{\text{Total deaths during the same period}} \times 100$$

Calculations Used in Health Impact Assessment

Number needed to treat (NNT) is the number of patients needed to receive a treatment to prevent one bad outcome. The NNT calculated should be rounded up to the next highest number. Before the NNT can be calculated, the absolute risk reduction (ARR) must be identified.

$$\text{ARR} = \text{Incidence in exposed} - \text{Incidence in nonexposed}$$
$$\text{NNT} = 1/\text{ARR}$$

(continued)

EXHIBIT 4.1

The NNT can also be calculated in randomized trials using mortality rates:

$$NNT = 1/(\text{Mortality rate in untreated group} - \text{Mortality rate in treated group})$$

Disease impact number (DIN) is the number of those with the disease in question among whom one event will be prevented by the intervention.

$$\frac{1}{\left(ARR \times \begin{array}{c}\text{Proportion of people with the disease}\\\text{who are exposed to the intervention}\end{array}\right)}$$

Population impact number (PIN) is the number of those in the whole population among whom one event will be prevented by the intervention.

$$\frac{1}{\left(ARR \times \begin{array}{c}\text{Proportion of people with}\\\text{the disease who are exposed}\\\text{to the intervention}\end{array} \times \begin{array}{c}\text{Proportion of the total}\\\text{population with the disease}\\\text{of interest}\end{array}\right)}$$

Years of potential life lost (YPLL) is used for setting heath priorities. Predetermined standard age at death in the United States is usually 75 years.

$$YPLL (75) = 75 - \text{Age at death from a specific cause}$$

Add the years of life lost for each individual for specific cause of death = YPLL

Calculations Used in Screening Programs

Sensitivity is the ability of a screening test to identify accurately those persons with the disease.

$$\text{Sensitivity} = TP/(TP + FN)$$

Specificity reflects the extent to which it excludes the persons who do not have the disease.

$$\text{Specificity} = TN/(TN + FP)$$

	DISEASE	NO DISEASE
+ Test	TP	FP
− Test	FN	TN

FP, false positive; TP, true positive.

Source: Adapted from Fulton, J. S., Goudreau, K. A., & Swartzell, K. L. (2021). *Foundations of clinical nurse specialist practice* (3rd ed.). New York, NY: Springer Publishing Company.

INCIDENCE AND PREVALENCE

Incidence rates describe the occurrence of new events in a population over a period of time relative to the size of the population at risk. *Prevalence rates* describe the number of all cases of a specific disease or attribute in a population at a given point in time relative to the size of the population at risk. Incidence provides information about the rate at which new cases occur and is a measure of risk. For example, the formula for the incidence rate for influenza is as follows:

$$\frac{\text{Total number of people who are diagnosed with influenza in a community during 2023}}{\text{Population in that community at midyear of 2023}} \times 1{,}000 = \text{Rate per } 1{,}000$$

Incidence rates provide us with a direct measure of how often new cases occur within a particular population and provide some basis on which to assess risk. By comparing incidence rates among population groups that vary in one or more risk factors, the APRN can begin to get some idea of the association between risk factors and disease. If, in the earlier example of breastfeeding, the APRN discovers breastfeeding rates are significantly different among different ethnic groups, the characteristics of the groups can be compared and the causes for this disparity can be hypothesized and tested.

Period prevalence measures the number of cases of disease during a specific period of time and is a measure of burden. The formula for the period prevalence rate for influenza in 2023 is as follows:

$$\frac{\text{Total number of people who are influenza positive in a community during 2023}}{\text{Population in that community at midyear of 2023}} \times 1{,}000 = \text{Rate per } 1{,}000$$

In the formula given here, all newly diagnosed cases for the year plus existing cases are included. *Point prevalence* is defined as the number of cases of disease at a specific point in time divided by the number of people at risk at that specific point in time multiplied by a constant multiplier. An example of the use of point prevalence would be the information gathered from a survey in which an investigator asks questions such as who has diabetes, hypertension, epilepsy, or any other disease or event at that specific point in time. Prevalence, whether point or period, cannot give us an estimate of the risk of disease; it can only tell us about the burden of disease for a specified period of time. Prevalence is useful when comparing rates between populations but should be interpreted with caution. Diseases that are chronic will have a higher prevalence because at any given time, those with chronic disease will always have that disease. This can make it challenging to interpret prevalence rates as they do not tell us the risk of developing disease but they can be helpful when trying to determine resource needs for chronic diseases. With diseases that are short in duration, prevalence may not capture the true burden of disease for that population. Additionally, it is important to note that unidentified cases are not captured in either prevalence rates or incidence rates. Rates can only estimate the burden of disease, but they are the best way to draw comparisons using a common denominator.

An example of how prevalence rates are used in the literature is as follows:

> The CDC (2022c, 2022d) reported that the prevalence of obesity was 19.7% for U.S. children from 2017 to 2020. Hispanics (26.2%) and non-Hispanic Blacks (24.8%) had the highest age-adjusted prevalence of obesity, followed by non-Hispanic Whites (16.6%) and non-Hispanic Asians (9.0%). The prevalence of obesity was 12.7% among 2- to 5-year-olds, 20.7% among 6- to 11-year-olds, and 22.2% among 12- to 19-year-olds.

Obesity puts people at risk for many other serious chronic diseases and increases the risk of severe illness from coronavirus disease 2019 (COVID-19). Although children are less likely to develop severe cases of COVID-19 than adults, children who are obese are more likely to develop a severe case of COVID-19 than children of normal weight. In one study, obese children with COVID-19 had a 3.1 times higher risk of hospitalization (CDC, 2022e). Information on the prevalence of childhood obesity in the United States and its attendant risks has led to increased attention to factors that cause obesity. This has led to the development of new programs aimed at primary and secondary prevention.

MORTALITY RATES

Mortality rates, also known as death rates, can be useful when evaluating and comparing populations. As stated earlier, there are many factors that can affect the natural history of disease, and measuring mortality allows investigators to compare death rates among and within populations. The formula for mortality rate is as follows:

$$\frac{\text{Number of deaths in a population during a specified time}}{\text{Average population estimate during the specified time}} \times \text{Constant multiplier}$$

Mortality rates can be specific or broad in definition and can include any qualifiers for time, age, or disease type. It is important to include those specifics in your denominator to ensure that the population value used is the best estimate of the population at risk. For example, to look at the number of deaths in 2022 due to breast cancer in women aged 18 to 40, the denominator should *only* include the midyear population of women aged 18 to 40 in 2022. It is also important to include those women who died during that year in the denominator. Again, it is impossible to know exactly how many women in that age group are at risk using a midyear population, but the key is to use similar sources of measurement so that comparisons can be made, assuming similar sources are used to estimate the denominator.

Standardization of crude rates is an important consideration when comparing mortality rates among populations. Standardization is used to control the effects of age and other characteristics in order to make valid comparisons between groups. Age adjustment is an example of rate standardization and perhaps the most important one. No other factor has a larger effect on mortality than age. Consider the problem of comparing two communities with very different age distributions. One community has a much higher mortality rate for colon cancer than the other, leading investigators to consider a possible environmental hazard in that community, when in fact, that community's population is older, which could account for the higher mortality. Direct age adjustment or standardization allows a researcher to eliminate the age disparities between two populations by using a standardized population. This allows the researcher to compare mortality or death rates between groups by eliminating age differences between populations and comparing actual age-adjusted mortality rates to determine whether age truly plays a role in the crude unadjusted mortality rates.

There are two methods of age adjustment: direct, as mentioned earlier, and indirect. The direct method applies observed age-specific mortality or death rates to a standardized population. The indirect method applies the age-specific rates of a standardized population to the age distribution of an observed population and is used to determine whether one population has a greater mortality because of an occupational hazard or risk compared to the general population. (To learn how to perform age adjustment, refer to an advanced epidemiology text.)

The *case fatality rate* (CFR) is a measure of the severity of disease (such as infectious diseases) and can be helpful when designing programs to reduce the rate or disparity in the population. It should be noted that CFR is not a true rate as it has no explicit time implication but rather is a proportion of persons with disease who died from that disease after diagnosis. It is a measure of the probability of death among diagnosed cases. Its usefulness for chronic diseases is limited because the length of time from diagnosis to death can be long. CFR is also useful in determining when to use a screening test. Screening tests identify disease early so that an intervention or treatment can be initiated in the hopes of lessening the morbidity or mortality of that disease. Those diseases that are rapidly fatal may not necessarily be beneficial to screen unless the screening will allow for a cure or treatment to change the overall outcome or to prevent unnecessary spread of the disease. Screening is useful in identifying disease in asymptomatic individuals in whom further transmission of disease can be prevented or reduced, such as in HIV. CFRs, therefore, can be helpful for comparisons between study populations and can provide useful information that could help determine whether an intervention or treatment is working. The formula for CFR is as follows:

$$\text{Case fatality percent} = \frac{\text{Number of individuals dying during a specified period of time after disease onset or diagnosis}}{\text{Number of cases of that specific disease}} \times 100$$

CFR is usually expressed as a percentage; so in this case, one would multiply this rate by a constant multiplier of 100 to obtain the percentage of disease that is fatal. It is important in all of these rates to include those who have died from the disease in the denominator. Removing those who have died from the denominator falsely increases the CFR, making the disease appear more fatal or severe (Celentano & Szklo, 2018).

The *proportionate mortality ratio* is useful for determining the leading causes of death. The formula for proportionate mortality ratio is as follows:

$$\frac{\text{Number of deaths from a specified cause during specified time period}}{\text{Total deaths from all causes during the same specified time period}} \times 100$$

Again, this measure is usually reported as a percentage and reflects the burden of death due to a particular disease. This information is useful for policymakers who make decisions about the allocation of resources. (See Exhibit 4.1 for a list of these formulae.)

SURVIVAL AND PROGNOSIS

Mortality rates are very helpful when comparing groups and looking at disparities among populations. One cannot discuss mortality without having an understanding of survival and prognosis. Many diseases, particularly cancer, are studied over time, with attention placed on survival. Ideally, survival should be measured from the onset of disease until death, but the true onset of disease is generally unknown. Survival rates are usually calculated at various intervals from diagnosis or initiation of treatment. Prognosis is calculated using collected data to estimate the risk of dying or surviving after diagnosis or treatment begins. As mentioned earlier, CFRs give a good estimate of prognosis or severity of disease. However, they are best suited for acute diseases in which death occurs relatively soon after diagnosis. Survival analysis is better suited for chronic diseases or those diseases that take time to progress.

Survival time is generally calculated from the time of diagnosis or from the start of treatment. This can vary from patient to patient, as some patients may seek care immediately after symptoms present or may wait months to seek care. Some patients are diagnosed prior to symptom presentation after they screened positive on a screening test. Some may obtain a diagnosis immediately, whereas others may have poor access to care and diagnosis is delayed by weeks to months or even years. Once a diagnosis is made, treatment may or may not occur immediately. Additionally, some patients may die before diagnosis or treatment. Because these individuals are not represented in survival analysis, this can lead to a falsely increased survival time. With that said, one can see how difficult it is to establish a true survival time after diagnosis. However, we can estimate survival if we use a common denominator and consistent criteria for measurement.

Before we discuss how to calculate and interpret survival data, we must touch on two important concepts, lead time bias and overdiagnosis bias. *Lead time bias* is a phenomenon whereby a patient is diagnosed earlier by screening and appears to have increased survival due to screening but rather dies at the same time they would regardless of screening. In other words, the time from which a patient is diagnosed earlier from screening is the lead time, and the bias is the error that occurs as a result of concluding that screening leads to a longer survival after diagnosis. As can be seen in the following timeline

FIGURE 4.1

Timeline illustrating lead time bias.

| | Survival time | |
| Disease onset | Time of diagnosis treatment without screening | Death |

| | Lead time | |
| Disease onset | Screening early diagnosis treatment | Death |

| | Survival time | |
| Disease onset | Screening early diagnosis treatment | Death |

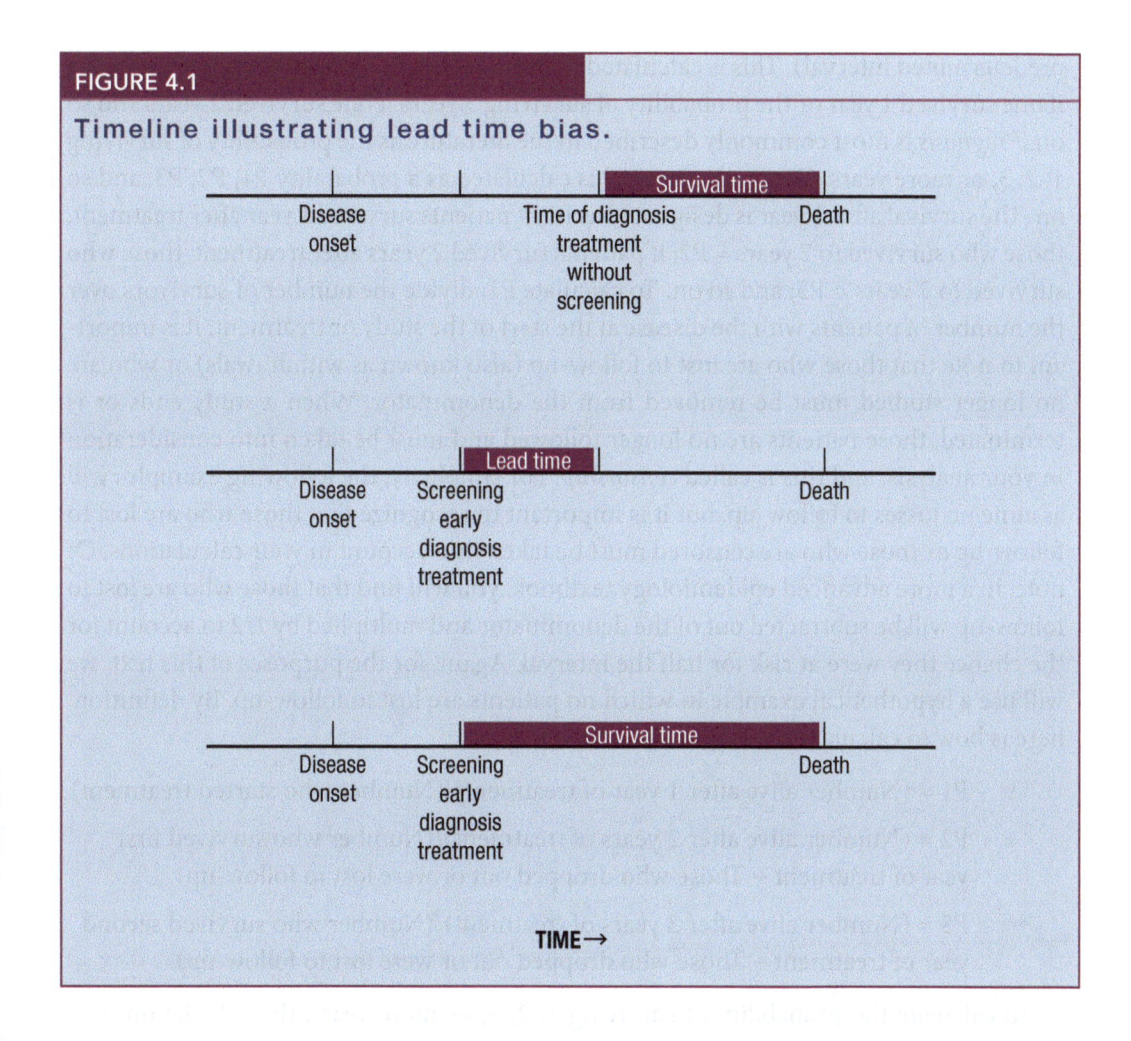

TIME →

(Figure 4.1), the survival time is longer when screening is implemented, but the ultimate time of death is unchanged. Although this is not true for all screening tests, it is important to recognize the phenomenon of lead time bias as it can affect the conclusions that are made regarding survival, which ultimately can affect a patient's perceived prognosis.

Overdiagnosis bias occurs as a result of making a diagnosis from screening for a disease or cancer that would not have manifested clinically or has a slow progression, such that the person dies from another etiology. This type of bias has the potential to increase undue stress in individuals and can also falsely increase survival times, especially for diseases with slow progression. In both these types of biases, there is no difference in overall mortality in those screened versus those who were not screened. With that said, considerations must also be made for those screening tests in which a false-negative test reassures a patient who may not seek care and ultimately develops cancer and potentially has decreased survival due to delay in diagnosis. All of these biases need to be taken into consideration when interpreting survival data.

Prognosis is calculated using survival rates. There are two methods of conducting survival analysis and estimating prognosis that are discussed. The first is the *actuarial method*, which measures the likelihood of surviving after each year of treatment (or a predetermined interval). This is calculated as follows: the probability of surviving 2 years if one survived 1 year or the probability of surviving 3 years if one survived 2 years and so on. *Prognosis* is most commonly described in the literature as the probability of surviving 1, 2, 3, or more years. Generally, survival is calculated as a probability P1, P2, P3, and so on. The survival after 1 year is designated as P1; if patients survived 1 year after treatment, those who survived to 2 years = P2; if patients survived 2 years after treatment, those who survived to 3 years = P3; and so on. To calculate P1, divide the number of survivors over the number of patients with the disease at the start of the study or treatment. It is important to note that those who are lost to follow-up (also known as withdrawals) or who are no longer studied must be removed from the denominator. When a study ends or is terminated, those patients are no longer followed and must be taken into consideration in your analysis, and this is called *censorship*. For simplicity, the following examples will assume no losses to follow-up, but it is important to recognize that those who are lost to follow-up or those who are censored must be taken into account in your calculations. Of note, in a more advanced epidemiology textbook, you will find that those who are lost to follow-up will be subtracted out of the denominator and multiplied by 1/2 to account for the chance they were at risk for half the interval. Again, for the purposes of this text, we will use a hypothetical example in which no patients are lost to follow-up. By definition, here is how to calculate P1, P2, and so on:

- P1 = (Number alive after 1 year of treatment)/(Number who started treatment)
- P2 = (Number alive after 2 years of treatment)/(Number who survived first year of treatment − Those who dropped out or were lost to follow-up)
- P3 = (Number alive after 3 years of treatment)/(Number who survived second year of treatment − Those who dropped out or were lost to follow-up)

To calculate the probability of surviving 1, 2, 3, or more years, the calculation is as follows:

P1 = Probability of surviving 1 year
P1 × P2 = Probability of surviving 2 years
P1 × P2 × P3 = Probability of surviving 3 years
P1 × P2 × P3 × P4 = Probability of surviving 4 years
P1 × P2 × P3 × P4 × P5 = Probability of surviving 5 years

Using data from Table 4.1, we can calculate and interpret these probabilities.

TABLE 4.1 Survival Rates After Treatment (Hypothetical Life Table of 100 Patients With No Patients Lost to Follow-Up)

	NUMBER SURVIVED				
	AFTER 1 YEAR	AT 2 YEARS	AT 3 YEARS	AT 4 YEARS	AT 5 YEARS
Cohort (N = 100)	88	76	55	47	33

In this example:

P1 = 88/100 = 0.88

P2 = 76/88 = 0.86

P3 = 55/76 = 0.72

P4 = 47/55 = 0.85

P5 = 33/47 = 0.70

Probability of surviving 1 year = 0.88

Probability of surviving 2 years = 0.88 × 0.86 = 0.76

Probability of surviving 3 years = 0.88 × 0.86 × 0.72 = 0.54

Probability of surviving 4 years = 0.88 × 0.86 × 0.72 × 0.85 = 0.46

Probability of surviving 5 years = 0.88 × 0.86 × 0.72 × 0.85 × 0.70 = 0.32

It is important to distinguish between the probability of surviving 5 years and the probability of surviving 5 years given that someone survived 4 years. Generally, the longer someone survives after treatment, the more likely that person will make it to the next year. Overall survival after 5 years is always a smaller number as the probability of surviving each year is multiplied against each year (Celentano & Szklo, 2018).

Note that the actuarial method can be used to look at outcomes other than survival or death as it can estimate probabilities of an outcome or event occurring, such as a treatment side effect (e.g., vomiting, headache) or recurrence of disease. Another important consideration is survival over time. When looking at survival rates measured over years, it is important that an APRN takes into account the improvements and advances in treatments over time. APRNs should consider comparing survival rates for earlier treatment regimens with those for newer regimens, as this can affect the validity of the overall survival if not taken into consideration. In addition, certain confounders (e.g., age, gender, ethnicity, socioeconomic status) may contribute to differences in survival rates and should be examined when performing a survival analysis (see Chapter 5, "Epidemiological Methods and Measurements in Population-Based Nursing Practice: Part II," for more on confounding). Recognition of these differences is a critical step for the evaluation of potential health disparities and is a perfect opportunity for an APRN to develop strategies to address the underlying issue causing those disparities.

In the literature, survival analysis using the actuarial method is plotted on a curve in which the *x*-axis represents time and the *y*-axis represents the number of survivors at each time interval. This is called a *survival curve* and represents the pattern of survival over predetermined time intervals. Using the data from the earlier example, the probabilities are plotted in a standardized survival curve (Figure 4.2).

The second type of survival analysis is the *Kaplan–Meier method*. This method is commonly used in medicine and is well suited for analyses of small and large populations, as well as comparisons between treatments or interventions. Although beyond the scope of

FIGURE 4.2

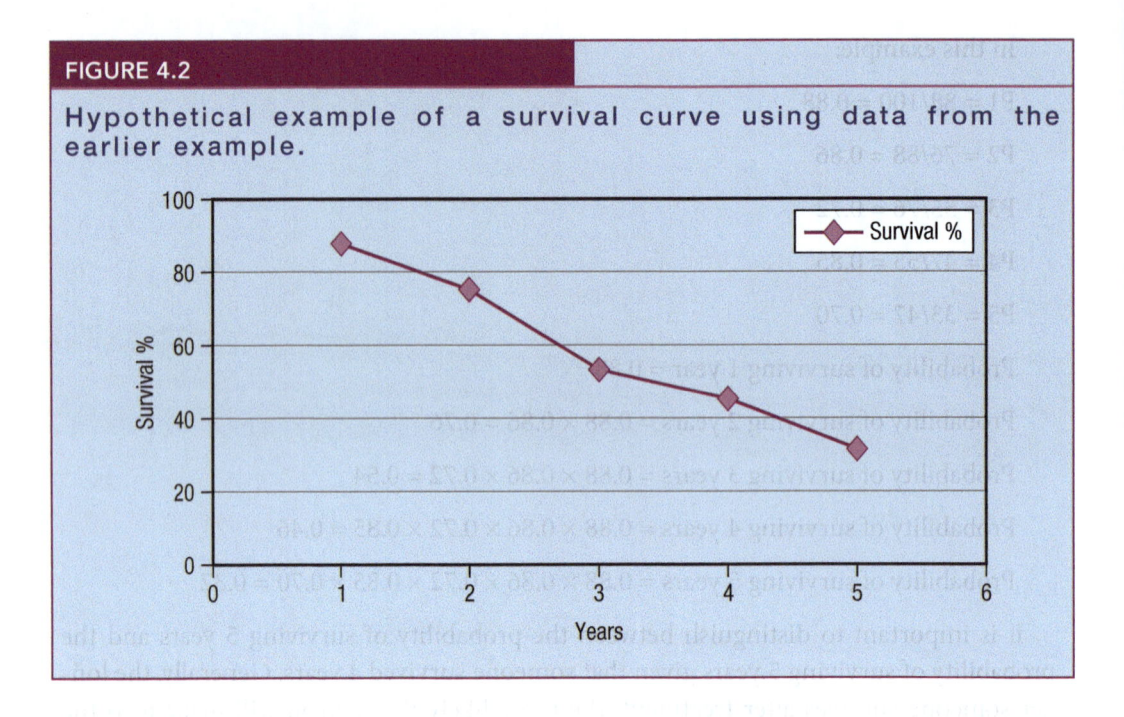

Hypothetical example of a survival curve using data from the earlier example.

this book, statistical analyses can be performed to compare treatments or interventions using tests of significance (log rank test) and logistic regression (proportional hazard models [Cox models]). As with any comparison trial, it is important to take into consideration the characteristics of those patients who are lost to follow-up because if they occur more frequently in one treatment group compared to another, this can affect the results. For example, if the majority of patients lost to follow-up are receiving treatment A and most of them can be characterized as impoverished with poor access to care, then this could skew the results of the remaining patients receiving treatment A. Thus, minimizing loss to follow-up or censored patients and/or maintaining similar losses with similar characteristics in each group is paramount to reducing bias and improving the strength of the study conclusions. This reiterates the importance of randomization, which will be discussed more thoroughly in Chapter 5, "Epidemiological Methods and Measurements in Population-Based Nursing Practice: Part II."

Kaplan–Meier curves are used to plot survival, and these plots represent a stepwise pattern of survival in which the increments of time are not standardized (e.g., 1 year, 5 years), but rather each step represents an event (e.g., time to death or an outcome of interest). Kaplan–Meier curves are seen more commonly in the literature and are a better estimate of survival as they also take into consideration patients who are lost to follow-up or are censored. These curves also allow for comparisons between different treatment regimens (Figure 4.3).

Kaplan–Meier curves are different from traditional survival curves in that they do not slope downward after each event but rather maintain a horizontal line until the next event (e.g., death) occurs, and then a downward vertical line is drawn until the new cumulative survival is reached and the steps are continued until the study is completed. At the time in which no deaths are occurring (also known as the death-free period), the cumulative

FIGURE 4.3

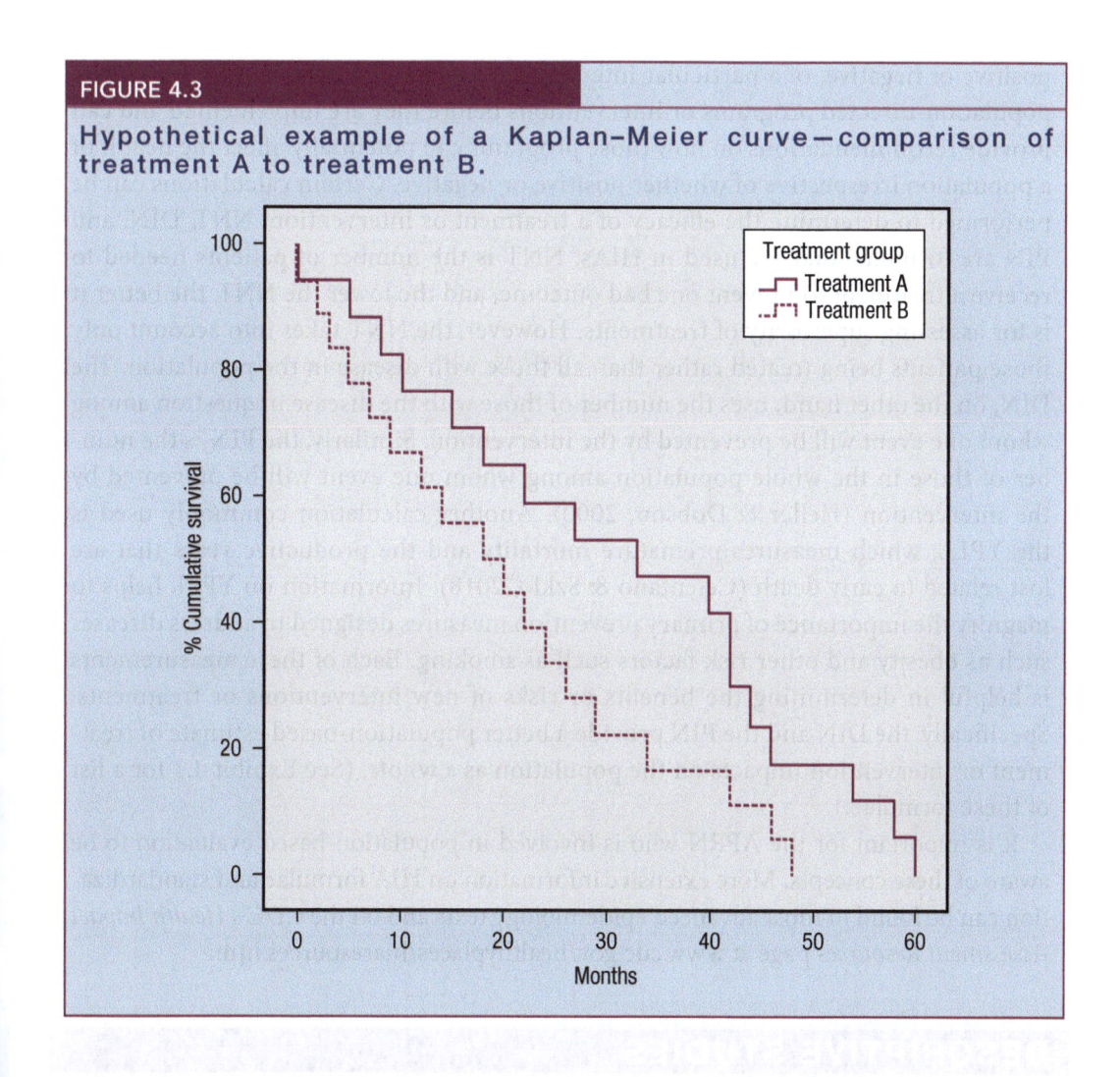

Hypothetical example of a Kaplan–Meier curve — comparison of treatment A to treatment B.

survival is maintained; however, hatch marks can be seen in these plots, which represent those lost to follow-up or censored during that interval (Jekel et al., 2007).

The importance of having the knowledge and skills to interpret and calculate survival data cannot be understated. APRNs can use survival data or outcome data in various ways. Most importantly, the evidence obtained from survival or outcome data can help APRNs to design and justify interventions to improve the quality of life for diseases such as cancer. Comparisons to other groups can be made by addressing outcomes of interest to determine whether certain interventions make a difference in the quality of life and ultimately impact the survival of those involved.

HEALTH IMPACT ASSESSMENT

As mentioned previously, rates can be used to describe the distribution of disease and other health-related states and events, but sometimes the APRN may be more concerned with knowing how data can be used to describe the relevancy of clinical practice. *Health impact assessment* (HIA) is the assessment of the potential health effects, positive or negative, of a particular intervention on a population. HIAs can evaluate population-directed programs or interventions before they are implemented and can provide recommendations on how those programs can potentially affect the health of a population irrespective of whether positive or negative. Certain calculations can be performed to determine the efficacy of a treatment or intervention. NNT, DIN, and PIN are formulae that are used in HIAs. NNT is the number of patients needed to receive a treatment to prevent one bad outcome, and the lower the NNT, the better it is for assessing superiority of treatments. However, the NNT takes into account only those patients being treated rather than all those with disease in the population. The DIN, on the other hand, uses the number of those with the disease in question among whom one event will be prevented by the intervention. Similarly, the PIN is the number of those in the whole population among whom one event will be prevented by the intervention (Heller & Dobson, 2000). Another calculation commonly used is the YPLL, which measures premature mortality and the productive years that are lost related to early death (Celentano & Szklo, 2018). Information on YPLL helps to magnify the importance of primary prevention measures designed to address diseases such as obesity and other risk factors such as smoking. Each of these measurements is helpful in determining the benefits or risks of new interventions or treatments. Specifically, the DIN and the PIN provide a better population-based estimate of treatment or intervention impacts on the population as a whole. (See Exhibit 4.1 for a list of these formulae.)

It is important for the APRN who is involved in population-based evaluation to be aware of these concepts. More extensive information on HIA formulae and standardization can be found in most advanced epidemiology texts and on the CDC's *Health Impact Assessment Resources* page at www.cdc.gov/healthyplaces/hiaresources.htm.

DESCRIPTIVE STUDIES

Descriptive epidemiology is used to describe the distribution of disease and other health-related states and events in terms of personal characteristics, geographical distribution, and time. There are four types of descriptive studies: case reports, case series, cross-sectional studies, and correlation or ecologic studies. The data used in descriptive studies are often readily available and can be retrieved from such sources as hospital records, census data, or vital statistics records.

CASE REPORTS AND CASE SERIES

Case reports are succinct written accounts of generally rare or unusual cases in which the treatment or management of the disease or condition is worth reporting. These are usually published to assist healthcare providers in the management of rare, unresearched, or undocumented cases. A case series is merely a report of a series of patients with similar diseases or conditions that describes their management or treatment in order to identify new strategies that may be helpful to treat patients with similar conditions. They also lead to future studies and can be helpful for APRNs, as they can use

CORRELATION STUDIES

Correlation studies are also referred to as ecologic studies and are used to conduct studies of aggregate or population characteristics. In ecologic studies, rates are calculated for characteristics that describe populations and are used to compare frequencies between different groups at the same time or the same group at different times. They are useful for identifying long-term trends, seasonal patterns, and event-related clusters. Because data are collected on populations instead of individuals, an event cannot be linked to an exposure in individuals, and the investigator cannot control for the effect of other variables. These types of studies lead to more rigorous studies that can control for variables of interest and look at individual data to determine whether an association truly exists. Correlation studies can only report that a correlation exists and cannot show an association exists as they compare population or aggregate data. An example of a correlation study would be one that shows a correlation between smoking by pregnant women and low birth weight babies. Without knowing individual data, one cannot determine whether smoking is the causative factor or if causation can be explained by the environmental, behavioral, and social characteristics of smokers versus nonsmokers (Celentano & Szklo, 2018).

A study by Pillai et al. (2013) provides an example of a correlation study. The authors used data from 143 countries to study the relationship between female literacy and maternal mortality. Their analysis reveals a significant negative relationship between female literacy rates and maternal mortality. Populations with a higher prevalence of literacy have lower maternal mortality rates, and populations with a lower prevalence of literacy have higher maternal mortality rates. The authors point out limitations to their study, most importantly the difficulty of controlling for known correlates with maternal mortality (such as access to healthcare services) due to a scarcity of cross-national data. These data show that a correlation exists between the variables, but not necessarily a causal one. There are many possible explanations for the relationship, including (but not exclusively) demographic and economic differences among the countries. Correlation studies must be interpreted with caution, but important information can be obtained from the trends that could identify disparities and lead to further studies and hypothesis testing.

CROSS-SECTIONAL STUDIES

In *cross-sectional studies*, also known as prevalence studies, both exposures and outcomes are collected simultaneously. These studies provide a "snapshot" at one point in time and thus exclude people who have died or who chose not to participate, which can introduce bias. Temporal relationships are difficult to determine in these studies as only prevalence can be determined and the risk of developing disease cannot be estimated. Many cross-sectional studies are surveys that sample a population and its various characteristics. They can be inexpensive and can provide timely descriptive data about a group under study, but again, they do not tell us about causality or the true risk of developing a certain outcome such as disease.

Perrodin-Njoku et al. (2022) conducted a cross-sectional study to understand the prevalence of health outcomes in a Black deaf and hard of hearing (DHH) adult sample (18 years of age and older) and compare it to a Black hearing sample. The authors used data from the primary Health Information National Trends Survey (HINTS)-American Sign Language survey data from Black DHH adults and secondary National Cancer Institute-HINTS English survey data from Black hearing adults. Self-reported data was gathered for all medical conditions as diagnosed by healthcare providers. The study showed that Black DHH adults had a higher likelihood for diabetes, hypertension, lung disease, cancer, and comorbidity compared to their hearing Black counterparts. The findings led the authors to conclude that DHH Black adults experience greater healthcare disparities than the general Black adult population. They believe that Black DHH individuals experience both racism and audism and recommend that anti-racist policies and the training of healthcare providers must address both anti-racist and sensory disabilities issues.

This study serves to illustrate both the advantages and disadvantages of cross-sectional studies. The study was carried out at one point in time using existing datasets. One limitation of the study was that it missed people whose healthcare conditions were not diagnosed/reported. The inability to control for or identify the significance of potentially important variables is a disadvantage of using a cross-sectional study design. With that said, a cross-sectional study is a fairly quick method to obtain descriptive data and can be useful in identifying prevalence rates for specified populations.

ANALYTIC EPIDEMIOLOGY

Analytic epidemiology looks at the origins and causal factors of diseases and other health-related events. Analytic designs are often carried out to test hypotheses formulated from a descriptive study. The goal of analytic epidemiology is to identify factors that increase or decrease risk. Risk is the probability that an event will occur. For example, a patient who is obese might ask, "What is the likelihood that I will develop diabetes if I do not lose weight?"

Although descriptive studies allow a basis for comparison and can provide the APRN with data to identify potential risk factors and differences among groups, study designs, such as a prospective cohort, need to be carried out in order to determine whether there is an association between an exposure and a disease and to determine the strength of that association. To do this, the APRN can compare exposed and nonexposed groups and follow them over time to see who develops an outcome (such as a specific disease) and who does not. Comparison is an essential component of population studies. Case–control studies can also allow for comparisons by retrospectively looking back in time to see what exposure or risk factors are associated with being a case or a control. Comparisons can also be made by following a group using treatment A compared to treatment B or treatment A can be compared to no treatment at all. There are multiple study designs, but we will focus only on the most common study designs and discuss the advantages and disadvantages that each one poses in practice.

COHORT STUDIES

Cohort designs can be either prospective or retrospective. In a prospective cohort design, the investigator begins with a defined population and then follows a group of individuals who were either exposed or nonexposed to a factor of interest and then follows both groups to compare the incidence of an outcome or disease. In a cohort study, one can look at multiple outcomes that develop from an exposure. In a retrospective cohort design, exposure is ascertained from past records and outcome is ascertained at the time the study begins. If an association exists between the exposure and the outcome, then the incidence rate in the exposed group will be greater than that in the nonexposed group. The ratio of these is the *relative risk* (RR), which is the incidence rate in the exposed group divided by the incidence rate in the nonexposed group. RR is a measure of the strength of an association between an exposure and an outcome or disease (Table 4.2).

If the RR is equal to 1 (the numerator equals the denominator), then the risk to the two groups is equal. If the RR is greater than 1 (the numerator is greater than the denominator), then the risk in the exposed group is greater than the risk in the nonexposed group and can be considered a positive association. If the RR is less than 1 (the denominator is greater than the numerator), then the risk in the exposed group is less than the risk in the nonexposed group and can be considered protective. An example of a protective association may be the association between exercise and heart disease. Exercise can actually reduce the risk of heart disease and has an RR of less than 1. Thus, it is considered a protective exposure.

Attributable risk (AR), absolute risk, or risk difference is the amount of risk that can be attributed to an exposure. For example, it is well-known that smoking can cause lung cancer, but lung cancer can also occur in nonsmokers. The amount of disease that is associated with risks/exposures other than smoking is called the *background risk*. In order to

TABLE 4.2 Calculation of RR and AR in a Cohort Study

	DISEASE	NO DISEASE	TOTALS	
Exposure	a	b	a + b	Inc exp = a/a + b
No Exposure	c	d	c + d	Inc nonexp = c/c + d
		RR = Inc exp/Inc nonexp		
		AR = Inc exp − Inc nonexp		
	AR proportion in the exposed population =	$\dfrac{\text{Inc exp} - \text{Inc nonexp}}{\text{Inc exp}}$		
	AR proportion in the total population =	$\dfrac{\text{Incidence in total population} - \text{Inc nonexp}}{\text{Incidence in total population}}$		

AR, attributable risk; Inc exp, incidence in the exposed; Inc nonexp, incidence in the nonexposed; RR, relative risk.

calculate the risk attributable to a particular exposure, subtract the incidence of disease (lung cancer) in the exposed group (smokers) minus the incidence of disease (lung cancer) in the nonexposed group (background risk). This value is considered the AR due to exposure (see Table 4.2). If an APRN wants to know how much risk of disease can be reduced by removing a risk factor, one can calculate the ARR, which is synonymous with the AR. The relative risk reduction (RRR) is calculated the same as the AR proportion. This can be confusing as these terms are interchanged in medicine and epidemiology, but it is important to recognize and understand how these terms are used and interpreted. An example of RRR would be described as: What percentage of motor vehicle deaths could be reduced if we could eliminate texting while driving? This RRR percentage is what is commonly reported in the news and can be very helpful for policymakers and for justification of funding. The AR can also be calculated as a proportion of the total population. For example, to determine the amount of lung cancer attributable to smoking in the total population (AR proportion), one would have to know the incidence in the total population (to review how to calculate the incidence in the total population, refer to an advanced epidemiology textbook). APRNs should be familiar with how to calculate and interpret RR and AR, as these values are reported commonly in the literature and reports such as the *MMWR*.

Cohort studies are best carried out when the investigator has good evidence that links an exposure to an outcome, when the time interval between exposure and the outcome is short, and when the outcome occurs relatively often. One of the major problems with cohort studies is that they can be time-consuming and expensive, especially if the cohort needs to be followed for a prolonged length of time. Diseases that are rare or that take many years to develop may be better suited for a case–control study as it can be difficult to follow participants for many years, especially if the outcome of interest is rare. The longer the time period, the more likely it is that participants will be lost to follow-up, and multiple exposures can potentially confound the relationship.

A prospective cohort study was carried out in in an urban, university-affiliated, level I trauma center (Sarangarm et al., 2017). The objective of the study was to compare the 30-day emergency department return rate between patients given a Take-Home Medication pack (THM) versus a standard paper prescription (SPP) prior to discharge. A total of 711 patients were included in the study, with 268 receiving a THM and 443 receiving a SPP. In comparison with the SPP group, the THM group was more likely to have an all-cause return (RR = 1.7, $P < .01$). The authors suggest that more research, preferably using a randomized clinical design, needs to be completed regarding the use of THMs to reduce emergency room revisits.

CASE–CONTROL STUDIES

In a *case–control* study, the APRN must first identify a group of individuals with the outcome of interest (cases). A second group is identified without the outcome of interest (controls). The proportion of those cases that have a history of exposures is then compared to the proportion of the cases that were not exposed, and the proportion

TABLE 4.3 Calculation of OR in a Case–Control Study

	CASES	CONTROLS
Exposure History	a	b
No Exposure History	c	d
Totals	a + c	b + d
	Proportion of cases exposed = a/a + c	Proportion of controls exposed = b/b + d
	OR = ad/bc	

OR, odds ratio.

of the controls that were exposed is compared to the proportion of the controls that were not exposed. The measure of the effect of exposure is expressed as an *odds ratio* (OR), which is the ratio of the odds of having been exposed if you are a case to the odds of having been exposed if you are not a case. If the exposure is not related to the disease or outcome, the OR is equal to 1. If the exposure is related to the disease or outcome, the OR is greater than 1, and if the OR is less than 1, the exposure is considered protective. To calculate the OR, construct a 2 × 2 table in which the columns represent the cases and controls and the rows represent the exposed and nonexposed populations. It is important to set up the table correctly. If it is not set up correctly, it will affect the interpretation and conclusions. Once the table is complete, multiply the cross products to obtain the result (see Table 4.3).

In a case–control study, if there is an association between an exposure and disease, the history of exposure should be higher in persons who have the disease (cases) compared to those who do not have disease (controls). It is important to keep in mind that the OR is not a calculation of risk and cannot predict which exposures/risk factors will develop into a case or disease. The fact that a person is obese may put that person at risk for diabetes, but it does not mean that that person will get diabetes. In case–control studies, one cannot calculate RR; therefore, we cannot conclude that if you are obese, you will develop diabetes, but rather, if your OR is greater than 1, you could conclude that those with diabetes (outcome) are more likely to be obese (risk factor/exposure).

Selection of cases and controls is an important step in case–control studies. Definite criteria should be used so that there is no ambiguity about how to distinguish between a case and a control. Exposure is not always all or nothing. Controls should resemble the cases as closely as possible except for the exposure to the factor under study. If the cases are drawn from a particular clinic, then ideally the controls should be drawn from the same clinic population. Matching is one method that can be used to select a sample so that potential confounders are distributed equally between the cases and controls. For example, if an APRN plans to evaluate an intervention to reduce burden among caregivers of dependent elderly in the home, it would be important to recognize the characteristics of the population studied prior to implementing the intervention. It is known that men and women have differing characteristics that affect their role as caregiver (Amankwaa, 2017). By matching for gender in the study, the APRN can eliminate this potentially confounding factor (gender). The problem with matching is that the investigator is not always aware of all of the potential confounding factors. It can be difficult to match each subject in a study, and in some cases, investigators can overmatch. When an investigator overmatches, one loses the ability to look at the matched variables as risk factors.

In case–control studies, the investigator begins with cases and controls and goes back retrospectively to look for exposures. In cohort studies, the investigator begins with exposed and nonexposed individuals and follows individuals over time to see who develops or does not develop an outcome or disease. Case–control studies allow the APRN to look at cases and the probability of having an exposure or risk factor. Cohort studies allow an APRN to follow a cohort over time to determine whether being exposed to a risk factor impacts the likelihood of developing a disease or diseases or improves outcomes (as in an intervention). If associations are found, further studies are necessary to determine causal links and to prevent ecologic fallacy. When examining the results of case–control and cohort studies, it is important for the APRN to consider whether or not all other explanations for an identified association have been eliminated. No single epidemiological study can satisfy all criteria for causality. The APRN needs to look at the accumulation of evidence, as well as the strength of individual studies.

RANDOMIZED CONTROLLED TRIALS

Randomized controlled trials (RCTs) or clinical trials are useful for evaluating treatments (including technology) and for assessing new ways of organizing and delivering health services. In population-based studies, the issue is often health promotion and disease prevention rather than treatment of an existing disease. Interventions can also be studied in RCTs, with the target involving defined populations rather than individuals and often involving educational, program, or policy interventions. When carefully designed, RCTs can provide the strongest evidence for evaluating treatments and interventions.

The basic design of an RCT is to assign subjects randomly to either receive the new treatment/intervention or not receive the new treatment/intervention. Inclusion and exclusion criteria for the participants must be precise and written in advance to eliminate any errors within the study or any future comparison studies. As with cohort studies, RCTs can compare more than two groups. Analysis is carried out to compare outcomes between the randomized groups. As mentioned earlier, comparisons can be made between different interventions, different treatments, or to a control group that has received no intervention or treatment.

There are many examples of how RCTs have been used to evaluate the effectiveness of interventions in specific groups of people. For example, they have been used to analyze the efficacy of a brief psychoeducation intervention added to treatment as usual in improving the rehospitalization rate at 3 and 6 months after discharge (Riera-Molist et al., 2023) and to assess the impact of the type of pushing used at delivery on the mother's medium-term pelvic floor function (Barasinski et al., 2023), as well as to examine the safety and efficacy of long-term exercise training in reducing physical functional loss in older adults with advanced chronic kidney disease (CKD) and comorbidity (Weiner et al., 2023). These studies illustrate how useful the randomized trial design is for testing a new intervention. RCTs are an excellent vehicle to provide evidence to enhance practice.

SAMPLE SIZE

Sample selection and sample size determination are critical steps in the research process. Sample size determination is necessary to identify the minimum number of subjects needed to enroll in a study to identify true differences and associations between groups and thus has implications for the investigators as they need to allocate ample resources based on sample size to carry out the study. Power analysis is used to determine sample size. There are several factors that influence the size of the sample: variance, significance, power, and effect size.

Variance

Variance is the variation about the mean. For example, if you are looking at a continuous variable such as blood pressure, the variance away from the mean is defined as s^2. Variance (s^2) is the square of the standard deviation (s). The standard deviation takes into account all blood pressure measurements and essentially sums the difference of each blood pressure measurement away from the mean (see a statistic textbook for more details). If you do not have data with which to calculate the standard deviation, you can review the literature or look at a pilot dataset to determine this number. A study that has very little variance (i.e., most of the values fall close to the mean) would require a smaller sample size than a study in which the blood pressure measurements have a very large range and a wider sigmoid curve.

Significance and Power

Significance is the probability that an observed difference or relationship exists and usually is defined as a *p*-value ($p < 0.05$). The smaller the *p*-value (e.g., $p < 0.01$), the larger the required sample size. *Power* ($1 - \beta$) is the capacity of the study to detect differences or relationships that actually exist in the population or the capacity to correctly reject a null hypothesis, that is, prevent a type II error. The larger the power required, the less likelihood of committing a type II error. Most studies use a power of 80% or 0.80, or if a more rigorous power is necessary (e.g., 90%), a larger sample size is required.

Effect Size

Effect size is the actual difference between groups and treatments that you hope to see in your study. One way to identify effect size is to review previous studies; another method is to conduct a pilot study. For example, if you are designing an educational intervention and want to see a 20% improvement of knowledge after the intervention,

20% is your effect size. If you want to see a smaller change in knowledge (e.g., 10%), then a larger sample will be required to detect a smaller effect or difference. In summary, effect sizes occur along a range of values. For example, if you want to see a 5% change in results of an outcome, you will need many more participants than if you want to see a 30% change.

Understanding what goes into power analysis is an important step in designing a study. Power analysis can be calculated using computer programs. There are many free software programs available on the Internet to assist with power analysis. Typing "sample size calculation" in a search engine will lead an APRN to many sites.

SCREENING

Screening is a tool used to detect disease in groups of asymptomatic individuals with the goal of reducing and/or preventing morbidity and mortality. Screening tests can be applied to groups of individuals or to high-risk populations. There are multiple examples of screening tests, including the Pap smear, the tuberculosis skin test (PPD test), the mammogram, and so on.

Determining whether a screening test is appropriate requires the APRN to address several aspects of the disease of interest. Screening is neither available nor appropriate for all diseases. In order for a screening program to be effective, certain criteria should be met. The target population needs to be identifiable and accessible and the disease should affect a sufficient number of people to make screening cost-effective. The preclinical period should be sufficient to allow treatment before symptoms appear so that early diagnosis and treatment make a difference in terms of outcome.

Finally, it is necessary for the screening test to be sensitive enough to detect most cases of the disease and to be specific enough to limit the number of false-positive tests. Screening tests should also be relatively inexpensive, be easy to administer, and have minimal side effects.

The *validity* of a screening test refers to its ability to accurately identify those who have the disease. Sensitivity and specificity are measures of a screening test's validity. *Sensitivity* is a measure of a screening test's ability to accurately identify disease when it is present. *Specificity* is a measure of a screening test's ability to correctly identify a person without disease with a negative test. The *positive predictive value* (PPV) is a measure of the probability of a positive test result when the disease is present. The *negative predictive value* (NPV) of a test is a measure of the probability that the disease is absent when there is a negative test (see Table 4.4).

Directing screening tests toward high-risk populations has many advantages. By screening populations with a higher disease prevalence, we can actually increase the PPV of that test. Screening low-prevalence populations can lead to more false positives, which can be costly and harmful to patients. Thus, selection of the disease to be tested and the patient population to be screened are both important to consider when designing a new test.

The APRN can evaluate the success of screening programs by looking at a variety of outcomes. For example, some of the outcomes that can be followed include the reduction

TABLE 4.4 Computing Sensitivity, Specificity, and Predictive Values in Screening Tests

	DISEASE	NO DISEASE	TOTALS	
+ Test	a	b	a + b	PPV = a/a + b
− Test	c	d	c + d	NPV = d/c + d
Totals	a + c	b + d		
	Sensitivity = a/a + c	Specificity = d/b + d		

NPV, negative predictive value; PPV, positive predictive value.

in overall mortality in screened individuals, a reduction in the CFR in screened individuals, an increase in the percentage of cases detected at earlier stages, a reduction in complications, and improvement of quality of life in screened individuals.

In 2018, the U.S. Preventive Services Task Force (USPSTF) released their final recommendations for cervical cancer screening (USPSTF, 2018). The complete recommendations can be found on the USPSTF website (www.uspreventiveservicestaskforce.org/uspstf/recommendation/cervical-cancer-screening). One of the recommendations for cervical cancer screening is that women aged 21 to 65 should get a Pap smear every 3 years. A second recommendation is that women aged 30 to 65 who wish to be screened less frequently can choose a combination of Pap smear and human papillomavirus (HPV) testing every 5 years. The Task Force does not recommend cervical cancer screening using HPV testing in women younger than age 30. This is because evidence indicates that the expected harms (such as false positives) in this age group outweigh the potential benefits. These recommendations are being updated as this book goes to print. Check the website for updates: www.uspreventiveservicestaskforce.org/uspstf/draft-update-summary/cervical-cancer-screening-adults-adolescents.

According to the Task Force, "since the implementation of widespread cervical cancer screening, there has been a dramatic reduction in cervical cancer deaths in the United States" (USPSTF, P4). For this reason, the Task Force urges healthcare providers to encourage women to be screened for cervical cancer, especially those who have never been screened or who have not been screened within the past 5 years. These guidelines provide an example of how evidence on the specificity and sensitivity of a screening test can be used to create more evidence-based clinical guidelines. Therefore, screening tests need to be tailored to the disease under investigation, and many factors need to be taken into consideration; for example, how many false negatives can be missed? How many false positives are acceptable? Can screening and early detection really make a difference in the outcome of the disease? Understanding these factors and balancing them with targeted screening in high-risk populations are important considerations in screening implementation. The USPSTF provides screening guidelines on a variety of disease states with recommendations (e.g., colorectal, prostate, and breast cancers). APRNs can visit their website located at www.uspreventiveservicestaskforce.org for the latest recommendations.

SUMMARY

The natural history of disease refers to the progression of a disease from its preclinical state to its clinical state, and knowledge of these stages provides a framework for understanding approaches to the prevention and control of disease. Primary prevention refers to the process of altering susceptibility or reducing exposure to susceptible individuals and includes general health promotion and specific measures designed to prevent disease prior to a person getting a disease. Primary prevention measures are generally carried out during the stage of susceptibility. With secondary prevention, it is sometimes possible to either cure a disease at a very early stage or slow its progression to prevent complications and limit disability. Secondary prevention measures are carried out during the preclinical or presymptomatic stage of disease. Tertiary prevention takes place during the middle or later stages of a disease (the clinical stage of disease) and refers to measures taken to alleviate disability and restore effective functioning.

The dynamic nature of disease calls for a sophisticated model for explaining causation. When designing interventions for populations, the APRN needs to keep in mind that disease develops as the result of many antecedent factors and not as a result of a single, isolated cause.

Descriptive epidemiology is used to describe the distribution of disease and other health-related states and events in terms of personal characteristics, geographical distribution, and time. It also helps APRNs design studies and measure mortality and prognosis. Analytic epidemiology looks at the origins and causal factors of diseases and other health-related events. Epidemiological methods can be used to identify populations at risk and to evaluate interventions provided to patient populations. Population-based evaluation and planning depend on understanding the many and varied factors that influence health and disease. APRNs can use their understanding of epidemiological methods in concert with their clinical expertise to develop policies and implement and evaluate new programs and interventions to improve population outcomes.

END-OF-CHAPTER RESOURCES

EXERCISES AND DISCUSSION QUESTIONS

EXERCISE 4.1 For the following scenarios, identify the type of study design: Answer a, b, c, or d.

a. Case–control study
b. Cohort study
c. Cross-sectional study
d. Ecologic study

_____ A study was done to look at childhood asthma and exposure to gas stoves in one suburban community. Prevalence rates of asthma for children living in homes with gas stoves were compared to prevalence rates of asthma for children who do not live in homes with gas stoves. The researchers found children living in homes with gas stoves had a higher prevalence rate of asthma than those not living in homes with gas stoves.

_____ Over a 2-month period, 10,000 patients with hepatitis will be categorized as alcoholic or nonalcoholic. Then over the next 20 years, new cases of liver cancer will be classified out of the 10,000.

_____ One thousand graduates of Doctor of Nursing Practice (DNP) programs are surveyed to determine level of job satisfaction and level of workplace independence.

_____ Over a 1-year period, all new cases of primiparous women with type 2 diabetes and a similar number of primiparous women without type 2 diabetes were asked if they have a history of gestational diabetes.

_____ Undergraduate students at three liberal arts universities are given a survey to measure caffeine consumption and levels of anxiety.

EXERCISE 4.2 The midyear population of Lawrence is 33,200. In 2023, 395 people in Lawrence were newly diagnosed with colon cancer. This brought the total number of active cases of colon cancer in Lawrence to 1,394. During 2023, 464 people in Lawrence died of colon cancer.

a. What was the incidence rate per 100,000 for colon cancer in 2023? (Round to nearest whole number for all answers in this exercise.)
b. What was the prevalence rate for colon cancer per 100,000 in 2023?
c. What was the CFR for colon cancer per 100 in 2023?

EXERCISE 4.3 The midyear population of City A is 1,000,000 people (355,100 old people and 644,900 young people), and during the year, 4,500 people died (3,550 old people and 950 young people). There were 250 people injured in car accidents during the same 1-year period (60 old people and 190 young people), and of these, 43 died (10 old people and 33 young people).

Using this information, compute the following:

a. The crude mortality rate per 1,000 (round to the nearest tenth)
b. The age-specific mortality rate per 1,000 for each age group (round to the nearest tenth)
c. The cause-specific mortality rate for car accidents per 1,000 (round to the nearest 100th)
d. The CFR for car accidents per 100 (round to the nearest tenth)
e. The proportionate mortality ratio for car accidents (round to the nearest whole number)

EXERCISE 4.4 A new rapid blood test was created to test for HPV in a community clinic. The following is a 2 × 2 chart which describes the results of the test. Answer questions a to g using the 2 × 2 chart.

	HPV	NO HPV	TOTALS
Positive (+) test	95	37	132
Negative (−) test	39	278	317
Totals	134	315	449

a. What is the sensitivity of this test?
b. What is the specificity of this test?
c. What is the PPV?
d. What is the NPV?
e. Describe in words the sensitivity of this test.
f. Describe in words the NPV.
g. What is the disease prevalence in this population?

R1 =
R0 =
R =

EXERCISE 4.5 An epidemiological study is conducted to learn about the relationship between asthma and hypertension. Suppose there are 65 cases of hypertension in 72,000 person-years in persons with asthma and 42 cases of hypertension in 312,000 person-years in those without asthma. (The overall rate in both groups combined = 107 cases in 384,000 person-years overall.) Use this information to answer questions a to b.

   a. Calculate the rate of hypertension in the asthma group ($R1$), in the no asthma group ($R0$), and overall (R). Express all rates in "per 100,000 person-years." (Round to nearest whole number.)
   b. Calculate and *interpret* the RR of hypertension associated with asthma.
   c. Calculate and *interpret* the AR of hypertension associated with asthma.

EXERCISE 4.6 You read about a new protocol (HTN T) that was used successfully to improve blood pressure control in an urban clinic population. A major feature of HTN T is the use of technology (such as text messaging) to communicate with patients. You work in a rural clinic and currently use protocol HTN 1. You wonder if HTN T would improve blood pressure control in your clinic population. Explain how you could use RCT to evaluate whether HTN T improves blood pressure control in your clinic population.

EXERCISE 4.7 You are reviewing the survival statistics from your hospital using a new treatment (treatment A) compared to the old treatment (treatment B) for breast cancer. The following table lists the number of survivors after each year of treatment for both treatments A and B. Answer the following questions using the table. Assume no patients were lost to follow-up.

TREATMENT A	NUMBER SURVIVED				
	AT 1 YEAR	AT 2 YEARS	AT 3 YEARS	AT 4 YEARS	AT 5 YEARS
Cohort ($N = 1,229$)	1,102	987	835	725	633

TREATMENT B	NUMBER SURVIVED				
	AT 1 YEAR	AT 2 YEARS	AT 3 YEARS	AT 4 YEARS	AT 5 YEARS
Cohort ($N = 1,179$)	1,084	886	755	602	544

   a. Calculate the survival rates for treatments A and B for each year after treatment: P1, P2, P3, P4, and P5.
   b. Calculate the probability of surviving for 1, 2, 3, 4, and 5 years cumulatively for each of the treatments.

c. Your administrator would like to know how the treatments compare to each other. You are asked for the following information:
    – What is the likelihood of surviving 5 years if you made it to 4 years of treatment for each of the treatments?
    – How does treatment A compare to treatment B for each year of survival after treatment?
    – Which treatment has the best 5-year survival rate?
d. Plot the survival curve for both treatments on the same graph.
e. Why might there be differences between these two treatments?
f. What are some potential confounders that may contribute to one treatment working better than the other?

EXERCISE 4.8 Explain the advantages and disadvantages of screening tests.

EXERCISE 4.9 Perform a search to determine the incidence, prevalence, and survival rates for one of the following cancers in your state: lung cancer, breast cancer, colon cancer, prostate cancer, and cervical cancer.

- Describe the screening recommendations for the cancer you selected.
- Describe the advantages and disadvantages of cancer screening for the cancer you selected.
- How do the incidence, prevalence, and survival rates in your state compared to the national rates.
- What are potential confounders for the cancer you selected?
- What disparities in cancer incidence, mortality, and survival were you able to determine from your search?

A robust set of instructor resources designed to supplement this text is located at http://connect.springerpub.com/content/book/978-0-8261-4377-8. Qualifying instructors may request access by emailing textbook@springerpub.com.

REFERENCES

Agaku, I. T., Nkosi, L., Agaku, Q. D., Gwar, J., & Tsafa, T. (2022). A rapid evaluation of the US Federal Tobacco 21 (T21) law and lessons from statewide T21 policies: Findings from population-level surveys. *Preventing Chronic Disease, 19,* E29. https://doi.org/10.5888/pcd19.210430

American Association of Colleges of Nursing. (2021). *The essentials: Core competencies for professional nursing education.* Author. Retrieved from https://www.aacnnursing.org/Essentials

Amankwaa, B. (2017). Informal caregiver stress. *ABNF Journal, 28*(4), 92–95.

Barasinski, C., Debost-Legrand, A., Savary, D., Bouchet, P., Curinier, S., & Vendittelli, F. (2023). Does the type of pushing at delivery influence pelvic floor function at 2 months postpartum? A pragmatic randomized trial-The EOLE study. *Acta Obstetricia et Gynecologica Scandinavica, 102*(1), 67–75. https://doi.org/10.1111/aogs.14461

Celentano, D. D., & Szklo, M. (Eds.). (2019). *Gordis epidemiology* (6th ed.). Elsevier.

Centers for Disease Control and Prevention. (2011). Decrease in smoking prevalence—Minnesota, 1999–2010. *Morbidity and Mortality Weekly Report, 60*(5), 138–141. Retrieved from http://www.ncbi.nlm.nih.gov/pubmed/21307824

Centers for Disease Control and Prevention. (2022a). *Smoking and tobacco use.* Retrieved from https://www.cdc.gov/tobacco/data_statistics/fact_sheets/health_effects/effects_cig_smoking/index.htm

Centers for Disease Control and Prevention. (2022b). *Morbidity and Mortality Weekly Report.* Retrieved from http://www.cdc.gov/mmwr/about.html

Centers for Disease Control and Prevention. (2022c). *QuickStats: Drug overdose death rates among persons aged ≥15 years, by age group and urban-rural status.* Retrieved from https://www.cdc.gov/mmwr/volumes/71/wr/mm7147a3.htm

Centers for Disease Control and Prevention. (2022d). *Overweight and obesity. Adult obesity facts.* Retrieved from https://www.cdc.gov/obesity/data/adult.html

Centers for Disease Control and Prevention. (2022e). *Overweight & obesity.* Retrieved from https://www.cdc.gov/obesity/data/obesity-and-covid-19.html

Framingham Heart Study. (2022). About the Framingham Heart Study. Retrieved from https://www.framinghamheartstudy.org/fhs-about/

Fulton, J. S., Goudreau, K. A., & Swartzell, K. L. (2021). *Foundations of clinical nurse specialist practice* (3rd ed.). Springer Publishing Company.

Harkness, G. (1995). *Epidemiology in nursing practice.* Mosby.

Heller, R. F., & Dobson, A. J. (2000). Disease impact number and population impact number: Population perspectives to measures of risk and benefit. *British Medical Journal, 321*(7266), 950–953. https://doi.org/10.1136/bmj.321.7266.950

Heller, R. F., & Page, J. (2002). A population perspective to evidence-based medicine: "Evidence for population health." *Journal of Epidemiology and Community Health, 56,* 45–47. https://doi.org/10.1136/jech.56.1.45

Jekel, J. F., Katz, D. L., Elmore, J. G., & Wild, D. M. J. (2007). *Epidemiology, biostatistics, and preventive medicine* (3rd ed.). Saunders Elsevier.

Kim, S. C., Martinez, J. E., Liu, Y., & Friedman, T. C. (2021). US Tobacco 21 is paving the way for a tobacco endgame. *Tobacco Use Insights, 14,* 1–6. https://doi.org/10.1177/1179173X211050396

Minnesota Department of Health. (2018). *The positive health impacts of raising tobacco taxes in Minnesota.* Retrieved from http://www.health.state.mn.us/divs/hpcd/tpc/topics/taxes.html

Patel, M., Simard, B. J., Benson, A. F., Donovan, E. M., & Pitzer, L. (2022). Measuring the impact of state and local Tobacco 21 policies in the U.S.: A longitudinal study of youth and young adults ages 15–21. *Nicotine & Tobacco Research: Official Journal of the Society for Research on Nicotine and Tobacco, 25*(4), 631–638. https://doi.org/10.1093/ntr/ntac248

Parkinson's Foundation. (2023). *Understanding Parkinson's.* Retrieved from Stages of Parkinson's | Parkinson's Foundation

Perrodin-Njoku, E., Corbett, C., Moges-Riedel, R., Simms, L., & Kushalnagar, P. (2022). Health disparities among Black deaf and hard of hearing Americans as compared to Black hearing Americans: A descriptive cross-sectional study. *Medicine, 101*(2), e28464. https://doi.org/10.1097/MD.0000000000028464

Pillai, V. K., Maleku, A., & Wei, F. H. (2013). Maternal mortality and female literacy rates in developing countries during 1970–2000: A latent growth curve analysis. *International Journal of Population Research, 2013,* 1–11. https://doi.org/10.1155/2013/163292

Riera-Molist, N., Riera-Morera, B., Roura-Poch, P., Santos-López, J. M., & Foguet-Boreu, Q. (2023). A brief psychoeducation intervention to prevent rehospitalization in severe mental disorder inpatients. *The Journal of Nervous and Mental Disease, 211*(1), 40–45. https://doi.org/10.1097/NMD.0000000000001567

Sarangarm, D., Sarangarm, P., Fleegler, M., Ernst, A., & Weiss, S. (2017). Patients given take home medications instead of paper prescriptions are more likely to return to emergency department. *Hospital Pharmacy, 52*(6), 438–443. https://doi.org/10.1177/0018578717717396

U.S. Preventive Services Task Force. (2018). *U.S. Preventive Services Task Force issues new cervical cancer screening recommendations*. Retrieved from https://www.uspreventiveservicestaskforce.org/Page/Name/us-preventive-services-task-force-issues-new-cervical-cancer-screening-recommendations

Weiner, D. E., Liu, C. K., Miao, S., Fielding, R., Katzel, L. I., Giffuni, J., Well, A., & Seliger, S. L. (2023). Effect of long-term exercise training on physical performance and cardiorespiratory function in adults with CKD: A randomized controlled trial. *American Journal of Kidney Diseases: The Official Journal of the National Kidney Foundation, 81*(1), 59–66. https://doi.org/10.1053/j.ajkd.2022.06.008

CHAPTER 5

EPIDEMIOLOGICAL METHODS AND MEASUREMENTS IN POPULATION-BASED NURSING PRACTICE: PART II

ANN L. CUPP CURLEY

INTRODUCTION

To provide leadership in evidence-based practice, advanced practice registered nurses (APRNs) require skills in the analytic methods that are used to identify population trends, prioritize needs, and evaluate outcomes and systems of care (American Association of Colleges of Nursing [AACN], 2021). APRNs need to be able to identify studies with strong designs and solid methodology, considering the factors that can affect study results. This chapter discusses the complexities of data collection and the strengths and weaknesses of study designs used in population research. Critical components of data analysis are discussed, including bias, causality, confounding, and interaction.

ERRORS IN MEASUREMENT

A dilemma that may occur with population research is the difficulty of controlling for variables that are not being studied but that may have an impact on the results. Finding a statistical association between an intervention and an outcome or an exposure and a particular disease is meaningful only if variables are correctly controlled, tested, and measured. The purpose of a well-designed study is to properly identify the impact of the variable (or variables) under study and to avoid bias and/or design flaws caused by another, unmeasured variable.

Statistics are used to analyze population characteristics by inference from sampling (Statistics, 2022, ahdictionary.com). They help us translate and understand data. Before we can begin to understand a measured difference between groups, we must identify the variation. But statistical analysis cannot overcome problems caused by a flawed study.

When a researcher draws the wrong conclusion because of a problem with the research methodology, the result is a type I or type II error, also referred to as *errors of inference*. A *type I error* occurs when a null hypothesis is rejected when in fact it is true. A *type II error* occurs when one fails to reject a null hypothesis when in fact it is false. Take, for example, an APRN who carries out a study to determine whether a particular intervention improves medication compliance in hypertensive patients. To keep the example simple, the intervention will simply be referred to as "Intervention A." A null hypothesis proposes no difference or relationship between interventions or treatments. In this case, the null hypothesis is as follows: There is no difference in medication compliance between hypertensive patients who receive Intervention A and those who receive no intervention. Let us assume that the APRN completes the study and carries out the statistical analysis of the data. The following conclusions are possible:

- There is no significant difference in medication compliance between the two groups.
- There is a significant difference in medication compliance between the two groups.

Now let us assume that the correct conclusion is number 1, but the APRN concludes that there is a difference in medication compliance between the two groups (rejects the null hypothesis when it is true). The APRN has committed a type I error. If the correct conclusion is number 2 but the APRN concludes that there is no difference in medication compliance between the two groups (fails to reject the null hypothesis when it is false), then a type II error has occurred (Table 5.1).

When using data or working with datasets, it is critical to understand that mistakes can occur where measurements are involved. There are two basic forms of error of measurement: *random error* (also known as nondifferential error) and *systematic error* (also known as bias). Random errors occur as the result of the usual, everyday variations that are expected and that can be anticipated during certain situations. The result is a fluctuation in the measurement of a variable around a true value. Systematic errors occur not as the result of chance but because of inherent inaccuracies in measurement. They are typically constant or proportional to the true value. Systematic error is generally considered the more critical of the two. It can be the result of either a weak study design or a deliberate distortion of the truth.

TABLE 5.1 Type I and Type II Errors

	RELATIONSHIP DOES NOT EXIST	RELATIONSHIP EXISTS
Conclude relationship does not exist (fail to reject null hypothesis)	Correct decision	Type II error (β)
Conclude relationship exists (reject null hypothesis)	Type I error (α)	Correct decision power ($1 - \beta$)

RANDOM ERROR

Random error measurements tend to be either too high or too low in about equal amounts because of random factors. Although all errors in measurement are serious, random errors are less serious than bias because they are less likely to distort findings. Random errors do, however, reduce the statistical power of a study and can occur because of unpredictable changes in an instrument used for collecting data or because of changes in the environment. For example, if one of three rooms being used to interview subjects became overheated occasionally during data collection, making the subjects uncomfortable, it could affect some of their responses. This effect in their responses is an example of a random error of measurement.

SYSTEMATIC ERROR

There are several types of systematic error or bias and all can impact the validity of study results. Bias can occur in many ways and is commonly broken down into two categories: selection and information bias. Such things as how the study design is selected, how subjects are selected, how information is collected, how the study is carried out (the conduct), or how the study is interpreted by investigators are all forms of potential bias. These problems can result in a deviation from the truth, which can lead to false conclusions.

Selection Bias

Selection bias occurs when the selected subjects in a sample are not representative of the population of interest or representative of the comparison group, and as a result, this selection of subjects can make it appear (falsely) that there is or is not an association between an exposure and an outcome. Selection bias is not simply an error in the selection of subjects for a study but rather the systematic error that occurs when selecting the subjects for a study (Celentano & Szklo, 2018). Nonprobability sampling (nonrandom sampling) is strongly associated with selection bias. In nonprobability sampling, members of a target population do not share equal chances of being selected for the study or intervention/treatment group. This can occur with studies using convenience samples or volunteers. People who volunteer to participate in a study may have characteristics that are different from people who do not volunteer, and this can impact the outcome of the results and is simply referred to as *volunteer bias*. Similarly, people who do not respond to surveys may possess characteristics different from those who do respond to surveys. Thus, it is important to characterize nonresponders as much as possible, as the characteristics of responders may be very different from those of nonresponders and can lead to errors in survey interpretation. The best way to avoid this type of bias is to keep it at a minimum, unless the characteristics of nonresponders can be identified and addressed. Another form of selection bias is *exclusion bias*, and this can occur when one applies different eligibility criteria to the cases and controls (Celentano & Szklo, 2018). *Withdrawal bias* can occur when people of certain characteristics drop out of a group at a different rate than they do in another group or are lost to follow-up at a different rate. This can also lead to systematic error in the interpretation of data. APRNs must be aware of these types of error early in their own study designs and also when critically appraising research conducted by others. All of these types of systematic error can have an impact on how data are interpreted; therefore, minimizing these types of error through careful assessment of subject selection and eligibility criteria and monitoring of characteristics in the populations of interest are critical for successful research and program implementation. Finally, probability sampling methods (random sampling) can be used to ensure that all members of a target population have an equal chance of being selected into a study, thereby eliminating the chance of selection bias (Merrill, 2017; Shorten & Moorley, 2014).

Information Bias

Information bias deals with how information or data are collected for a study. This includes the source of data that are collected, such as hospital records, outpatient charts, or national databases. Many of these types of data are not collected for research purposes, so they may be incomplete, inaccurate, or contain information that is misleading. This can complicate data analysis as the information abstracted from these sources may be incorrect and can lead to invalid conclusions. *Measurement bias* is a form of information bias and occurs during data collection. It can be caused by an error in collecting information for an exposure or an outcome. Calibration errors can occur when using instruments to measure outcomes. This type of bias can also occur when an instrument is not sensitive enough to measure small differences between groups or when interventions are not applied equally (e.g., blood pressure measurements taken using the wrong cuff size). Information bias also includes how the data are recorded and classified. This can lead to *misclassification bias*, in which a control may be recorded as a case or a case is classified as having an exposure or exposures that they did not actually have. Misclassification bias can be subdivided into differential and nondifferential. For example, *differential misclassification* occurs when a case is misclassified into exposure groups more often than controls. In this case, this type of bias usually leads to the appearance of a greater association between exposure and the cases than one would find if this bias was not present (Celentano & Szklo, 2018). In *nondifferential misclassification*, the misclassification occurs as a result of the data collection methods such that a case is entered as a control or vice versa. In this situation, the association between exposure and outcome may be "diluted," and one may conclude there is not an association when one really exists (Celentano & Szklo, 2018). Another example of misclassification bias occurs when members of a control group are exposed to an intervention. This results in *contamination bias*. An example would be a nurse who floats from the floor where hourly rounding is being carried out to a control floor where no rounding is supposed to occur, but the nurse carries out hourly rounding on the control floor. In this case, contamination bias minimizes the true differences that would have been seen between groups. However, these cases should not be reassigned; in fact, any unexpected or unplanned crossover that occurs should be analyzed in the original group to which it was assigned by the investigator. This is known as the *intent-to-treat principle*. For example, patients who are assigned to one group or another and crossover intentionally or accidentally to the other group should be analyzed according to their original assignment. *Intent to treat* simply means that you assign patients to the original group you intended to treat them in from the start of the study, regardless of the treatment they received.

If information is obtained from interviews, there can be bias introduced based on how the questions are asked or there may be variance between interviewers in how the questions are prompted to the subject. *Recall bias* happens when subjects are asked to remember or recall events from the past. For example, people who experience a traumatic event in their lives may recall events of that day more accurately and with more detail than someone asked to recall events from a day without significance. *Reporting bias* occurs when a subject may not report a certain exposure, as they may be embarrassed or not want to disclose certain personal information, or the subject may report certain things to gain approval from the investigator (Celentano & Szklo, 2018). The effects of bias can impact a study in two ways: it can make it appear that there is a significant effect when one does not exist (type I error), or there is an effect but the results suggest there is no effect (type II error; see Table 5.1).

Finally, an APRN needs to be aware of both publication bias and citation bias (additional types of information bias), particularly when carrying out systematic reviews or meta-analyses. *Publication bias* refers to the tendency of peer-reviewed journals to publish a higher percentage of studies with significant results than those studies with nonsignificant or negative statistical results. *Citation bias* refers to the practice of selective citation of articles based on their results.

Publication bias has been identified and studied for decades (Ayorinde et al., 2020; Joober et al., 2012; Mlinarić et al., 2017; Song et al., 2009). Song et al. (2009) completed a meta-analysis to determine the odds of publication by study results. Although they identified many problems that were inherent in studying publication bias (e.g., they pointed out that studies of publication bias may be as vulnerable as other studies to selective publication), they concluded that "[t]here is consistent empirical evidence that the publication of a study that exhibits significant or 'important' results is more likely to occur than the publication of a study that does not show such results" (p. 11).

Duyx et al. (2017) conducted a meta-analysis of citation bias. They found that articles that report statistically significant results are cited more often than articles that report nonsignificant results. They also found that this occurs more often in the biomedical sciences than the natural sciences. As has been found in studies on publication bias, these authors warn that citation bias can lead to an overrepresentation of positive results and unfounded beliefs.

There are several issues related to these two types of information bias. They can give readers a false impression about the impact of an intervention, can lead to costly and futile research, can distort the literature on a topic, and can be unethical. People who participate in research studies (subjects) are often told that their participation will lead to a greater understanding of a problem. There is a breach of faith when the results of these studies are not published and shared in the scientific community (Joober et al., 2012; Siddiqi, 2011). The publication and citation of both categories of research is ethical and provides a more balanced and objective view of current evidence.

In summary, bias must be recognized and addressed early in the study design. Ultimately, bias should be avoided, when possible, but if it is recognized, it should be acknowledged in the interpretation of results and addressed in the study discussion.

CONFOUNDING

Confounding occurs when it appears that a true association exists between an exposure and an outcome but this association is confounded by another variable or exposure. An interesting study by Matsumoto et al. (2010) raised questions about the potential confounding effect of weather on differences found among communities in Japan. They investigated the rural–urban gap in stroke incidence and mortality by conducting a cohort study that included 4,849 men and 7,529 women in 12 communities. On average, subjects were followed for 10.7 years. Information on geographical characteristics (such as population density and altitude), demographic characteristics (including risk factors for stroke), and weather information (such as rainfall and temperature) were obtained and analyzed using logistic regression. The researchers discovered a significant association between living in a rural community and stroke, independent of risk factors. However, further analyses revealed that the actual link may be between the weather and stroke. They proposed that the difference seen in the incidence of stroke in these communities may be related not to living in a rural versus an urban community but to the weather differences between communities. Low temperatures are known to cause an increase in coagulation factors and plasma lipids, and therefore, differences in weather could have an impact on the incidence of stroke. They cite the small number of communities as a limitation of the study, and for this reason, they did not generalize their findings. But they did raise an important point. It is important to be aware of the many variables (e.g., biological, environmental) that may confound a relationship in population studies (Matsumoto et al., 2010).

Identification of confounding or other causes of spurious associations is important in population studies. A *confounder* is a variable that is linked to both a causative factor or an exposure and the outcome. There are many examples of confounders, such as age, gender, and socioeconomic status. Confounding occurs when a study is performed and it appears from the study results that an association exists between an exposure and an outcome, when, in fact, the association is between the confounder and the outcome. Another example of confounding might occur if an APRN carried out a study to determine whether there is a relationship between age and medication compliance without controlling for income. Younger, working patients might be more compliant not because of the age factor but because they have the resources to buy their medications. If confounding is ignored, there can be long-term implications, as the APRN may implement interventions for medication compliance with education programs aimed at older patients without considering problems related to income. The intervention would ultimately not succeed because the relationship is false or not causal due to confounding. Confounders must be known risk factors for the outcome and must not be affected by the exposure or the outcome (Celentano & Szklo, 2018). Confounding, although difficult to avoid, must be recognized and accounted for in studies.

There are some techniques that an investigator can use to reduce the effects of confounding variables. Random assignment to treatment and nontreatment groups can reduce confounding by ensuring each group has similar shared characteristics that otherwise might lead to spurious associations. In the earlier example, if you were concerned about the socioeconomic status and education level, you may stratify early on for those characteristics and randomly assign from each of those groups so that they are equally represented in your intervention and nonintervention groups. When random assignment is not possible, the matching of cases and controls for possible confounding variables can improve equal representation of subjects and can minimize the effect of confounding. Investigators can match groups or individuals. Group matching allows groups with similar characteristics of interest to be matched to each other. Each group should share a similar proportion of the characteristics of interest. Usually, cases should be selected first, and the control group should be selected with similar proportions of the characteristics of interest (Celentano & Szklo, 2018).

In individual matching, each individual case is matched to a control with similar characteristics of interest. This is referred to as *matched pairs*. One has to be careful not to match cases and controls for too many characteristics, as it can be difficult to find a control, or the control may be too similar to the case and true differences may not be able to be demonstrated in the analysis phase. Using strict inclusion and exclusion criteria also can be helpful and should be applied similarly for comparison groups. There are limitations to the latter two methods.

Although it is possible to match for known confounding variables, there may be other unknown confounding variables that cannot be controlled for and, if not recognized, can impact study conclusions. If the study groups are matched for gender, then gender cannot be evaluated in the final analysis. Additionally, if the study is matched for too many variables, this can also limit the study as all of the matched variables cannot be studied, and this may limit the ability to make valid conclusions. There is a similar problem with inclusion and exclusion criteria as both criteria should be applied the same to each of the study groups. The method for analyzing data can also help reduce problems related to confounding.

Multivariable regression, for example, can measure the effects of multiple confounding variables. This method is useful only when the variables are recognized and acknowledged. Recognition of confounders requires a basic understanding of the relationship between an exposure and a disease or an outcome and can also be identified by performing a stratified analysis first. Once confounders are determined, then these variables can be added in and removed from the model, one at a time. Interaction needs to be assessed, and the exposure–disease relationship is determined. These inferential methods estimate the contribution of each variable to the outcome while holding all other variables constant in the model. The objective is to include a set of variables that are theoretically or actually correlated with both the intervention and the outcome to reduce the bias of treatment effect. Therefore, the goal of regression analysis is to identify causal relationships by recognizing the confounders to ensure found relationships are real and not spurious (Kahlert et al., 2017; Kellar & Kelvin, 2013; Starks et al., 2009).

INTERACTION

Whenever two or more factors or exposures are being studied simultaneously, the possibility of interaction exists. *Interaction* occurs when one factor impacts another such that one sees a greater or lesser effect than would be expected by one factor alone. *Synergism* occurs when the combined effect of two or more factors is greater than the sum of the individual effects of each factor. And, conversely, the opposite or negative impact can be seen with *antagonism* of factors. One example of synergism is seen with the interaction of exercise and diet. The combination of these two factors can reduce the risk of heart disease more than each factor alone. Synergistic models can have an additive effect in which the effect of one factor or exposure is added to another or can have a multiplicative effect in which the effect of one factor multiples the effect of another factor. For example, epidemiologists identified an interactive effect between cigarettes and alcohol; these two factors together have a multiplicative effect on the risk of developing digestive cancers (National Cancer Institute, 2021). There are many synergistic effects that can be found in clinical practice, especially as they pertain to drugs. First-generation antihistamines, such as chlorpheniramine, have a synergistic effect on opioids such as codeine. Patients are warned not to take them in combination as the sedative effects are more significant when taken together. APRNs who carry out investigations need to be aware of the potential interactions when examining the effects of multiple exposures on an outcome. A discussion on how to determine whether a model is multiplicative or additive can be found in more detail in an advanced epidemiology textbook, but a basic understanding is necessary for interpreting the different outcomes that can occur from multiple exposures.

There are clearly many sources of error that can occur while conducting a study. The informed APRN needs to identify and acknowledge these types of errors. Therefore, it is essential that APRNs recognize when errors occur and how they can impact a study and should be familiar with measures that can be taken to avoid or minimize errors.

RANDOMIZATION

Randomized controlled trials (RCTs) are considered inherently strong because of their rigorous design. Random selection of a sample and random assignment to groups are objective methods that can be used to prevent bias and produce comparable groups. Random assignment helps to minimize bias by ensuring that every subject has an equal chance of being selected and that results are more likely to be attributed to the intervention being tested and not to some other extraneous factor such as how subjects were assigned to the treatment or control group. It is impossible to know all the characteristics that could influence results. The random assignment of subjects to different treatment groups helps to ensure that study groups are similar in the characteristics that might affect results (e.g., age, gender, ethnicity, and general health).

BLINDING

Another problem encountered in research occurs when investigators or subjects themselves affect study results. This can happen when a researcher's personal beliefs or expectations of subjects influence their interpretation of the outcome. Sometimes observers can err in measuring data toward what is expected. If subjects know or believe that they are given a placebo or the nonexperimental treatment, it may cause them to exaggerate symptoms that they would dismiss if given the experimental treatment. These actions by both investigators and subjects are not necessarily intentional; they can occur subconsciously.

The best way to eliminate or minimize this type of bias is to use a *single-blind* or a *double-blind* study design. In a double-blind study, both the subjects and the investigators are blinded, that is, unaware of which group is receiving the experimental treatment or intervention. Sometimes, it is impossible to blind the investigator because of the nature of the treatment, in which case a single-blind design, in which the subjects are unaware of which group they are in, can be used. If blinding cannot be used, measures need to be taken that ensure that study groups are followed with strict objectivity.

DATA COLLECTION

As mentioned earlier, how data are collected and analyzed can lead to bias when conducting a study. The training of investigators to ensure that data are collected uniformly from all subjects and the use of a strict methodology for data collection and analysis contribute to a strong study design. Objective criteria should be used for the collection of all data. Strict inclusion and exclusion criteria should be developed in writing so that there are no questions as to what criteria are to be applied to the study. Avoiding subjective criteria is important as it can lead to inconsistent application of criteria. For example, if you chose "ill appearance" as an exclusion criterion, it may be difficult to apply this criterion uniformly as each APRN may have different levels of experience making this assessment. Objective criteria, such as heart rate greater than 120 beats per minute, respiratory rate greater than 24 breaths per minute, or oxygen saturations less than 90%, are easy to apply uniformly. Of course, even those criteria can be incorrectly assessed by someone who is inexperienced; however, one can see that these types of data are more easily reproducible within and between studies. One way to assess reliability between raters in a study is by using the *kappa statistic*. This statistic tests how reliable different investigators or data collectors are in their assessment or interpretation of data beyond what one would expect by chance alone.

$$kappa = \frac{(\text{Percent agreement observed}) - (\text{Percent agreement expected by chance alone})}{100\% - (\text{Percent agreement expected by chance alone})}$$

If you were to evaluate two observers without any training, you would expect them to agree a certain percentage of the time, and that percentage represents the chance of agreement, usually around 50%. Using the kappa statistic, you can estimate how reliable this agreement is by subtracting out the percentage expected by chance alone. In general, any kappa below 0.60 indicates inadequate agreement among the raters and little confidence should be placed in the study results. These values, although not perfect, can give an investigator an assessment of how well observers are agreeing with each other in their data interpretation (Celentano & Szklo, 2018; McHugh, 2012). The kappa statistic appears frequently in the literature, and the APRN should be familiar with its use and limitations.

One of the first steps in data analysis is to compare the demographic information of each of the groups studied to ensure that they are matched for important characteristics and that they represent the population of interest. Frequencies of data can be generated and compared for similarities and differences. This should be done early on so that any imbalance between groups is addressed before it becomes a problem in the analysis stage. This reiterates the importance of generating strict inclusion and exclusion criteria that can be followed with minimal error.

CAUSALITY

Ernst Mach, an Austrian professor of physics and mathematics and a philosopher, argued that all knowledge is based on sensation and that all scientific measurements are dependent on the observer's perception. He proposed that "in nature there is no cause and effect" (Huttemann, 2013, pp. 101–122). This is a relevant quote to begin a discussion of causality because causality is a complex issue faced by all investigators. A single clinical disease can have many different "causes," and one cause can have several clinical consequences. Causality becomes even more complex when we begin to look at chronic diseases. Chronic diseases can have multiple etiologies. Cardiac disease, for example, has multiple causes, such as genetic predisposition, obesity, smoking, lack of exercise, poor diet, or any combination of these factors.

A useful definition of causation for population research is that an increase in the causal factor or exposure causes an increase in the outcome of interest (e.g., disease). With that said, if an association is found between an exposure and an outcome, then the next question is "Is it causal?" There are many theories of causation, some of which have been addressed in Chapter 4, "Epidemiological Methods and Measurements in Population-Based Nursing Practice: Part I," but no one theory can explain entirely the complex interactions of an exposure with the development of disease or an outcome.

There are multiple criteria that can help determine causality. No one criterion in and of itself determines causality, but each one may help strengthen the argument for or against causality. One important criterion is the determination of a statistical *strength of association*. Statistics are used to test hypotheses: Is an exposure or risk factor present significantly more often in a population with the disease than without? If a new intervention is put into place, is there a significant improvement in the targeted outcome? The strength of association is measured by such things as relative risk and attributable risk. Another criterion is the confirmation of a *temporal relationship*: The suspected exposure or risk factor needs to occur before the disease or outcome. For example, a person needs to smoke before they develop lung cancer to attribute lung cancer to smoking as a potential causal agent. To show a causal relationship requires the elimination of all known *alternative explanations,* and an experienced investigator will seek out other potential explanations to explain why such a relationship may not exist (Celentano & Szklo, 2018; Katz et al., 2013).

Two additional important considerations are scientific plausibility and the ability to replicate findings. *Scientific plausibility* refers to coherence with our current body of knowledge as it relates to the phenomenon under study, that is, do the results make sense based on what we know about the phenomenon? For example, is it biologically plausible that exposure to cigarette smoke (e.g., benzene, nicotine, tar) could convert normal cells into cancer cells? Additionally, the ability to *replicate findings* in different studies and in different populations provides strong evidence that a causal association exists. Other criteria for causation include the *dose-response* relationship. For example, with increasing exposure (e.g., smoking), one can see increasing risk of disease (e.g., lung cancer). Similarly, if one has a *cessation of exposure*, one would expect a cessation or reduction of disease. Finally, another criterion worth mentioning is consistency with other knowledge. This criterion takes into consideration knowledge of other known factors (e.g., environmental changes, product sales, behavioral changes) that may indicate a causal relationship. For example, if a law is passed that prohibits smoking in public places, it may result in fewer cases of smoking-related diseases reported in area hospitals. These criteria, in concert with a strong study design and methodology, can assist an APRN in determining the likelihood of causality when an association is found between an exposure and an outcome (Celentano & Szklo, 2018).

Causes can be both direct and indirect. An example of a direct cause would be an infectious agent that causes a disease. Pertussis (whooping cough, a bacterial infection) is caused by *Bordetella pertussis*. The disease is a direct cause of the organism. Toxic shock syndrome is an example of an indirect cause. Although the staphylococcal organism and its toxins are the direct cause of the syndrome, the indirect cause (and the first factor that was identified) is tampons.

As is evident from the coronavirus disease 2019 (COVID-19) pandemic, even the infectious disease process is not simple. Both the host and the environment can have an impact on the infectious disease process. Characteristics of the host (e.g., age, previous exposures, general health, and immune status) can influence the development of the disease. Environmental conditions also play a role. Crowded living conditions contribute to the rapid spread of infectious diseases, as maintaining a safe distance from infected people can be difficult, if not impossible. Seasons can also be a factor, as people are more likely to gather indoors during cold months. Some diseases such as influenza are most prevalent during certain times of the year. Infectious disease departments document these seasonal trends during the year, and they are available for healthcare providers to review. Such information can assist in antibiotic selection, hospital staffing, and educational campaigns to ensure immunizations or prevention programs are put into place. Awareness of seasonal fluctuations in certain diseases, trends in drug resistance, or changes in the community that affect the overall management of a patient are important in an APRN's practice. By following these trends, the APRN can better assess the needs of the community and ensure that appropriate resources are available to address the fluctuations that occur naturally in all communities.

SCIENTIFIC MISCONDUCT (FRAUD)

Scientific misconduct includes (but is not limited to) gift authorship, data fabrication and falsification, plagiarism, and conflict of interest. It can have an impact on researchers, patients, and populations (Karcz & Papadakos, 2011). No one wants to believe that there are investigators who commit fraud by deliberately distorting research findings, but it does happen. Unfortunately, in some cases, the fraud is intentional; in other instances, it occurs via a series of missteps from methodology to analysis. As mentioned earlier, multiple forms of bias or confounding can be introduced into a study, and these, if ignored, can lead to spurious results. Intentionally ignoring these issues, especially without addressing them as a limitation, can be fraudulent. The review process in a prominent peer-reviewed journal and/or evidence that the protocol was approved by an institutional review board (IRB) minimizes the occurrence of such problems but cannot completely ensure the accuracy and/or ethical conduct of that research.

Perhaps one of the most infamous cases of fraud involved a well-respected peer-reviewed journal. In 1998, *The Lancet* published an article written by Andrew Wakefield and 12 others that implied a link between the measles-mumps-rubella (MMR) vaccine and autism and Crohn's disease. Although epidemiologists pointed out several study weaknesses, including a small number of cases, no controls, and reliance on parental recall, it received wide notice in the popular press. It was 7 years before a journalist uncovered the fact that Wakefield altered facts to support his claim and exploited the MMR scare for financial gain. *The Lancet* retracted the paper in 2010 (Godlee et al., 2011). A series of articles in the *British Medical Journal* (Deer, 2011) revealed how Wakefield and his associates distorted data for financial gain. Before this article was retracted, it caused widespread fear among parents and accelerated an anti-vaccine movement that many blame for the resurgence of infectious diseases among children and the reluctance of many people to be vaccinated against infectious diseases such as influenza and COVID-19.

In 2006, a writer for *The New York Times* (Interlandi, 2006) wrote an article that described a case of fraud that involved a formerly tenured professor at the University of Vermont. Dr. Eric Poehlman was tried in a federal court and found guilty. He was sentenced to 1 year and 1 day in jail for fraudulent actions that spanned 10 years. His misconduct included using fraudulent data in lectures and in published papers and using these data to obtain millions of dollars in federal grants from the National Institutes of Health (NIH). He pleaded guilty to fabricating data on obesity, menopause, and aging. Interlandi's article, which includes a very detailed account of Dr. Poehlman's actions and his downfall, documents how a "committed cheater can elude detection for years by playing on the trust—and self-interest—of his or her junior colleagues" (p. 3).

It is safe to say that most researchers carry out their research with scrupulous attention to detail and with integrity, but APRNs need to be aware that instances such as those mentioned do happen. As stated in Chapter 4, "Epidemiological Methods and Measurements in Population-Based Nursing Practice: Part I," it is important that when an APRN is making decisions related to population-based evaluation, the decisions need to be based on a sound methodological framework that includes ethical considerations of the effect of the research on the population. It is also important that APRNs are aware that fraud occurs in research and that they should be vigilant not only in how they carry out research but also in how they critically review the results of studies by other investigators.

STUDY DESIGNS

There is no perfect study design; however, there are strategies that can be used to decrease the threat of bias and increase the likelihood that hypotheses are answered accurately. The awareness that bias and confounding can cause a threat to the validity of study results is important and may be unavoidable; however, recognizing these limitations and addressing them within a study is even more critical. The design of high-quality and transparent studies creates a good foundation for evidence-based practice. Table 5.2 outlines the strengths and weaknesses of study designs used in population research.

TABLE 5.2 Strengths and Weaknesses of Study Designs

TYPE OF STUDY	STRENGTHS	WEAKNESSES
Randomized controlled trials	• Lower likelihood of confounding variables • Minimize bias in treatment assignment • Able to control intervention or treatment	• Labor intensive • Costly • Lengthy • Sometimes impractical or unethical to conduct
Cohort designs	• Able to identify confounding and address it in the study • Able to control exposure • Able to calculate relative risk and incidence rates • Can study multiple outcomes	• Labor intensive • Costly • Lengthy
Case–control studies	• Inexpensive • Shorter time to completion • Able to study variables with long latency or impact periods • Provides a means to compare groups • Able to calculate odds ratios • Able to study rare or fatal diseases • Can study multiple exposures	• Risk of bias and confounding variables • Sometimes unable to measure or determine exposure • Selection bias • Measurement error • Recall bias • Cannot assess risk
Cross-sectional studies	• Able to calculate prevalence of population studied • Assesses exposures and outcomes at one time • Provides a snapshot of study population • Inexpensive	• Risk of confounding variables • Selection bias • Cannot control for or identify the significance of potentially important variables • Cannot assess risk

RANDOMIZED CONTROLLED TRIALS

When carefully designed, RCTs can provide the strongest evidence for the effectiveness of a treatment or intervention. Subjects are randomly assigned to either the intervention group (which will receive the experimental treatment or intervention) or the control group (which will receive the nonexperimental treatment or no intervention). Inclusion and exclusion criteria for the participants must be precise and spelled out in advance.

RCTs are considered strong designs because of their ability to minimize bias; however, if the randomization is not executed in a truly random manner, then the design can be flawed, or if the data are not reported consistently, then errors can lead to invalid conclusions. Consolidated Standards of Reporting Trials (CONSORT) is a method that has been developed to improve the quality and reporting of RCTs. It offers a standard way for authors to prepare reports of trial findings, facilitate their complete and transparent reporting, and aid their critical appraisal and interpretation (CONSORT, 2018). The CONSORT checklist items focus on reporting how the trial was designed, analyzed, and interpreted; the flow diagram displays the progress of all participants through the trial (CONSORT, 2018). An update of the guidelines was published in September 2022 (Butcher et al., 2022). The CONSORT guidelines are endorsed by many professional journals and editorial organizations. They are part of an effort to improve the quality, transparency, and reporting of research that is conducted to make better clinical decisions. The CONSORT website is under construction as this book goes to print.

RCTs are believed to provide the most reliable scientific evidence, but they can be expensive, time-consuming, and sometimes difficult to conduct for ethical reasons. There are general guidelines that APRNs can follow when conducting a study to provide a framework for a quality design. They are as follows:

- Formulate an answerable research question (see Chapter 6, "Applying Evidence at the Population Level").
- Complete an extensive review of the literature to determine what is currently known about the problem and to provide a sound theoretical background (see Chapter 6, "Applying Evidence at the Population Level").
- Select a study design that will best answer the research question.
- Choose a study design that is feasible in terms of both time and money.
- Once a design is chosen, plan every step of the research process before beginning the study (e.g., determination of inclusion and exclusion criteria, selection of primary and secondary outcomes of interest).
- Ensure that comparison groups are as similar as possible; stratify for possible confounders early on to avoid making false conclusions.
- Determine sufficient sample size to ensure the study has adequate power for result interpretation.
- Use objective criteria for the collection of all data.

- Train all investigators to ensure that data are collected uniformly.
- Choose the appropriate methods for data analysis.
- Provide sufficient and clear details of the study in papers and presentations to allow others to understand how the study was carried out and to allow them to assess for possible biases (e.g., provide an audit trail).

COHORT STUDIES

Cohort designs can be either prospective or retrospective. In a prospective cohort design, the investigator selects a group of individuals who were exposed to a factor of interest and compares it to a group of nonexposed individuals and follows both groups to determine the incidence of an outcome (e.g., disease). This type of design should be carried out when the APRN has good evidence (a sound theoretical base) that links an exposure to an outcome. A well-designed, prospective cohort study has the potential to provide better evidence than a poorly designed RCT. One of the major problems with cohort studies is that they can be time-consuming and expensive if the cohort needs to be followed for a prolonged period, and the longer the time frame involved, the more likely that participants can and will be lost to follow-up. This potential loss of subjects can result in withdrawal bias, particularly when people with certain characteristics drop out of one group at a different rate than that of another group or are lost to follow-up at different rates. Both occurrences can lead to spurious results or results that are difficult to generalize. For example, subjects who participate for the duration of a study may be healthier than those who drop out, leading to potential characteristic differences between groups that may affect the final analysis. These types of differences can falsely dilute observed differences between groups or falsely strengthen results and should be avoided when possible.

When conducting a cohort study, investigators should provide detailed information on the following: subjects' data that are lost or incomplete, subjects' rates of withdrawal or loss to follow-up, characteristics of subjects that are lost to follow-up or who have withdrawn from the study, and, when possible, reasons for the dropouts. They should also include detailed descriptions of the groups that are included in the analysis of outcomes (e.g., age, gender, family history, and severity of disease).

Des Jarlais et al. (2004) first presented the Transparent Reporting of Evaluations with Nonrandomized Designs (TREND) in the *American Journal of Public Health*. These guidelines provide a framework for the design and reporting of nonrandomized studies in order to facilitate research synthesis. The TREND checklist has 22 steps and was designed for use as an evaluation tool of nonrandomized behavioral or public health intervention studies. The TREND statement and checklist are available through the Centers for Disease Control and Prevention website: www.cdc.gov/trendstatement/index.html. These types of studies should include a defined intervention and research design that provides for an assessment of the efficacy or effectiveness of the intervention. The TREND guidelines provide APRNs with a comprehensive checklist for designing studies and writing research reports.

CASE STUDY

An APRN employed by a large hospital system as a clinical specialist read a news brief on a Really Simple Syndication (RSS) that described the problem of nonventilator hospital-acquired pneumonia (NVHAP). NVHAP had recently been identified as an ongoing issue by the infectious disease department where they worked. Intrigued by what they read in the short synopsis, they accessed the full article. The author of the article identified NVHAP as the most common hospital-acquired infection (HAI) and explained that the infection is often caused by bacteria from the mouth that proliferate on unbrushed teeth and is aspirated into the lungs. Bedridden and immobile patients are at highest risk. Studies were cited that support the use of interventions to reduce germs in the mouth as an effective method to prevent NVHAP (Kelman, 2022). Wanting to know more about the evidence behind the recommended interventions, the APRN acquired copies of two of the cited studies.

Lacerna, C., Patey, D., Block, L., Naik, S., Kevorkova, Y., Galin, J. , . . ., Witt, D. (2020). A successful program preventing nonventilator hospital-acquired pneumonia in a large hospital system. *Infection Control & Hospital Epidemiology, 41*(5), 547–552.

Giuliano, K. K., Penoyer, D., Middleton, A., & Baker, D. (2020). 93. Enhanced oral care as prevention for non-ventilator hospital acquired pneumonia. *Open Forum Infectious Diseases, 7*(Suppl. 1), S177–S178.

The APRN decides that based on their readings, there is sufficient evidence to carry out a quality improvement project (QIP) in the hospital system to decrease the rate of NVHAP. Using the information garnered from the two studies mentioned above, they design an intervention to address the risk factors for NVHAP and choose a prospective case-control design. They then write a detailed proposal and approach the Research Council to discuss implementation of the QIP.

What should the intervention include? What are the strengths and weaknesses of the design? Identify some of the systematic errors that could occur.

CASE–CONTROL STUDIES

In a *case–control* study, the investigator first identifies a group of individuals with the attribute of interest (cases), and a second group is identified without the attribute of interest (controls). Cases and controls can be matched individually or as a group for variables that might cause confounding (e.g., age, gender, and ethnicity), or they can be unmatched. If unmatched, then each group should have similar characteristics. As mentioned earlier, matching can be on an individual level or group level. In Chapter 4, "Epidemiological Methods and Measurements in Population-Based Nursing Practice: Part I," we defined the odds ratio (OR) in case–control studies as the odds of being an exposed case compared to the odds of being an exposed control (ad/bc). This is the calculation for an unmatched study. However, when we calculate the OR for a matched pairs study (e.g., matching of individual pairs for a variety of characteristics), we need to take into consideration only those situations in which cases have different exposures. We

TABLE 5.3A 2 × 2 Table for Calculating Odds Ratio in an Unmatched Case–Control Study

	CASES	CONTROLS
Exposed Cases	a	b
Nonexposed Cases	c	d
	OR = ad/bc (unmatched pairs)	

OR, odds ratio.

TABLE 5.3B 2 × 2 Table for Calculating Odds Ratio in a Matched Pairs Case–Control Study

	EXPOSED CONTROLS	NONEXPOSED CONTROLS
Exposed Cases	a	b
Nonexposed Cases	c	d
	OR = b/c (matched pairs)	

OR, odds ratio.

are not interested in comparing cases with controls if both are exposed (as in "a") or are unexposed (as in "d"). Therefore, the OR for a matched case–control study is calculated as b/c. Also, of note in a matched case–control study, the 2 × 2 table is set up differently as individual cases are matched to individual controls (Tables 5.3A and 5.3B).

Case–control studies tend to be inexpensive and relatively quick to complete, but they have several weaknesses. Because subjects in the groups are not randomly assigned, associations found in the analysis may be the result of exposure to another, unknown variable. To decrease the likelihood of bias, definite criteria should be used so that there is no ambiguity about how to distinguish between a case and a control. Controls should resemble the cases as closely as possible except for exposure to the factor under study. If the cases are drawn from a medical surgical unit in an acute care hospital, then ideally the controls should be drawn from the same population. Matching, as previously described, is one method that can be used so that potential confounders are distributed equally between the cases and controls. A problem with case–control studies is that data are usually abstracted from medical records that are not designed for collection of research material; data obtained from medical records may be limited and may not provide adequate or accurate information on exposures. For example, data collected from medical records may be incomplete (e.g., missing diagnoses), may use old diagnostic criteria, or may be coded or entered incorrectly. Additionally, if abstracting data from interviews, biases, such as recall bias or reporting bias, may play a role in how data are recorded and ultimately can affect the interpretation and final conclusions of a study.

DATABASES

Databases have become ubiquitous in the healthcare field, and their use is growing. Many of the larger and better-known databases are discussed throughout this text. There is a good reason for their frequent mention. Nurses in all fields and in all positions enter data electronically into databases of some kind. Managers use databases to assess the level of satisfaction of their patient population and nursing staff. Direct care nurses use data to assess the performance of their units on important patient care indicators (such as falls) and record patient information into electronic health records that may be linked with larger databases or registries. Departments dedicated to quality improvement track infection rates, readmission rates, and other identified indicators of quality of care. Health departments track infectious diseases as well as other indicators linked to population health.

Some databases are for a single site (e.g., one acute care hospital or one community), but it is becoming increasingly common for databases to be linked or for databases to include information at the state, regional, and national level (e.g., trauma registries that log all incoming trauma data from all trauma centers in the state). State and federal regulatory agencies, such as the Agency for Healthcare Research and Quality (AHRQ) and the Centers for Medicare and Medicaid Services (CMS), are requiring healthcare providers to report specific patient safety indicators. Some of these data, such as those compiled by CMS, are being posted for public view. Other organizations, such as the American Nurses Credentialing Center (ANCC), are requiring data entry for accreditation by programs, such as Magnet®, and setting performance standards using benchmarks.

Nursing care data that are captured using technology can be aggregated, analyzed, and benchmarked. The information can provide APRNs with a clear picture of the population that they serve and help to guide decisions for the provision of services.

Successful databases are created collaboratively. Members of the healthcare team who will be entering and using the data need to work together with technicians who understand systems. And the creation of a workable database is just a beginning. Once the data are entered, they need to be analyzed and checked for accuracy (*data editing*). Posting data that are summarized and benchmarked using graphs and trend lines on shared drives that are accessible to direct care nurses, as well as nurse leaders, brings the information to people who directly impact care and helps nurses to identify areas for improvement. Nurses at all levels should be involved in data management and analysis.

SUMMARY

APRNs need to be able to identify and design studies with strong methodology and designs and understand the factors that can influence study results. One problem with population research is that it is difficult to identify and control for variables that are not part of the study but that may have an effect on the results. When a researcher analyzes data in a study and draws the wrong conclusion, the result is a type I or type II error, also referred to as errors of inference. A type I error occurs when a null hypothesis is rejected when in fact it is true. A type II error occurs when a null hypothesis is not rejected when in fact it is false. There are two kinds of error of measurement—random error and systematic error. It is essential that APRNs are aware how these errors can occur, how they can impact a study, and what measures can be taken to avoid or minimize them. RCTs are considered the gold standard in population research and offer the best protection for preventing bias, but they are not always feasible. Well-designed cohort and case–control studies are acceptable alternatives when RCTs are not an option.

Databases are increasingly used in healthcare. Aggregated data provide valuable information about population groups that can be used to direct care and establish evidence for clinical guidelines. APRNs should work closely with technology experts in the planning, implementation, and use of databases in order to maximize their ability to analyze data in an accurate and systematic manner. Strong methodology and data collection with a sound research design are the foundation for an excellent study/intervention that ultimately can contribute to evidence-based practice.

END-OF-CHAPTER RESOURCES

EXERCISES AND DISCUSSION QUESTIONS

EXERCISE 5.1 An APRN carries out a study to determine if a new media campaign (Intervention M) improved vaccination rates in their community.

- What is the null hypothesis?

The APRN carries out the study and concludes that "Vaccination rates did not improve significantly following implementation of Intervention M." In fact, vaccination rates *did* improve significantly following implementation of Intervention M.

- What type of error has the APRN committed?

EXERCISE 5.2 In a small pilot study, ten women with liver cancer and ten women with no apparent disease were contacted and asked whether they had hepatitis B. Each woman with cancer was matched by age, ethnicity, weight, and parity to a woman without cancer. The results are shown in the following table.

PAIR NUMBER	LIVER CANCER	NO LIVER CANCER
1	Hepatitis B	Hepatitis B
2	Hepatitis B	No Hepatitis B
3	Hepatitis B	No Hepatitis B
4	No Hepatitis B	No Hepatitis B
5	No Hepatitis B	No Hepatitis B
6	Hepatitis B	Hepatitis B
7	Hepatitis B	No Hepatitis B
8	No Hepatitis B	Hepatitis B
9	Hepatitis B	No Hepatitis B
10	No Hepatitis B	No Hepatitis B

a. Construct the 2 × 2 table for **matched** pairs.
b. Calculate the estimated odds ratio for a matched-paired analysis.
c. Interpret this statistic.
d. What is the purpose of matching cases and controls?

EXERCISE 5.3 You are working in a health center at a large university and are concerned about an increase in the incidence of antibiotic-resistant gonorrhea in the student population that you serve. Before you launch an educational campaign aimed at both your staff and the university community, you need to establish the severity of the problem.

- Identify a database at the local, state, or national level that can help you obtain the necessary information.
- How can you determine the incidence and prevalence of gonorrhea in your community?
- What are some of the potential errors that can occur in the reporting of gonorrhea to a local, state, or national database?
- How might this affect your interpretation of the data?
- What are some of the barriers to reporting in your community?

You determine from your investigation that there is a significant problem in your community.

- Describe how you would address the increasing rate of gonorrhea in the population that you serve.
- What type of study design would you use to evaluate the effectiveness of your intervention?
- What are potential confounders?

EXERCISE 5.4 You are a manager on a medical unit in a community hospital. You are concerned about a recent increase in falls with injury on your unit. You have not had any recent changes in staffing or patient mix and acuity.

- How might you assess this situation?
- Where might you find the data in your hospital to support your concern?
- What type of study could you perform to identify the cause(s) for the increase in falls with injury?
- How will you select your population of study?
- How will you select a control group or comparison group?
- What are potential errors in measurement that you may encounter?

A robust set of instructor resources designed to supplement this text is located at http://connect.springerpub.com/content/book/978-0-8261-4377-8. Qualifying instructors may request access by emailing textbook@springerpub.com.

REFERENCES

American Association of Colleges of Nursing. (2021). *The essentials: Core competencies for professional nursing education*. Author. Retrieved from https://www.aacnnursing.org/Essentials

Ayorinde, A. A., Williams, I., Mannion, R., Song, F., Skrybant, M., Lilford, R. J., & Chen, Y.-F. (2020). Assessment of publication bias and outcome reporting bias in systematic reviews of health services and delivery research: A meta-epidemiological study. *PLoS One, 15*(1), e0227580. https://doi.org/10.1371/journal.pone.0227580

Butcher, N. J., Monsour, A., Mew, E. J., Chan, A.-W., Moher, D., Mayo-Wilson, E., Terwee, C. B., Chee-A-Tow, A., Baba, A., Gavin, F., Grimshaw, J. M., Kelly, L. E., Saeed, L., Thabane, L., Askie, L., Smith, M., Farid-Kapadia, M., Williamson, P. R., Szatmari, P., …, Offringa, M. (2022). Guidelines for reporting outcomes in trial reports: The CONSORT-Outcomes 2022 Extension. *JAMA, 328*(22), 2252–2264. https://doi.org/10.1001/jama.2022.21022

Celentano, D. D., & Szklo, M. (Eds.). (2018). *Gordis epidemiology* (6th ed.). Elsevier.

CONSORT. (2018). *Transparent reporting of trials*. Retrieved from http://www.consort-statement.org

Deer, B. (2011). How the case against the MMR vaccine was fixed. *British Medical Journal, 342*, 77–82. https://doi.org/10.1136/bmj.c5347

Des Jarlais, D., Lyles, C., Crepaz, N., & the TREND Group. (2004). Improving the reporting quality of nonrandomized evaluations of behavioral and public health interventions: The TREND statement. *American Journal of Public Health, 94*(3), 361–366. https://doi.org/10.2105/AJPH.94.3.361

Duyx, B., Urlings, M. J. E., Swaen, G. M. H., Bouter, L. M., & Zeegers, M. P. (2017). Scientific citations favor positive results: A systematic review and meta-analysis. *Journal of Clinical Epidemiology, 88*, 92–101. https://doi.org/10.1016/j.jclinepi.2017.06.002

Giuliano, K. K., Penoyer, D., Middleton, A., & Baker, D. (2020). 93. Enhanced oral care as prevention for non-ventilator hospital acquired pneumonia. *Open Forum Infectious Diseases, 7*(Suppl. 1), S177–S178. https://doi.org/10.1093/ofid/ofaa439.403

Godlee, F., Smith, J., & Marcovitch, H. (2011). Wakefield's article linking MMR vaccine and autism was fraudulent. *British Medical Journal, 342*, 64–66. https://doi.org/10.1136/bmj.c7452

Huttemann, A. (2013). A disposition-based process-theory of causation. In S. Mumford & M. Tugby (Eds.), *Metaphysics and science*. Oxford University Press.

Interlandi, J. (2006, October 22). An unwelcome discovery. *The New York Times*. Retrieved from http://www.nytimes.com/2006/10/22/magazine/22sciencefraud.html

Joober, R., Schmitz, N., Annable, L., & Boksa, P. (2012). Publication bias: What are the challenges and can they be overcome? *Journal of Psychiatry & Neuroscience, 37*(3), 149–152. https://doi.org/10.1503/jpn.120065

Kahlert, J., Gribsholt, S. B., Gammelager, H., Dekkers, O. M., & Luta, G. (2017). Control of confounding in the analysis phase—An overview for clinicians. *Clinical Epidemiology, 9*, 195–204. https://doi.org/10.2147/CLEP.S129886

Karcz, M., & Papadakos, P. J. (2011). The consequences of fraud and deceit in medical research. *Canadian Journal of Respiratory Therapy, 47*(1), 18–27.

Katz, D., Elmore, J. G., Wild, D. M. G., & Lucan, S. C. (2013). *Jekel's epidemiology, biostatistics, preventive medicine, and public health* (4th ed.). Elsevier Saunders.

Kellar, S. P., & Kelvin, E. A. (2013). *Munro's statistical methods for health care research* (6th ed.). Wolters Kluwer/Lippincott Williams & Wilkins.

Kelman, B. (2022, July). *Hospital-acquired pneumonia is killing patients. There's a simple way to stop it.* Kaiser Health News. Retrieved from https://www.nbcnews.com/health/health-news/hospital-acquired-pneumonia-killing-patients-simple-way-stop-rcna37330

Lacerna, C., Patey, D., Block, L., Naik, S., Kevorkova, Y., Galin, J., Parker, M., Bettes, R., Parodi, S., & Witt, D. (2020). A successful program preventing nonventilator hospital-acquired pneumonia in a large hospital system. *Infection Control & Hospital Epidemiology, 41*(5), 547–552. https://doi.org/10.1017/ice.2019.368

Matsumoto, M., Ishikawa, S., & Kajii, E. (2010). Rurality of communities and incidence of stroke: A confounding effect of weather conditions? *Rural and Remote Health, 10*, 1493. Retrieved from http://www.rrh.org.au

McHugh, M. (2012). Interrater reliability: The kappa statistic. *Biochemia Medica, 22*(3), 276–282. https://doi.org/10.11613/BM.2012.031

Merrill, R. M. (2017). *Introduction to epidemiology* (7th ed.). Jones and Bartlett Learning.

Mlinarić, A., Horvat, M., & Šupak Smolčić, V. (2017). Dealing with the positive publication bias: Why you should really publish your negative results. *Biochemia Medica, 27*(3), 030201. https://doi.org/10.11613/BM.2017.030201

National Cancer Institute. (2021). *Alcohol and cancer risk.* Retrieved from https://www.cancer.gov/about-cancer/causes-prevention/risk/alcohol/alcohol-fact-sheet#how-does-the-combination-of-alcohol-and-tobacco-affect-cancer-risk

Shorten, A., & Moorley, C. (2014). Selecting the sample. *Evidence-Based Nursing, 17*(2), 32–33. https://doi.org/10.1136/eb-2014-101747

Siddiqi, N. (2011). Publication bias in epidemiological studies. *Central European Journal of Public Health, 19*(2), 118–120. Retrieved from https://doi.org/10.21101/cejph.a3581

Song, F., Parekh-Bhurke, S., Hooper, L., Loke, Y. K., Ryder, J. J., Sutton, A. J., Hing, C. B., & Harvey, I. (2009). Extent of publication bias in different categories of research cohorts: A meta-analysis of empirical studies. *BMC Medical Research Methodology, 9,* 79. Retrieved from http://web.ebscohost.com/ehost/pdfviewer/pdfviewer?hid=110&sid=01961f3d-cd2e-4770-86af-bc7107e2f85e%40sessionmgr113&vid=4

Starks, H., Diehr, P., & Curtis, J. R. (2009). The challenge of selection bias and confounding in palliative care research. *Journal of Palliative Medicine, 12*(2), 181–187. https://doi.org/10.1089/jpm.2009.9672

Statistics. (2022). In *AHDictionary*.com. Retrieved February 20, 2023, from American Heritage Dictionary Entry: statistics (ahdictionary.com)

CHAPTER 6

APPLYING EVIDENCE AT THE POPULATION LEVEL

VERA KUNTE

INTRODUCTION

Nurses in advanced practice have an obligation to improve the health of the populations they serve by providing evidence-based care. In their latest updated education framework *The Essentials: Core Competencies for Professional Nursing Education,* the American Association of Colleges of Nursing (2021) lists core competencies for entry-level and advanced-level nursing programs. Evidence-Based Practice (EBP), one of the eight featured concepts of the new *Essentials,* is integrated within most domains for the advanced nursing practice level, especially Domain 1: Knowledge for Nursing Practice and Domain 3: Population Health. Advanced practice registered nurses (APRNs) are educated in research and critical appraisal at the graduate level and possess both scientific knowledge and clinical expertise. These specialized abilities prepare the APRN to demonstrate the importance of EBP to others and to facilitate the incorporation of such evidence into practice (Clarke et al., 2021).

In this chapter, the APRN will learn how to gather, appraise, and synthesize information in order to design interventions that are based on evidence to improve population health. APRNs need a sound knowledge of research methodology to support an EBP. They also require a wide array of knowledge gleaned from the sciences and the ability to translate that knowledge quickly and effectively to benefit patients (Ylimäki et al., 2022). The goal of this chapter is to summarize the skills required for EBP and to provide specific examples of how APRNs use these skills to improve population outcomes.

Evidence is defined as facts or observations that support a conclusion or assertion. Melnyk and Fineout-Overholt (2019) define *EBP* as a paradigm and lifelong problem-solving approach to clinical decision-making that involves the conscientious use of the best available evidence (including a systematic search for and critical appraisal of the most relevant evidence to answer a clinical question) with one's own clinical expertise and patient values and preferences to improve outcomes for individuals, groups, communities, and systems (p. 753).

A related concept is *best practices* which refers to providing high-quality care based on evidence to achieve optimal outcomes (Ten Ham-Baloyi et al., 2020). APRNs require several skills to become practitioners of evidence-based care and to improve clinical outcomes. They must be able to identify clinical problems, recognize patient safety issues, compose clinical questions that provide a clear direction for study, conduct a search of the literature, appraise and synthesize the available evidence, and successfully integrate new knowledge into practice. The APRN plays an important role in this complex process of incorporating EBP into policies and standards of care to improve population outcomes. In population-based care, there is additional complexity in determining the values and needs of diverse groups of people. Making decisions related to population-based health requires consideration of the effects of the intervention on the population as a whole. Balancing the overall needs of groups of people with the rights of individuals requires careful and thoughtful consideration. A sound EBP provides a foundation to better assess and meet those needs based on current evidence.

ASKING THE CLINICAL QUESTION

There are many situations that drive clinical questions. Clinical practice and observation, as well as information obtained by reading the professional literature, can lead nurses to ask questions such as "Why is this happening?" "Would this approach to care work in my clinical practice?" or "What can we do to improve this outcome?" An APRN who reads an article about an innovation in practice that leads to an improvement in a population outcome might wonder whether such an intervention would work in another setting. The observation that the readmission rates for a particular diagnosis are increasing, or that rates for a particular disease are higher in one population than in another, or that patient satisfaction scores for a particular group of patients are lower can all lead to a search of the literature for evidence to change and improve outcomes. It may also lead to further research to improve outcomes or the implementation of new interventions to change outcomes. But before the search can begin, it is important that clinical questions are defined clearly and in a way that can be effectively answered and applied to practice.

Clinical questions should be written in a format that provides a clear direction for examination. PICO is a popular framework used to develop clinical questions. The acronym stands for population "studied, intervention, comparison, and outcome". Sometimes, practitioners use PICOT, in which the "T" stands for "time frame." When framing a qualitative question, the acronym SPIDER (sample, phenomenon of interest, design, evaluation, and research type) may be used (Ubeda, 2022). As you formulate your PICO question, it is helpful to describe the type of question you are asking to better define your research method. Is this an intervention, diagnosis, etiology, or prognosis type of question? (Lansing Community College Library, 2019, Table 6.1).

TABLE 6.1 PICOT Questions, Types of Evidence, and Databases

Type of Clinical Question	Primary Research	Synthesized Research (Secondary Literature)	Other Evidence (Secondary Literature)
	Use CINAHL and MEDLINE to find the following: • RCT • Controlled trials • Case-control studies • Cohort studies • Descriptive studies • Qualitative studies • Instrument development research	Use Cochrane Collection Plus, CINAHL Plus, and MEDLINE to find the following: • Systematic reviews • Meta-analyses	Use CINAHL Plus, MEDLINE, Joanna Briggs Institute, nursing, healthcare, and government organizations to find the following: • Clinical practice guidelines • Use published clinical articles (not research based), peer institution practices, expert clinician practices to find the following: • Expert opinion
Therapy "What is the best treatment or intervention?"	RCT, controlled trials	Systematic reviews	Clinical practice guidelines
Prevention "How can I prevent this problem?"	RCT, controlled trials	Systematic reviews	Clinical practice guidelines

(continued)

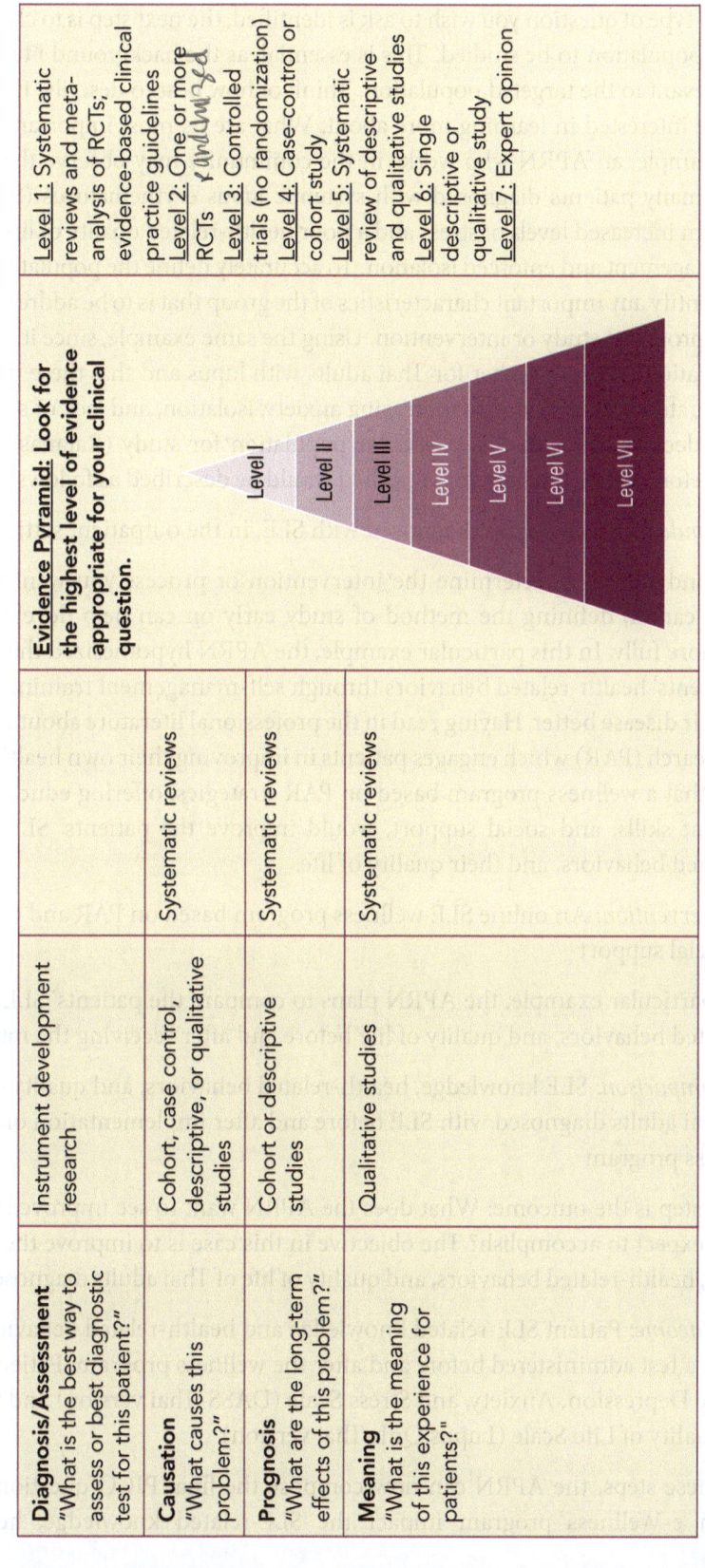

6 APPLYING EVIDENCE AT THE POPULATION LEVEL 133

		Evidence Pyramid: Look for the highest level of evidence appropriate for your clinical question.	Level 1: Systematic reviews and meta-analysis of RCTs; evidence-based clinical practice guidelines Level 2: One or more randomized RCTs Level 3: Controlled trials (no randomization) Level 4: Case-control or cohort study Level 5: Systematic review of descriptive and qualitative studies Level 6: Single descriptive or qualitative study Level 7: Expert opinion
Diagnosis/Assessment "What is the best way to assess or best diagnostic test for this patient?"	Instrument development research	Systematic reviews	Level I Level II Level III Level IV Level V Level VI Level VII
Causation "What causes this problem?"	Cohort, case control, descriptive, or qualitative studies	Systematic reviews	
Prognosis "What are the long-term effects of this problem?"	Cohort or descriptive studies	Systematic reviews	
Meaning "What is the meaning of this experience for patients?"	Qualitative studies		

CINAHL, Cumulative Index to Nursing and Allied Health Literature; PICOT, population studied, intervention, comparison, outcome, and time frame; RCT, randomized controlled trial.

Source: Used with permission of Lansing Community College Library. (2019). What is PICOT? Retrieved from libguides.lcc.edu/c.php?g=167860&p=6198388

Once the type of question you wish to ask is identified, the next step is to clearly describe the patient population to be studied. This is essential, as the background literature search must be relevant to the targeted population. Think of how best to describe the population that you are interested in learning more about. What are its most important characteristics? For example, an APRN who works in the community may observe that during the pandemic, many patients diagnosed with systemic lupus erythematosus (SLE) or lupus suffered from increased levels of stress and a poor health-related quality of life due to poor disease management and enforced isolation. To accurately define the population, an APRN needs to identify any important characteristics of the group that is to be addressed or examined in the proposed study or intervention. Using the same example, since it is known that the complication rates are higher for Thai adults with lupus and that these patients experience high rates of distress due to increasing anxiety, isolation, and lack of social support, the APRN decides to target this particular population for study (Ratanasiripong et al., 2023). Therefore, the population to be studied would be described as follows:

- *Population:* Thai adults diagnosed with SLE, in the outpatient setting

The second step is to determine the intervention or process you want to study. As mentioned earlier, defining the method of study early on can help develop the PICO question more fully. In this particular example, the APRN hypothesized that by improving the patients' health-related behaviors through self-management training, they would manage their disease better. Having read in the professional literature about Participatory Action Research (PAR) which engages patients in improving their own health, the APRN postulates that a wellness program based on PAR strategies, offering education, disease management skills, and social support, would improve the patients' SLE knowledge, health-related behaviors, and their quality of life.

- *Intervention:* An online SLE wellness program based on PAR and offering social support

In this particular example, the APRN plans to compare the patients' SLE knowledge, health-related behaviors, and quality of life before and after receiving the intervention.

- *Comparison:* SLE knowledge, health-related behaviors, and quality of life of Thai adults diagnosed with SLE before and after implementation of the wellness program

The last step is the outcome: What does the APRN want to see improved? What does the APRN expect to accomplish? The objective in this case is to improve the SLE-related knowledge, health-related behaviors, and quality of life of Thai adults diagnosed with SLE.

- *Outcome:* Patient SLE-related knowledge and health-related behaviors based on a test administered before and after the wellness program. Patient scores on the Depression, Anxiety, and Stress Scale (DASS-Thai version) and the Lupus Quality of Life Scale (Lupus QoL-Thai version)

Using these steps, the APRN can now compose the final PICO question: "How will a 3-month e-Wellness program impact the SLE-related knowledge, health-related behaviors, and quality of life of Thai adults diagnosed with SLE, in an outpatient setting?" (Ratanasiripong et al., 2023). Development of the PICO question provides the APRN with a better understanding of the clinical problem, allows for specific measures to be introduced, and provides the foundation for a well-designed study. The next step is to perform a thorough and comprehensive literature review.

THE LITERATURE REVIEW

The literature search should further define and clarify the clinical problem; summarize the current state of knowledge on the subject; identify relationships, contradictions, gaps, and inconsistencies in the literature; and, finally, suggest the next step in solving the problem (American Psychological Association [APA], 2020). The search for the literature can be conducted by the APRN, or they can engage the assistance of a research librarian if available. Librarians are educated to find and access information and are excellent resources for assisting with literature reviews. Navigating databases in order to find relevant information can be a complex process. The searcher needs to use the correct terms, search the correct databases, and use a well-designed and systematic search strategy. The searcher should also document each step of the process in order to provide an audit trail and avoid duplication of work. An audit trail provides transparency to the breadth and depth of the strategies used to find the evidence and allows others to follow the decision-making process (Carcary, 2020). In the absence of a librarian, there are steps that the APRN can take to increase the likelihood of a successful search.

In order to find the most relevant literature to inform decision-making, the searcher should use key terms from the PICO question (i.e., population studied, intervention, comparison, and outcomes of interest). The first step is to search each key term separately and then to take steps to refine the search. The APRN should use at least two databases for the literature search. Access to some databases requires a subscription, while others are free. Cochrane is an international organization that provides up-to-date systematic reviews (currently more than 7,500). It can be accessed through its website, www.cochrane.org, that requires a subscription in many countries, including the United States. For a complete list of countries with free access, go to the Cochrane page at www.cochranelibrary.com/help/access. Some of the content is free. For example, access to summaries or older versions of the reviews can be accessed without a subscription, but for access to full systematic reviews, currently, a paid subscription is required. However, by 2025, the organization aims to achieve universal open access to all reviews immediately upon publication (Cochrane, 2023). PubMed is a free resource which includes MEDLINE and is the U.S. National Library of Medicine (NLM) journal literature search system. It includes more than 29 million citations for biomedical literature from MEDLINE, journals, and online books and includes citations from full-text content (NLM, 2022). Free online training on how to use resources at PubMed is available at learn.nlm.nih.gov/documentation/training-packets/T0042010P.

JBI (formerly known as the Joanna Briggs Institute) and the Cumulative Index to Nursing and Allied Health Literature (CINAHL) are excellent databases that both require a subscription. JBI, which includes the JBI EBP Database, is a global, not-for-profit, membership-based organization located within the University of Adelaide, Australia, and can be accessed at jbi.global. Students receive a discounted subscription rate to JBI. CINAHL is a comprehensive resource for nursing and allied health literature which is owned and operated by EBSCO. CINAHL is the basic database, and access to four other versions is also offered, CINAHL with Full Text, CINAHL Plus with Full Text, CINAHL Complete, and CINAHL Ultimate. The main difference among the versions is the variety of added content (EBSCO, 2023).

Searches of a single key word can result in a very large number of articles. For example, a CINAHL search for full-text articles using the key word "lupus" yielded a list of 22,825 articles. Including more than one concept in the search is more likely to provide relevant and useful articles. *Boolean logic* is the term used to describe certain logical operations that are used to combine search terms in many databases. Using the Boolean connector AND narrows a search by combining terms; it will retrieve documents that use the two keywords (e.g., *lupus and quality of life*) and can narrow the search. In CINAHL, using *lupus AND quality of life* reduced the number to 595 articles. Using OR, on the other hand, broadens a search to include results that contain either of the words that are typed in the search. OR is a good tool to use when there are several common spellings or synonyms of a word. An example in this case would be *lupus OR systemic lupus erythematosus*. Using NOT will narrow a search by excluding certain search terms. NOT retrieves documents that contain one but not the other of the search terms entered and is appropriate to use when a word is used in different contexts. An example would be *quality of life NOT mental health*. Parentheses indicate relationships between search terms. When they are used, the computer will process the search terms in a specified order and also combine them in the correct manner. For example, *(lupus OR systemic lupus erythematosus) AND quality of life* combines these terms to get the most relevant results. A search conducted in the full-text database of CINAHL using these words and connectors yielded 615 articles.

There are other methods that can be used to make searches more relevant and useful. Specifying limits, such as English language only, peer-reviewed journals only, randomized controlled trials (RCTs) only, and a date range, can narrow a search and increase the relevance of the information retrieved. Keep in mind that the more limits that are placed on the search, the fewer the results. A search using *(lupus OR systemic lupus erythematosus) AND quality of life, full text only, English only, limited to articles published in the past 5 years* yielded 184 articles. However, it is recommended that the initial search is broad and explored before restricting the search limits, as this could lead to information bias. For this PICO question, the following key words were used, both alone and in combinations: lupus, systemic lupus erythematosus, quality of life, QoL, Asian, Thailand, health behaviors, education, participatory action research, perceived stress, and self-care.

A search of electronic databases does not complete the search for the most current known evidence about a topic. A hand search of current and relevant journals may reveal information that has not yet been entered into an electronic database. Studies can also appear in publications other than journals, such as books, and in noncommercial "grey" literature like government reports, conference proceedings, monographs, working papers, and unpublished doctoral dissertations (Hoffecker, 2020). Projects and reports that are completed by specialized organizations, such as foundations and professional membership groups, may appear only on websites. Internet searching can help locate such resources and can scan organizational websites of professional and specialized organizations such as the Lupus Foundation, the American Public Health Association, the American Nurses Association, and the Robert Wood Johnson Foundation. The APRN should also consider contacting experts who may know of important findings and recent discoveries in a particular field. A technique known as snowballing (citation tracking using citation databases such as Science Citation Index Expanded, Social Sciences Citation Index, and Arts and Humanities Citation Index) might also be helpful (Briscoe et al., 2020). After reviewing the literature, many references that may not have been discovered in an Internet search can be found by simply reviewing the references of collected literature.

Finally, although not as popular as they once were, Really Simple Syndication (RSS) feeds provide a convenient way for subscribers to obtain constantly updated information (see also Chapter 7, "Using Information Technology to Improve Population Outcomes"). These function as another version of a database. Rather than searching individual websites, APRNs can browse content, summaries of content, headlines, and/or links to information quickly and in one place from an aggregator that automatically downloads the new data to the user. Sites such as PubMed allow subscribers to customize the information for which they want alerts. Several free RSS feed aggregators or feed readers like Feedly (feedly.com) or Feedreader Online (feedreader.com) are available to find and organize feeds for news, websites, podcasts, and more.

During the literature search, APRNs should keep in mind the difference between primary and secondary sources. Primary sources are those materials or documents created during the time under study and directly experienced by the writer. For example, an original article written by researchers that summarizes the methods and findings of a study carried out by them is an example of a primary source. Other examples of primary sources are letters, diaries, and speeches. Secondary sources interpret and analyze primary sources. An example is a news article announcing a new scientific discovery. A key here is that secondary sources generally analyze and interpret the findings in primary sources and this can lead to bias. It is always advisable to use primary sources when seeking evidence for a change in practice.

ASSESSING THE EVIDENCE

Once a list of articles is obtained, the next step is to assess and synthesize the evidence. Appraising evidence for its usefulness can be a challenge. While reviewing the evidence, the APRN needs to ask some fundamental questions that address the relevance of information such as "How confident am I that the relationships and knowledge in this particular study will apply to the situation in question?" (Alajami, 2021). To determine whether the evidence discovered is enough to drive a practice change, it is important to ask "Is the evidence strong enough to use the results?", "Are the findings applicable to my setting?", and "If I adopt the practice, what will be the impact on the target population?" (Yancey, 2019). It is also essential to examine the *efficacy* (evidence of an effect under ideal conditions, such as double-blind, RCTs) and *effectiveness* (evidence of what actually works in practice) of the findings and of the study. In summary, during the process of determining which studies to include in a synthesis, the APRN needs to ask not only "Does this intervention work?" and "For whom does this intervention work?" but also "When, why, and how does it work?"

Since all published evidence is not completed with equal rigor, the value of published articles varies on a continuum from the lowest to the highest value. A search can potentially find an enormous number of articles, but not all articles may be useful. Because there is often a limited amount of time that is available to assess and synthesize the evidence, it is helpful to have a method that provides guidance as to which articles might be the most valid and useful. After conducting an extensive search of sources, the APRN must establish criteria for inclusion and exclusion of studies. Selecting studies that fit the set criteria will ensure that the evidence discovered is relevant to the clinical question (Popenoe et al., 2021). The inclusion/exclusion criteria may specify date, language, or geographical restrictions or the type of participants, type of research design, or clinical setting as appropriate. For example, if the APRN is seeking to address the needs of older adults in the outpatient setting, then studies related to inpatients and children are excluded.

A *systematic review* is a comprehensive summary of the best available evidence on a particular topic at the time the review was written (Polit & Beck, 2021). There are several organizations that provide guidelines and resources for the conduct of systematic reviews. Many of these help healthcare professionals keep pace with the professional literature by maintaining a database of completed systematic reviews. Information on some sources is listed in Table 6.2. These reviews are completed using strict inclusion and exclusion criteria and aim to include as much of the research that is relevant to the clinical question being asked as possible. The overall objective of an appraisal is to assess the general strength of the evidence in relation to the particular issue being studied. The Evidence for Policy and Practice Information and Coordinating Centre at the Institute of Education, University College London (2023), describes in detail the method used for conducting a comprehensive systematic review on its website (see Table 6.2).

To begin the appraisal, it is helpful to use a table to summarize and group the information according to key areas. Table 6.3 is an example of a tool that can be used to document the critical elements of the evidence such as the design of the study, the study population, and the outcomes. It provides the APRN with a standardized method for evaluating the important points gleaned from the literature search; it can also serve as an audit trail, so others can judge the rigor and quality of the review. An important step in the research review process is the organization and grading of the evidence. A hierarchical level of evidence is a useful way to rank evidence according to its strength and to remove subjectivity from the assessment. Evidence is graded based on scientific merit, and the strength of the evidence is determined by the rigor of the study design used by investigators to minimize bias. Hierarchies of evidence vary, as organizations use different inclusion criteria and ranking systems. Some established hierarchies of evidence include Cochrane, the American Academy of Pediatrics, the Oxford Centre for

TABLE 6.2 Online Resources for Evidence-Based Practice

ORGANIZATION	DESCRIPTION	WEB LINK
Cochrane	Cochrane is an independent, not-for-profit organization.	www.cochrane.org
	Systematic reviews are published in the Cochrane Library. Summaries and abstracts are free of charge; a subscription is required for full use of the library resources.	
	Publishes the *Cochrane Handbook for Systematic Reviews of Intervention* (training.cochrane.org/handbook)	
JBI (formerly Joanna Briggs Institute), Australia	JBI is a global organization that promotes evidence-based decisions to improve health and healthcare.	jbi.global
	The JBI EBP Database is an online resource that includes 4500+ JBI Evidence Summaries, Recommended Practices, and Best Practice Information Sheets. Access to this and the two journals, JBI Evidence Synthesis and JBI Evidence Implementation, are available exclusively on Ovid®.	
CRD, University of York, UK	The CRD is part of the NIHR.	www.york.ac.uk/inst/crd
	The CRD makes available systematic reviews on health and public health questions.	
	Access is available to archived records of the DARE and NHS EED, and guidelines for undertaking systematic reviews HTA database is currently being produced by the INAHTA (database.inahta.org)	
The EPPI Centre at the UCL Institute of Education, University College London	The EPPI Centre is part of the Social Science Research Unit at the UCL Institute of Education, University College London.	eppi.ioe.ac.uk/cms
	Provides the main findings, technical summary, or full technical reports of individual EPPI Centre Systematic Reviews.	
	Available online: EPPI Centre Methods for Conducting Systematic Reviews at www.betterevaluation.org/sites/default/files/Methods.pdf	
U.S. NLM	PubMed (which includes MEDLINE) is the NLM literature search system; it includes more than 35 million citations for biomedical literature from MEDLINE, journals, and online books and includes citations from full-text content.	www.nlm.nih.gov
	PubMed Central is a web-based repository of biomedical journal literature providing free, unrestricted access to more than 8.3 million full-text articles.	
	Publishes and provides the following: systematic reviews, meta-analyses, reviews of clinical trials, evidence-based medicine, consensus development conferences, and guidelines.	

TABLE 6.3 Example of Tool for Evidence-Based Practice Literature Review and Synthesis

CLINICAL QUESTION:

TITLE OF ARTICLE	AUTHORS WITH CREDENTIALS	QUESTION	STUDY DESIGN	LEVEL OF EVIDENCE	DESCRIPTION OF SAMPLE	MEASURES	RESULTS

CRD, Centre for Reviews and Dissemination; DARE, Database of Abstracts of Reviews of Effects; EPPI, Evidence for Policy and Practice Information; HTA, Health Technology Assessment; INAHTA, International Network of Agencies for Health Technology; JBI, Joanna Briggs Institute; JBI EBP, Joanna Briggs Institute Evidence-Based Practice; NHS EED, National Health Service Economic Evaluation Database; NIHR, National Institute for Health Research; NLM, National Library of Medicine.

Evidence-Based Medicine, and JBI. The Centre for Reviews and Dissemination (CRD) at the University of York (2008) includes study designs like case-control and cohort studies that are often used in population research. Nearly 50 different hierarchies of evidence have been identified (Vere & Gibson, 2020). Generally, systematic reviews and RCTs are ranked as best evidence (studies providing the most reliable evidence), while those offering less reliable evidence, like observational studies, are ranked lower.

Most hierarchies of evidence classify the levels in a descending order with RCTs at the top and case studies at the bottom (Figure 6.1). However, there are instances, as in population-based research, where it is not ethical or practical to conduct an RCT. Also, professional groups, like nursing and occupational therapy, have been critical of traditional hierarchies which do not value qualitative research. The levels of evidence developed by the Oncology Nursing Society and the American Association of Critical-Care Nurses (AACN) include both qualitative studies and expert opinion. The AACN classifies its levels in descending order, with the highest level of evidence in Level A and the lowest in Level M (Table 6.4).

A word of caution, while evidence hierarchies rate the strength of the evidence, one can only determine the quality of the evidence by examining the quality and limitations of each individual study. By first evaluating the strength of the evidence and then critiquing individual studies, the practitioner can "ensure that the evidence is credible and appropriate for inclusion into practice" (Peterson et al., 2014, p. 59).

The inclusion of different study designs in a systematic review can provide valuable insight as it has a direct impact on the complexity of the information. For example, although qualitative studies are not classified as high levels of evidence, they can still provide an APRN with important information to better understand observed phenomena. The findings of qualitative studies offer answers to different types of questions and help describe complex human interactions. A classic example is Beck's (1993) qualitative

FIGURE 6.1

Hierarchy of study designs. Note: This list is not exhaustive but covers main study designs. Names and definitions may differ.

STRENGTH OF EVIDENCE: STRONGER → WEAKER

EXPERIMENTAL STUDIES

Secondary preappraised research
Multiple studies are reviewed, and the results are summarized

- **Systematic reviews:** A form of research that uses systematic methods to identify, appraise and summarize the findings of all relevant individual studies that answer a specific research question.
- **Meta-analyses:** Statistical methods are used to summarize the data of these similar individual studies.

Randomized controlled trials
Participants are randomly assigned to two or more groups. The groups are treated according to their assignment and the outcomes of interest are compared.

- **Randomized cross-over trials:** All participants receive all the interventions, it is the sequence of interventions that is randomized. For example, in a two-arm cross-over trial, one group receives intervention A before intervention B, and the other group receives intervention B before intervention A.
- **Cluster randomized trials:** Clusters of people are randomized to different interventions. For example, whole clinics or geographical locations may be randomized to receive particular interventions, rather than individuals.

Quasi-experimental studies
The main distinction between randomized and quasi-experimental studies is that random assignment is not used to create the comparison groups.

- **Nonrandomized controlled studies:** Individuals are allocated to a concurrent comparison group, using methods other than randomization.
- **Before-and-after study:** The outcomes in study participants are compared before and after the introduction of an intervention. The before-and-after comparisons may be in the same sample of participants or in different samples.
- **Interrupted time series:** Multiple observations are made over time that are 'interrupted,' usually by an intervention or treatment.

NONEXPERIMENTAL STUDIES

Observational studies
The *natural* variation in interventions or exposure among participants is investigated to explore the effect of the interventions or exposure on health outcomes.

- **Cohort study:** Groups of participants who did and did not receive an intervention or exposure are identified. The groups are followed over time and the outcomes of interest are compared.
- **Case-control study:** Persons from the same population with an outcome of interest (cases), are compared to those without the same outcome (controls) to evaluate the association between exposure, intervention and the outcome.
- **Case series:** A number of cases of an intervention and the outcome are described. There are no control groups, and no comparison is made.

Source: Adapted from Centre for Reviews and Dissemination. (2008). *Systematic reviews: CRD's guidance for undertaking reviews in healthcare.* York: University of York. With permission from Centre for Reviews and Dissemination, University of York, UK.

TABLE 6.4 2012 American Association of Critical-Care Nurses Levels of Evidence with Revisions to 2008 Hierarchy

CATEGORY	LEVEL	DESCRIPTION
Experimental evidence	A	Meta-analysis or metasynthesis of multiple controlled studies with results that consistently support a specific action, intervention, or treatment (systematic review of a randomized controlled trial)
	B	Evidence from well-designed controlled studies, both randomized and nonrandomized, with results that consistently support a specific action, intervention, or treatment
	C	Evidence from qualitative, integrative reviews, or systematic reviews of qualitative, descriptive, or correlational studies or randomized controlled trials with inconsistent results
Recommendations	D	Evidence from peer-reviewed professional organizational standards, with clinical studies to support recommendations
	E	Theory-based evidence from expert opinion or multiple case reports
	M	Manufacturer's recommendation only

Source: Peterson, M. H., Barnason, S., Donnelly, B., Hill, K., Miley, H., Riggs, L., & Whiteman, K. (2014). Choosing the best evidence to guide clinical practice: Application of AACN levels of evidence. *Critical Care Nurse, 34*(2), 58–68. Used with permission ©2014 by the American Association of Critical-Care Nurses, all rights reserved.

study that used grounded theory to explore the phenomenon of postpartum depression. Because it was a qualitative study, the results were not generalized to the population of all women with postpartum depression. Instead, Beck's research offered the reader vivid descriptions of the women in her study and an insight into how she derived the evocative theme of "teetering on the edge" to effectively illustrate the women's experience.

VALIDITY

Once the APRN has completed evidence collection, each individual study needs to be appraised for the internal and external validity of the design. A hallmark of good research is that it is carried out by researchers who are aware of the existence of error and who design studies in such a way that errors are minimized. Table 6.3 is a useful tool to facilitate the appraisal of evidence by providing a method to organize the individual aspects or components of the study. The APRN uses this information to examine the soundness of the design, conduct an analysis of the study (internal validity), and to determine how well the study results can be applied to other settings and populations (external validity) (Jung et al., 2022).

When appraising the quality of a study, the APRN should attempt to assess how accurate the findings are and whether they are of relevance in the particular setting or population of interest. The appraisal should include the appropriateness of the study design to the research question, the risk of bias, the overall quality of the methods used to carry out the study, the outcome measure, the quality of the intervention, appropriateness of the analysis, the quality of the research report, and the generalizability of the results. When appraising a qualitative study, the APRN evaluates its credibility and trustworthiness by reviewing the methods of observation, data collection, reporting strategies, and audit trails (Moorley & Cathala, 2019). The APRN may choose to perform an *integrative review* (Lubbe et al., 2020) where qualitative evidence is synthesized with quantitative findings on a specific topic to generate a new perspective or interpretation. Chalmers and Cowdell (2021) explain that both methodologies are equally important, as "all good research has value, what is important is that the right method is used to answer the question" (p. 45).

APRNs are often intimidated when faced with evaluating the data analysis section in a research article. An important fact to keep in mind is that statistical significance is not synonymous with proof and that sometimes overemphasis is placed on statistically significant findings. It is equally important to evaluate the clinical significance of the results and how they affect treatment outcomes. Researchers report a statistical significance when they are confident that the difference they found between groups is real and not likely to be caused by chance. When determining clinical significance, however, the treatment benefit or amount of meaningful clinical improvement in treated individuals is assessed (Sharma, 2021). When evaluating the evidence, one should consider both the statistical and clinical significance before implementing a practice change. The APRN should review the results section of a research report carefully to determine whether or not the method of analysis used by the researcher answers the research question(s) or hypothesis and provides enough information to support the interpretation of the results.

TRANSPARENCY

Transparency is another important concept for consideration during the appraisal of research publications. Transparency in research is a reflection of both the accountability and the integrity of the investigator(s). Clarity about the research methods and techniques used ensures the rigor of the research study and the validity of its outcomes (Mellor, 2021). It should be possible, for example, for the study and results to be replicated by others. There should also be a disclosure of relationships that have the potential to cause a conflict of interest. A conflict of interest may occur when a researcher's objectivity is impacted by economic (ownership of stocks or shares), commercial (payouts by companies), or personal interests (when a researcher's status may be impacted by the results of the research) (APA, 2020). For example, an investigator with ties to a company that is closely related to the area of research may stand to profit from steering the results in a particular direction. Even when investigators disclose their conflicts of interest, the APRN should critically review the research for potential bias.

RESEARCH SYNTHESIS

The literature review not only provides a historical account of past work in the area of interest but also supports or refutes the necessity for ongoing study. The background for any study is founded on a thorough and comprehensive literature review. It serves as a justification for current research goals and introduces the reader to important past studies that have similar outcomes of comparison. Although not all studies will have an array of historical evidence in the literature, review of similar study designs or interventions can still provide a strong justification if the background is well researched.

The overall purpose of the example described earlier was to determine whether an online self-management program for Thai adults diagnosed with SLE would improve their knowledge of SLE, their disease related health behaviors, and their quality of life. The literature search demonstrated that in Asian populations, especially in Thailand, the incidence of SLE was higher; the disease was more severe and caused more organ damage, and the mortality rate was higher among this group. Research showed that besides medications, programs that offered physical exercise and psychological interventions had a marked benefit on fatigue, depression, and the overall quality of life of these patients. However, literature on interventions for SLE patients in Thailand was very limited at the time of the literature review, and very few studies evaluated the effect of the interventions on their mental health and quality of life. Table 6.5 provides a portion of the research synthesis that was completed by Ratanasiripong et al. (2023) using the sample PICO question. The literature review identified a gap in knowledge and highlighted the significance of the problem, justifying the need for the pilot study.

Following the review, the APRN, in consultation with the Thai SLE Foundation, created an e-Wellness program to support SLE patients in Thailand who were distressed by the social isolation caused by the pandemic. This one group, pretest-posttest study was conducted for 3 months in 2021. The e-Wellness program consisted of social support and lifestyle and stress management. Social support was provided by an online support group via a smartphone app and was led and monitored by two SLE Foundation leaders. The participants were trained to use Zoom and received 90-minute weekly workshops for 3 weeks. The workshops focused on SLE education, disease self-management, and mental health management. Prior to implementation of the e-Wellness program (pretest) and again 3 months after the last workshop (posttest), the participants completed a Physical and Psychosocial Health Assessment (PPHA) which included demographics, an SLE-related knowledge and health behavior survey, and the DASS-Thai version and the Lupus QoL-Thai version scales.

Ratanasiripong et al. report that the results in this study are consistent with other studies discovered during the literature review. Post implementation of the e-Wellness program, participants had improved SLE-related knowledge scores; exercised more; had improved medication compliance; and reported reduced sun exposure, increased hours of sleep, and lower stress. The quality-of-life scores for domains of pain, intimate relationship, burden to others, emotional health, and fatigue showed statistically significant improvement. The overall outcomes of the e-Wellness program are promising and demonstrate the effectiveness of an innovative approach to assist SLE patients in managing their own health. To build on the program success, Ratanasiripong et al. recommend that the Thai SLE Foundation include online exercise and cosmetic training in the program and, for those patients who do not have internet access, to offer similar inperson wellness programs. The summation of this work from literature review, to research synthesis, to pilot project is an excellent example of how APRNs can use this approach to design interventions to improve population outcomes.

TABLE 6.5 Tool Used to Assess Literature Review: Interventions, Purpose, Populations, and Outcomes

TITLE/AUTHOR	DESCRIPTION OF INTERVENTION	PURPOSE AND POPULATIONS	OUTCOMES ACHIEVED
1. Carter, E. E., Barr, S. G., & Clarke, A. E. (2016). The global burden of SLE: prevalence, health disparities and socioeconomic impact. *Nature Reviews. Rheumatology. 12*(10), 605–620.	Article exploring the worldwide incidence, prevalence, and socioeconomic impact of SLE	The authors seek to understand the factors responsible for variations in the global burden of SLE.	Indications that SLE develops more frequently, has a more severe disease course, causes more organ damage, and has a higher mortality among Asian and Aboriginal populations and individuals of African ancestry than in White individuals
2. Case, S., Sinnette, C., Phillip, C., Grosgogeat, C., Costenbader, K. H., Leatherwood, C., Feldman, C. H., & Son, M. B. (2021). Patient experiences and strategies for coping with SLE: A qualitative study. *Lupus, 30*(9), 1405–1414.	Qualitative study that used trained moderator-led focus groups, each lasting 90 minutes, to explore psychosocial aspects, medications, transitions to adulthood, and doctor–patient relationship of patients with SLE.	The study aimed to explore the illness experience and to qualitatively assess patient-identified influences and strategies to improve the care experience. Participants recruited were 13 adults with SLE from two medical centers.	Patients identified common challenges, modifying influences, and coping strategies based on personal experiences. A strong patient–provider relationship and trust in the medical team emerged as key modifiable factors.
3. Chang, A., Winquist, N. W., Wescott, A. B., Lattie, E. G., & Graham, A. K. (2021). Systematic review of digital and non-digital non-pharmacological interventions that target quality of life and psychological outcomes in adults with systemic lupus erythematosus. *Lupus, 30*(7), 1058–1077.	Systematic review using PRISMA guidelines of research on diet, physical activity, and psychological and course-based interventions on SLE	Aim was to examine the efficacy of non-pharmacological interventions for improving psychological outcomes and/or QoL in patients with SLE. Included 23 studies, 21 RCTs, and two quasi-experimental studies	Non-pharmacological interventions improved QoL and psychological outcomes and were delivered in traditional settings or remotely.

(continued)

TABLE 6.5 **Tool Used to Assess Literature Review: Interventions, Purpose, Populations, and Outcomes** (*continued*)

TITLE/AUTHOR	DESCRIPTION OF INTERVENTION	PURPOSE AND POPULATIONS	OUTCOMES ACHIEVED
4. da Hora, T. C., Lima, K., & Maciel, R. R. B. T. (2019). The effect of therapies on the quality of life of patients with systemic lupus erythematosus: A meta-analysis of randomized trials. *Advances in Rheumatology, 59*(1), 34–34	A systematic review with a meta-analysis of RCTs was conducted comparing patients who received cognitive therapy, physical activity, medications, and/or herbal therapy.	The aim of the study was to evaluate the effect of various therapies on the quality of life of patients with SLE. Seven studies were included in this meta-analysis.	This systematic review suggests that interventions improve QoL in patients with SLE, being most evident in cognitive behavioral therapy. Because the samples were so small, repeat individual studies with large samples are recommended.
5. Drenkard, C., & Lim, S. S. (2019). Update on lupus epidemiology: Advancing health disparities research through the study of minority populations. *Current Opinion in Rheumatology, 31*(6), 689–696.	Current descriptive epidemiological studies in the United States provide very accurate estimates of the burden and mortality of SLE across diverse demographic groups.	The current review focuses on recent population-based studies that examine the burden of lupus to address existing health disparities.	SLE strikes disproportionately more people from racial and ethnic minorities. They are also at increased risk of developing severe manifestations; mortality is higher, and death occurs at a younger age.
6. Fangtham, M., Kasturi, S., Bannuru, R. R., Nash, J. L., & Wang, C. (2019). Non-pharmacologic therapies for systemic lupus erythematosus. *Lupus, 28*(6), 703–712.	A systematic review of RCTs compared the effects of non-pharmacological therapy to medical therapy in improving fatigue, depression, and QoL in patients with SLE.	A review was conducted to determine the effects of non-pharmacological therapies on patients with SLE to inform practice. Fifteen studies involving 846 patients met the inclusion criteria.	Exercise and psychological interventions are useful adjuncts to medical therapy in improving pain, depression, and QoL in SLE patients.

(*continued*)

7. Fernandez-Ruiz, R., Masson, M., Kim, M. Y., Myers, B., Haberman, R. H., Castillo, R., Scher, J. U., Guttmann, A., Carlucci, P. M., Deonaraine, K. K., Golpanian, M., Robins, K., Chang, M., Belmont, H. M., Buyon, J. P., Blazer, A. D., Saxena, A., & Izmirly, P. M. (2020). Leveraging the United States epicenter to provide insights on COVID-19 in patients with systemic lupus erythematosus. *Arthritis & Rheumatology 72*(12), 1971–1980.	SLE patients were recruited from several sources in New York City. Patients were >18 years and completed a REDCap-based questionnaire. Patients were contacted weekly for 7 weeks to track changes in COVID-19 status. Data on hospitalized and deceased patients were collected from medical records.	Aim of the study was to analyze associations of comorbidities and medications on infection outcomes in patients with SLE affected by COVID-19. Two hundred and twenty-six patients were included, 41 with confirmed COVID-19, 42 symptomatic with no testing, and 124 asymptomatic.	Of the SLE patients with confirmed COVID-19, hospitalization was required in 59%, and among them, 10% were admitted to the ICU, all of whom died. Hospitalized patients tended to be older, non-White, Hispanic, have higher BMI, and with at least one comorbidity. Predictive variables for hospitalization were same as the general population.
8. Pereira, M. G., Duarte, S., Ferraz, A., Santos, M., & Fontes, L. (2020). Quality of life in patients with systemic lupus erythematosus: The mediator role of psychological morbidity and disease activity. *Psychology, Health & Medicine, 25*(10), 1247–1257.	Cross-sectional study that surveyed participants about their disease state and QoL. Instruments used were demographic and clinical questionnaire, SLE Activity Questionnaire, Fatigue Severity Scale, Body Image Scale, and WHOQOL-BREF.	One hundred and four women from two hospitals participated. The aim of the study was to analyze the relationship between psychological morbidity, body image, and disease severity and the QoL in patients with SLE.	More disease activity, fatigue, psychological morbidity, and a poor body image were associated with lower QoL, in all domains. There were no associations between age, disease duration, and the domains of QoL.
9. Lu, M.-C., & Koo, M. (2021). Effects of exercise intervention on health-related quality of life in patients with systemic lupus erythematosus: A systematic review and meta-analysis of controlled trials. *Healthcare (Basel), 9*(9), 1215.	Randomized and nonrandomized controlled trials published up to July 2021 were examined. The PICO question was used as follows: (P) = in patients with SLE; (I) = exercise; (C) = usual care; and (O) = quality of life.	This study aimed to examine the effects of exercise interventions on health-related QoL in patients with SLE. Of the 1158 articles retrieved, nine were included for systematic review. Five were RCTs and assessed using meta-analysis.	The systematic review and meta-analysis supported that exercise, compared to usual care, improved the health-related QoL in patients with SLE.

(continued)

TABLE 6.5 Tool Used to Assess Literature Review: Interventions, Purpose, Populations, and Outcomes (*continued*)

TITLE/AUTHOR	DESCRIPTION OF INTERVENTION	PURPOSE AND POPULATIONS	OUTCOMES ACHIEVED
10. Ratanasiripong, N. T., & Ratanasiripong, P. (2020). Predictive factors of quality of life among systemic lupus erythematosus patients in Thailand: A web-based cross-sectional study. *Quality of Life Research, 29*(9), 2415–2423.	This was a cross-sectional study that used survey methods to gather demographic information and the DASS and LupusQoL to gather data on the participants.	This study aimed to assess mental health status and explore factors associated with the disease-specific QOL among (SLE) patients in Thailand. Six hundred and fifty members of the SLE club were surveyed.	Lower education and income were associated with higher depression and anxiety. Number of symptoms, stress, anxiety, and depression were predictors of quality of life.

BMI, body mass index; COVID-19, coronavirus disease 2019; DASS, Depression, Anxiety, Stress Scale; LupusQoL, Lupus Quality of Life Scale; PICO, population studied, intervention, comparison, and outcome; PRISMA, Preferred Reporting Items for Systematic Reviews and Meta-analyses; REDCap, Research Electronic Data Capture; RCT, randomized controlled trial; SLE, systemic lupus erythematosus; QoL, quality of life; WHOQOL-BREF, World Health Organization Quality of Life Assessment Brief Version.

Source: From Ratanasiripong, N., Cahill, S., Crane, C., & Ratanasiripong, P. (2023). The outcomes of an e-wellness program for lupus patients in Thailand: A participatory action research approach. *Journal of Preventive Medicine & Public Health.*

INTEGRATION OF EVIDENCE INTO PRACTICE

Often, time lags occur when applying new research findings to clinical practice. The time period between the discovery that an intervention works and the application of that new knowledge into actual practice can take up to 15 years (Khan et al., 2021). In 1999, the American Society of Anesthesiologists (ASA) published evidence-based guidelines for preoperative fasting in healthy patients undergoing elective procedures. Moving away from the accepted tradition of nothing by mouth (NPO) after midnight, the ASA advocated fasting periods of 2 hours for clear liquids, 6 hours for a light meal (tea and toast), and 8 hours for heavier meals before elective surgery. Crenshaw and Winslow (2002) conducted a study to determine how well the ASA guidelines were being followed. They interviewed 155 patients in one hospital about their preoperative fasting, comparing preoperative fasting instructions, actual preoperative fasting, and ASA-recommended fasting durations for liquids and solids. They found that the majority of patients continued to receive instructions to remain NPO after midnight for both liquids and solids, whether they were scheduled for early or late surgery. They also discovered that, on average, the patients fasted from liquids and solids for 12 hours and 14 hours. These fasts were significantly longer than those recommended by the ASA. Clearly, in this case, the authors discovered a significant lag time between the generation of new knowledge and the implementation of that knowledge into practice.

A follow-up study in 2004 sought to evaluate the effects of the implementation of a preoperative fasting policy and the education of healthcare practitioners on preoperative fasting practices at their facility. Unfortunately, the authors found that the traditional practice of allowing NPO after midnight persisted (Crenshaw & Winslow, 2008). The authors identified the difficulty of changing entrenched traditions as one reason that preoperative fasting in excess of evidence-based recommendations persisted.

Since the publication of the original preoperative fasting guidelines (ASA, 1999), the ASA has published two updates (ASA, 2011, 2017) reiterating the adverse effects of prolonged fasting and maintaining the previously recommended fasting periods. Yet, in a recent study, despite claiming strict adherence to current ASA guidelines, over 50% of anesthetists reported enforcing strict fasting, disallowing even clear fluids after midnight (Merchant et al., 2020). The researchers relate an interesting anecdote about Dr. Maltby, a physician on the team responsible for the early seminal research endorsing 2-hour fasting requirements for clear liquids. Recently, Dr. Maltby fasted for more than 20 hours preoperatively when his elective surgery was postponed to accommodate an emergency. Even after all these years, many facilities still cling to outdated protocols, with the average preoperative NPO time for patients hovering around 10 hours (Bassa et al., 2021).

In order to effect change, the APRN needs to understand why these time intervals exist between the development of new knowledge and the incorporation of that knowledge into practice. Globally, studies that have examined APRNs' knowledge, attitudes, practices, and barriers to integrating evidence in their nursing care report similar results (Crawford et al., 2023; Labrague et al., 2019). As reported in prior studies, these researchers found that nurses in all areas of care overwhelmingly report positive attitudes toward EBP. But nurse interest in EBP does not translate into implementation. Across borders, implementation of EBP is still low, and the challenges cited include environmental and organizational barriers like time constraints, work overload, and lack of resources and management support. Personal barriers include lack of knowledge and critical appraisal skills and resistance to change. A systematic review summarizing EBP practices of community/public health nurses revealed that less than 25% of nurses reported that they had accessed databases or used research in clinical practice (Li et al., 2019). In their mixed-methods study, Crawford et al. (2023) reported that "Fear and Resistance to Change" (p. 31) was not only a major personal theme but it also cuts across all the identified qualitative themes. Unfortunately, they report that the reasons, such as concerns about increased workload, older staff still practicing out of nursing school textbooks, and an unwillingness to let go of the traditional way of doing things, have remained the same.

Tradition is a difficult barrier to overcome. Nurses need to question practices based on tradition and instead use evidence whenever possible to guide nursing practice. Besides education, nurses need mentors to improve their evidence retrieval skills and to promote evidence implementation into daily practice (Wang et al., 2021). Depending on the focus of their advanced degrees, APRNs are experts who can assume the roles of highly skilled practitioners and/or leaders and educators in their respective clinical fields. APRNs are uniquely situated to be trusted opinion leaders and mentors to help bring about practice change and influence patient outcomes. They can challenge clinical staff to identify and remove barriers to evidence-based practice. Because they receive advanced education in research, APRNs can be the much-needed nurse scientist/nurse expert to guide staff nurses in developing PICO questions, searching and synthesizing the literature, and changing practice interventions to reflect current knowledge.

MODELS OF EVIDENCE-BASED PRACTICE

Several models have been created to facilitate the implementation of evidence-based practice. They provide an organized approach to integrate evidence into practice and sustain the change. A practice model ensures that professional nursing practice is consistent and minimizes practice variations that often increase risk and create gaps in care. Some examples of the EBP models in use are the Advancing Research and Clinical Practice through Close Collaboration (ARCC©) Model, the Johns Hopkins Nursing Evidence-Based Practice (JHNEBP) model, the Chronic Care Model (CCM), and the Iowa Model Revised: Evidence-Based Practice to Promote Excellence in Healthcare (Iowa Model). The overriding characteristic of each is that it provides a structured method for incorporating best evidence into practice.

The focus of the ARCC model is to bring research experts together with direct care nurses to integrate research into practice. Developed by Bernadette Melnyk and the faculty of the School of Nursing at the University of Rochester in 1999, it was originally designed to bring academic communities together with acute and community-based healthcare organizations. The APRN, as mentor, plays a prominent role in the ARCC model, as one of its key components is educating and coaching nursing staff on evidence-based practice. Fineout-Overholt et al. (2004) conducted a study to test this model in two pediatric units at acute care facilities. The authors identified the following crucial factors for implementing evidence-based practice: administrative support, creation of a clear role for nurses that includes evidence-based practice, adequate infrastructure (such as computer resources and databases), evidence-based practice mentors to work directly with direct care nurses, time and money to carry out studies, and creation of an evidence-based practice culture. In this study, direct care nurses valued the importance of APRN mentorship in bringing about practice change as opposed to simply being told what to do. The authors stress that APRN mentors facilitate and sustain a culture of evidence-based practice by working closely with direct care nurses. Several studies support the ARCC model which has since been implemented in a number of healthcare organizations worldwide (Melnyk & Fineout-Overholt, 2019).

Similar to the ARCC model, the origin of the JHNEBP model is found in a successful partnership between academia and a healthcare institution. This model was developed in collaboration with the Johns Hopkins Hospital and the Johns Hopkins University School of Nursing. In this model, the three-step PET (**p**ractice question, **e**vidence, and **t**ranslation) process provides the framework to incorporate best evidence into clinical practice (Dang et al., 2021). The essential cornerstones of the model are practice, education, and research, with evidence at its core.. The JHNEBP model encourages critical thinking and provides a framework to guide nurses as they seek and find the best available evidence to improve patient outcomes.

The CCM (ACT Center, 2023) employs a holistic approach to chronic disease management through the use of evidence-based practice. It summarizes the basic elements for improving care in health systems at the community, organization, practice, and patient levels. It has six components: the healthcare delivery system, community, patient self-management support, decision support, delivery system design, and clinical information system. The emphasis of this model is on health promotion. Tillman (2020) implemented a pilot program to test the effectiveness of the CCM in improving health outcomes for uninsured high-risk diabetic patients who attended a free clinic in the city. Patients who participated in the 4-month diabetes self-management program had significantly lower hemoglobin A1C when compared to their preprogram baseline values. Patients also showed reductions in their blood pressure and lipid levels and reported high satisfaction with the program. This was an ambitious project that included all six elements of the CCM; the researchers credited the intense community commitment and volunteer support from physicians, nurse practitioners, local pharmacies, and the YMCA for its success.

The Iowa Model was first developed in 1994 "to serve as a guide for nurses and other healthcare providers to use research findings for improvement of patient care" (Titler et al., 2001, p. 498). Responding to the advances in healthcare and user feedback, the Iowa Model Collaborative (2017) revised the Iowa Model to streamline the process and make it easy to use. Important features of the Iowa Model Revised are decision points and feedback loops that are characteristic of the ongoing process of improving care through research and evidence-based practices. The revised model begins with the identification of problems or change opportunities. It continues with a stepwise approach, ending with dissemination of the project results to share lessons learned, internally and externally, with other organizations. The following case study illustrates how an inpatient stroke unit used this practice model in collaboration with its population health department and community partners to revise existing care coordination practices and improve patient outcomes.

CASE STUDY

USE OF THE IOWA MODEL TO IMPROVE POST-STROKE CARE TRANSITIONS FOR PATIENTS AND THEIR FAMILIES

Identify triggers/opportunities
The APRN Stroke Coordinator and members of the Stroke Committee at a community hospital noted variations in their quality metrics for acute stroke patients, with 90-day readmission rates reaching as high as 24%. This was concerning as the hospital is recognized as a Joint Commission Comprehensive Stroke Center at one campus and as a Joint Commission Advanced Primary Stroke Center at another. Both provide comprehensive care to acute stroke patients in the community.

Identify purpose, determine priority
The Centers for Medicare and Medicaid Services (CMS) Bundled Payments for Care Improvement Advanced (BPCI Advanced) Model offers providers incentives for the delivery of efficient, high-quality, affordable care for stroke patients. Since the hospital was enrolled in the BPCI-A program, reducing the 90-day readmission rates for stroke patients was a top organizational priority.

Form team
An interprofessional Stroke Care Collaboration team was created which included stroke coordinators, a nurse practitioner, the care transitions manager and the director of population health and care management (both nurses), and representatives from rehabilitation services and the department of medicine.

Assemble, appraise, and synthesize the evidence
A literature review provided information on current practice and gaps in care transitions for stroke patients. In addition, it revealed best evidence to improve the coordination of care for patients from the time of their hospital admission to their discharge to the home and finally into the community.

Determine if the evidence is sufficient
Key findings supporting the change included the following:

- Coordination of care is imperative especially in the post-acute phase to provide efficient care and improve patient outcomes (Matchar et al., 2015).
- High-quality communication with a timely transfer of pertinent patient information at every stage, between all care providers, prevents fragmentation and successfully transitions stroke patients from acute care to rehabilitation and into the community (Miller et al., 2018).
- Early supported discharge (ESD) is effective in shortening length of stays, reducing rates of rehospitalization, and improving patient and caregiver satisfaction (Fisher et al., 2016).

This information was summarized and discussed with team members who met biweekly to create a coordinated plan of care to optimize the transition of stroke patients to home and community and reduce hospital readmission rates.

(continued)

Pilot change and carryout study
The Stroke Collaboration Team, in collaboration with post-acute care providers, acute rehabilitation facilities, and home health agencies, developed a comprehensive program to improve communication and coordinate care between all facilities, patients, and their caregivers. They established the criteria for ESD to the community, expedited delivery of home health and outpatient services, and initiated advanced care planning. In the hospital, a multidisciplinary team of nurses, rehabilitation services, and care management conducted daily rounds using multiple standardized tools to assess patients' eligibility for ESD, including the availability of caregiver support at home. A dedicated care transitions nurse then followed ESD patients for 90 days. Communication was maintained with rehabilitation services and home health agencies to identify issues and intervene early to ensure patient compliance with stroke orders, medication and rehabilitation regimens, and follow-up visits.

Determine whether the change is appropriate for adoption in practice
Post-implementation, quality outcomes, and resource utilization measures for patients showed marked improvement. Although clinical and demographic characteristics of the pre- and post-implementation patient groups were similar, the 90-day hospital readmission rate dropped significantly from 23.4% to 9.3%. On average, post-acute care cost decreased by $16,608 per patient, resulting in a substantial reduction in the 90-day cost per episode. The team concluded that the enhanced coordination of post-acute services facilitates patients' care transitions after a stroke.

Sustain practice change, monitor structure, process, and outcome data
The Stroke Care Collaboration Team reviews quality metrics and outcomes for the BPCI-A program quarterly. The coordination of care program is evaluated and revised and updated as needed. Readmission rates are reviewed regularly and any upticks in the rates are addressed. Communication with post-acute care providers, including rehabilitation facilities and home health agencies, is emphasized. The organization has maintained its designations as Comprehensive Stroke Center and Advanced Primary Stroke Center.

Disseminate results
The APRN Stroke Coordinator and other members of the Stroke Team have presented the results of this project at hospital-based events and in hospital newsletters. Results were also disseminated externally via poster presentations at regional institutions and at the International Stroke Conference in California.

Source: Adapted from Sanfillippo, G., Olkowski, B. F., Schumacher, H. C., Dafilou, D. K., Bowski, C. M., Gilli, M., & Demirjian, J. (2020, February). Unbundling care transitions and cost after stroke: Results from the BPCI-Advanced Program. Poster presentation at the International Stroke Conference 2020, Los Angeles, California.

With the increased emphasis on the adoption of evidence-based practice, there are now many more EBP models with freely available resources. Ultimately, APRNs need to determine which practice model will best suit their needs. Tucker et al. (2021) compared three established models/frameworks and found that despite different approaches, all share key attributes like the use of an EBP mentor, organizational support, evaluation of the evidence, selecting appropriate strategies, and monitoring outcomes. They caution that the selection of an EBP model is not "a one size fits all" and that APRNs desiring practice change should consider that "each model/framework has unique features and benefits that should be evaluated for the best fit for an organization, individual, or group. The best fit may depend on the nature of the setting, healthcare team, and practice change" (p. 79). The researchers also provide resources to aid the APRN in selecting the best practice model relevant to their work setting.

SUMMARY

The use of research evidence to guide practice can lead to the implementation of interventions that will improve population outcomes, but this is a complex process. The ability to identify clinical problems and issues, ask clinical questions in a format that allows for study, conduct a search of the literature, appraise and synthesize the available evidence, and successfully integrate new knowledge into practice requires specialized skills and knowledge. This process can be challenging and time consuming. Researchers have identified many barriers to evidence-based practice, including the lack of belief by practicing nurses that research can make a real difference. APRNs are uniquely positioned to influence nursing practice through their roles as leaders, educators, and clinical experts. This chapter described some of the basic skills needed to integrate and synthesize information in order to design interventions that are based on evidence to improve population health. APRNs need to use their specialized knowledge and advanced practice roles to identify the barriers to evidence-based practice and build the capacity to implement change. They also require the ability to engage individuals, teams, and organizations in the process. By adopting a culture of evidence-based practice in the work environment, APRNs have the opportunity to facilitate change that can lead to improved quality of care and enhanced population outcomes.

END-OF-CHAPTER RESOURCES

EXERCISES AND DISCUSSION QUESTIONS

EXERCISE 6.1 Describe in your own words a clinical problem you would like to examine.

- Explain why you think it is important to address this problem.

EXERCISE 6.2 Write a clinical question using the PICO format.

EXERCISE 6.3 Carry out a literature review for the PICO question you wrote in Exercise 6.2.

- Establish criteria for inclusion and exclusion of studies.
- Synthesize and appraise the information using the sample tool in Table 6.3.

EXERCISE 6.4 Which practice model would you use to implement an evidence-based change in your practice area?

- Provide a rationale for your choice of model.
- Describe how you would apply the model to address your PICO question.

A robust set of instructor resources designed to supplement this text is located at http://connect.springerpub.com/content/book/978-0-8261-4377-8. Qualifying instructors may request access by emailing textbook@springerpub.com.

REFERENCES

ACT Center. (2023). *The chronic care model*. Retrieved March 1, 2023, from https://www.act-center.org/application/files/1616/3511/6445/Model_Chronic_Care.pdf

Alajami, A. (2021). Critiquing the past for solidifying the future: Understanding the synthesizing facet of reviewing the social studies: Critical approach. *Current Research in Behavioral Sciences, 2*, 100047. https://doi.org/10.1016/j.crbeha.2021.100047

American Psychological Association. (2020). *Publication manual of the American psychological association* (7th ed.). https://doi.org/10.1037/0000165-000

American Association of Colleges of Nursing. (2021). *The essentials: Core competencies for professional nursing education*. https://www.aacnnursing.org/Portals/42/AcademicNursing/pdf/Essentials-2021.pdf

American Society of Anesthesiologists. (1999). Practice guidelines for preoperative fasting and the use of pharmacologic agents to reduce the risk of pulmonary aspiration: Application to healthy patients undergoing elective procedures. *Anesthesiology, 90(3)*, 896–905. https://doi.org/10.1097/00000542-199903000-00034

American Society of Anesthesiologists. (2011). Practice guidelines for preoperative fasting and the use of pharmacologic agents to reduce the risk of pulmonary aspiration: Application to healthy patients undergoing elective procedures, an updated report by the American Society of Anesthesiologists Committee on Standards and Practice Parameters. *Anesthesiology, 114(3)*, 495–511. https://doi.org/10.1097/ALN.0b013e3181fcbfd9

American Society of Anesthesiologists. (2017). Practice guidelines for preoperative fasting and the use of pharmacologic agents to reduce the risk of pulmonary aspiration: Application to healthy patients undergoing elective procedures, an updated report by the American Society of Anesthesiologists Task Force on Preoperative Fasting and the Use of Pharmacologic Agents to Reduce the Risk of Pulmonary Aspiration. *Anesthesiology, 126*(3), 376–393. https://doi.org/10.1097/ALN.0000000000001452

Bassa, R., McGraw, C., Leonard, J., McGuire, E. L., Banton, K., Madayag, R., Tanner, A. H., Lieser, M., Harrison, P. B., & Bar-Or, D. (2021). How long are mechanically ventilated patients fasted prior to surgery? An exploratory study examining preoperative fasting practices across trauma centres. *Journal of Perioperative Practice, 31*(7–8), 261–267. https://doi.org/10.1177/1750458920936058

Beck, C. T. (1993). Teetering on the edge: A substantive theory of postpartum depression. *Nursing Research, 42*(1), 42–48. https://doi.org/10.1097/00006199-199301000-00008

Briscoe, S., Bethel, A., & Rogers, M. (2020). Conduct and reporting of citation searching in Cochrane systematic reviews: A cross-sectional study. *Research Synthesis Methods, 11*(2), 169–180. https://doi.org/10.1002/jrsm.1355

Carcary, M. (2020). The research audit trail: methodological guidance for application in practice. *Electronic Journal of Business Research Methods, 18*(2), 166–177. https://doi.org/10.34190/JBRM.18.2.008

Centre for Reviews and Dissemination. (2008). Systematic reviews: CRD's guidance for undertaking reviews in health care. University of York. Retrieved from http://www.york.ac.uk/inst/crd/index_guidance.htm

Chalmers, J., & Cowdell, F. (2021). What are quantitative and qualitative research methods? A brief introduction. *Dermatological Nursing, 20*(2), 45–48.

Clarke, V., Lehane, E., Mulcahy, H., & Cotter, P. (2021). Nurse practitioners' implementation of evidence-based practice into routine care: A scoping review. *Worldviews on Evidence-Based Nursing, 18*(3), 180–189. https://doi.org/10.1111/wvn.12510

Cochrane. (2023). *Our open access strategy.* https://www.cochrane.org/about-us/our-open-access-strategy

Crawford, C. L., Rondinelli, J., Zuniga, S., Valdez, R. M., Tze-Polo, L., & Titler, M. G. (2023). Barriers and facilitators influencing EBP readiness: Building organizational and nurse capacity. *Worldviews on Evidence-Based Nursing, 20*(1), 27–36. https://doi.org/10.1111/wvn.12618

Crenshaw, J. T., & Winslow, E. H. (2002). Preoperative fasting: Old habits die hard. *The American Journal of Nursing, 102*(5), 36–44. https://doi.org/10.1097/00000446-200205000-00033

Crenshaw, J. T., & Winslow, E. H. (2008). Preoperative fasting duration and medication instruction: Are we improving? *AORN Journal, 88*(6), 963–976. https://doi.org/10.1016/j.aorn.2008.07.017

Dang, D., Dearholt, S., Bissett, K., Ascenzi, J., & Whalen, M. (2021). *Johns Hopkins evidence-based practice for nurses and healthcare professionals: Model and guidelines* (4th ed.). Sigma Theta Tau International.

EBSCO. (2023). *CINAHL databases.* Retrieved from https://www.ebsco.com/products/research-databases/cinahl-database

Fineout-Overholt, E., Levin, R. F., & Melnyk, B. M. (2004). Strategies for advancing evidence-based practice in clinical settings. *The Journal of the New York State Nurses Association, 35*(2), 28–32.

Fisher, R. J., Cobley, C. S., Potgieter, I., Moody, A., Nouri, F., Gaynor, C., Byrne, A., & Walker, M. F. (2016). Is stroke early supported discharge still effective in practice? A prospective comparative study. *Clinical Rehabilitation, 30*(3), 268–276. https://doi.org/10.1177/0269215515578697

Hoffecker, L. (2020). Grey literature searching for systematic reviews in the health sciences. *Serials Librarian, 79*(3–4), 252–260. https://doi.org/10.1080/0361526X.2020.1847745

Iowa Model Collaborative. (2017). Iowa model of evidence-based practice: Revisions and validation: Iowa model-revised. *Worldviews on Evidence-Based Nursing, 14*(3), 175–182. https://doi.org/10.1111/wvn.12223

Jung, A., Balzer, J., Braun, T., & Luedtke, K. (2022). Identification of tools used to assess the external validity of randomized controlled trials in reviews: A systematic review of measurement properties. *BMC Medical Research Methodology, 22*(1), 100. https://doi.org/10.1186/s12874-022-01561-5

Khan, S., Chambers, D., & Neta, G. (2021). Revisiting time to translation: Implementation of evidence-based practices (EBPs) in cancer control. *Cancer Causes & Control, 32*(3), 221–230. https://doi.org/10.1007/s10552-020-01376-z

Labrague, L. J., McEnroe-Petitte, D., D'Souza, M. S., Cecily, H. S. J., Fronda, D. C., Edet, O. B., Ibebuike, J. E., Venkatesan, L., Almazan, J. U., Al Amri, M., Mirafuentes, E. C., Cayaban, A. R. R., Al Yahyaei, A., & Bin Jumah, J. A. (2019). A multicountry study on nursing students' self-perceived competence and barriers to evidence-based practice. *Worldviews on Evidence-Based Nursing, 16*(3), 236–246. https://doi.org/10.1111/wvn.12364

Lansing Community College Library. (2019, June). *What is PICOT?* Retrieved from https://libguides.lcc.edu/c.php?g=167860&p=6198388

Li, S., Cao, M., & Zhu, X. (2019). Evidence-based practice: Knowledge, attitudes, implementation, facilitators, and barriers among community nurses-systematic review. *Medicine, 98*(39), e17209. https://doi.org/10.1097/MD.0000000000017209

Lubbe, W., Ham-Baloyi, W. ten, & Smit, K. (2020). The integrative literature review as a research method: A demonstration review of research on neurodevelopmental supportive care in preterm infants. *Journal of Neonatal Nursing: JNN, 26*(6), 308–315. https://doi.org/10.1016/j.jnn.2020.04.006

Matchar, D. B., Nguyen, H. V., & Tian, Y. (2015). Bundled payment and care of acute stroke: What does it take to make it work? *Stroke, 46*(5), 1414–1421. https://doi.org/10.1161/STROKEAHA.115.009089

Mellor, D. (2021). Improving norms in research culture to incentivize transparency and rigor. *Educational Psychologist, 56*(2), 122–131. https://doi.org/10.1080/00461520.2021.1902329

Melnyk, B. M., & Fineout-Overholt, E. (2019). *Evidence-based practice in nursing and healthcare: A guide to best practice* (4th ed.). Wolters Kluwer Health

Merchant, R. N., Chima, N., Ljungqvist, O., & Kok, J. N. J. (2020). Preoperative fasting practices across three anesthesia societies: Survey of practitioners. *JMIR Perioperative Medicine, 3*(1), e15905. https://doi.org/10.2196/15905

Miller, K. K., Lin, S. H., & Neville, M. (2019). From hospital to home to participation: A position paper on transition planning poststroke. *Archives of Physical Medicine and Rehabilitation, 100*(6), 1162–1175. https://doi.org/10.1016/j.apmr.2018.10.017

Moorley, C., & Cathala, X. (2019). How to appraise qualitative research. *Evidence-Based Nursing, 22*(1), 10–13. https://doi.org/10.1136/ebnurs-2018-103044

Peterson, M. H., Barnason, S., Donnelly, B., Hill, K., Miley, H., Riggs, L., & Whiteman, K. (2014). Choosing the best evidence to guide clinical practice: Application of AACN levels of evidence. *Critical Care Nurse, 34*(2), 58–68. https://doi.org/10.4037/ccn2014411

Polit, D., & Beck, C. T. (2021). *Nursing research: Generating and assessing evidence for nursing practice* (11th ed.). Wolters Kluwer Health.

Popenoe, R., Langius-Eklöf, A., Stenwall, E., & Jervaeus, A. (2021). A practical guide to data analysis in general literature reviews. *Nordic Journal of Nursing Research, 41*(4), 175–186. https://doi.org/10.1177/2057158521991949

Ratanasiripong, N., Cahill, S., Crane, C., & Ratanasiripong, P. (2023). The outcomes of an e-wellness program for lupus patients: A participatory action research approach. *Journal of Preventive Medicine & Public Health, 56*(2), 154–163. https://doi.org/10.3961/jpmph.22.491

Sharma, H. (2021). Statistical significance or clinical significance? A researcher's dilemma for appropriate interpretation of research results. *Saudi Journal of Anaesthesia, 15*(4), 431–434. https://doi.org/10.4103/sja.sja_158_21

Ten Ham-Baloyi, W., Minnie, K., & van der Walt, C. (2020). Improving healthcare: a guide to roll-out best practices. *African health sciences, 20*(3), 1487–1495. https://doi.org/10.4314/ahs.v20i3.55

Tillman, P. (2020). Applying the chronic care model in a free clinic. *Journal for Nurse Practitioners, 16*(8), e117–e121. https://doi.org/10.1016/j.nurpra.2020.05.016

Titler, M. G., Kleiber, C., Steelman, V. J., Rakel, B. A., Budreau, G., Everett, L. Q., Buckwalter, K. C., Tripp-Reimer, T., & Goode, C. J. (2001). The Iowa model of evidence-based practice to promote quality care. *Critical Care Nursing Clinics of North America, 13*(4), 497–509. https://doi.org/10.1016/S0899-5885(18)30017-0

Tucker, S., McNett, M., Mazurek Melnyk, B., Hanrahan, K., Hunter, S. C., Kim, B., Cullen, L., & Kitson, A. (2021). Implementation science: Application of evidence-based practice models to improve healthcare quality. *Worldviews on Evidence-Based Nursing, 18*(2), 76–84. https://doi.org/10.1111/wvn.12495

Ubeda, S. R. G. (2022). How to build and assess the quality of healthcare-related research questions. *Global Journal on Quality and Safety in Healthcare, 5*(2), 39–43. https://doi.org/10.36401/JQSH-21-17

Vere, J., & Gibson, B. (2021). Variation amongst hierarchies of evidence. *Journal of Evaluation in Clinical Practice, 27*(3), 624–630. https://doi.org/10.1111/jep.13404

Wang, M., Zhang, Y., & Guo, M. (2021). Development of a cadre of evidence-based practice mentors for nurses: What works? *Worldviews on Evidence-Based Nursing, 18*(1), 8–14. https://doi.org/10.1111/wvn.12482

Yancey, N. R. (2019). Evidence-based practice in nursing for teaching-learning: But is it really nursing? *Nursing Science Quarterly, 32*(1), 25–28. https://doi.org/10.1177/0894318418807929

Ylimäki, S., Oikarinen, A., Kääriäinen, M., Holopainen, A., Oikarainen, A., Pölkki, T., Meriläinen, M., Lukkarila, P., Taam-Ukkonen, M., & Tuomikoski, A.-M. (2022). Advanced practice nurses' experiences of evidence-based practice: A qualitative study. *Nordic Journal of Nursing Research, 42*(4), 227–235. https://doi.org/10.1177/20571585221097658

CHAPTER 7

USING INFORMATION TECHNOLOGY TO IMPROVE POPULATION OUTCOMES

LAURA P. ROSSI AND ALYSSA E. ERIKSON

INTRODUCTION

Innovative technologies are now evolving to improve the timely and effective use of information to deliver patient-centered health care. For healthcare providers, it means improved access to tools that support clinical guidance in diagnosis, care planning, and monitoring. For patients and the general public, it means improved access to information to facilitate informed decisions about treatment and self-care management. New technology is also changing the way healthcare is delivered. Healthcare providers can remotely monitor physiologic and behavioral patterns of patients in real time. Virtual healthcare visits are becoming routine as a means of increasing access to consultation and specialized healthcare. This has been especially important for patients living in rural areas, as well as those burdened by age or chronic illness. From computers to smartphones, the recent explosion in technology constantly offers patients and their healthcare providers new opportunities to stay connected and manage care (Elenko et al., 2015). A proliferation of software applications is now available to provide scientific, as well as self-help, information. Devices monitor and track many activities of daily life, symptoms of health problems, and related responses. Communication devices are also now routinely integrated into the care delivery process to improve health team functioning with clinical decision aids, alerts for critical findings, and handoffs. Similarly, patients and families can also communicate more conveniently with healthcare providers directly through a variety of portals to obtain information, including procedural preparation, test results, and follow-up advice.

In direct care roles, advance practice registered nurses (APRNs) can maintain communication with patients and/or other healthcare providers as part of ongoing care. Information can be exchanged via teleconferencing, webcasts, podcasting, and social media accounts, to name just a few. Many platforms also exist to guide the collection of data to assess the impact of this technology on the quality-of-care delivery. Domain 7: Informatics and Healthcare Technologies for APRNs requires attention to the various information and communication technology tools used in the care of patients, communities, and populations (American Association of Colleges of Nursing, 2021). APRNs provide a unique and essential lens into how technology can be used to redesign care and assure nursing care is accessible and available where it is needed. This chapter describes the available technology to facilitate the analysis and improvement of care delivery processes, in particular, to assure the delivery of nursing care is visible and linked to improvements in individual and population health outcomes.

USING TECHNOLOGY IN CARE DELIVERY FOR POPULATIONS

A number of technologies are mainstream in healthcare to support ongoing collection of clinical data and routine care delivery. Numerous data elements, sources, and strategies are available in daily practice to address the health needs of individuals and populations over time. In this section, a summary of the resources that APRNs can use to improve population outcomes is provided.

ELECTRONIC HEALTH RECORDS AND HEALTH INFORMATION EXCHANGE

Electronic health records (EHR) systems are now in widespread use following the federal EHRs incentive programs designed to promote health information exchange (HIE) in the United States. Since that time, the transition to EHRs has transformed healthcare and significantly impacted professional practice. Clinicians can also be more efficient in documentation using templates to address regulatory and billing requirements. Ideally, these efficiencies potentially increase the time available for direct patient care. Electronic documentation also provides a convenient means for retrieving data in real time during a patient encounter to view patient progress and plan for follow-up. Aggregated data can provide insight into the trends in population needs and experiences that can alert or provide decision support for clinicians. Finally, the convenience and efficiency of aggregating data can support quality improvement efforts and original research. Identification of patterns has the potential to detect variations in patient needs that are unexplained by a medical diagnosis and/or a patient's stated reason for seeking healthcare. This detection of patterns can provide essential information to understand the effectiveness of care interventions and the need for staffing and other healthcare resources (Castellan et al., 2017; D'Agostino et al., 2019; Jones et al., 2010). Sanson et al. (2017) reviewed the available literature and found this data helpful in evaluating factors affecting patient outcomes, health service utilization, and health system performance.

Although EHRs are fully integrated into the healthcare system, the promise of EHRs has not been fully realized for many reasons (Honavar, 2020). Variability in vendor products and implementation across health systems has revealed many differences in the available fields, screens structures, and visibility of data. The sheer volume of data available can affect the clinician's ability to view and synthesize information in the clinical decision-making process. Template redundancies and lengthy problem lists can also contribute to cognitive overload. The tendency to drift into drop-downs and simple checklists does not consistently capture the patient's narrative which can lead to misdiagnosis and other clinical judgment errors.

While drop-down menus and checklists have the potential to improve efficiencies for nursing documentation, the lack of coherence in data collection structures can make care planning challenging during ongoing encounters with a single patient, as well as during movement across practice settings. Total reliance on a review of systems structures often fails to capture the patient's narrative about their activities of daily living and goals for care. The lack of standardized language among nurses makes it difficult to aggregate and consistently articulate the health concerns being addressed by nurses, which impedes the development of evidence demonstrating nursing's impact on the outcomes of care for individuals and/or populations (Rossi et al., 2023).

The introduction of big data models using artificial intelligence and machine learning now requires that nurses work together globally to assure nursing's unique disciplinary focus is captured in a consistent manner. A systematic review by Tastan et al. (2014) revealed the North American Nursing Diagnosis Association-International (NANDA-I), Nursing Interventions Classification (NIC), Nursing Outcomes Classification (NOC), or some combination of those three standardized nursing terminologies represented the predominant languages used in clinical practice. Less commonly used but recognized classifications included the Omaha System, the International Classification for Nursing Practice, the Clinical Care Classification/Home Health Care Classification, the Perioperative Nursing Data Set, and the Nursing Minimum Data Set. Many have also advocated for a standardized assessment structure for nursing using Gordon's functional health patterns (see Table 7.1) to assure data to support clinical decision-making by nurses is easily visible to guide care planning (Banister et al., 2022; Rossi et al., 2023).

The American Nursing Association (ANA, 2018) had recognized standardized languages and encourages their adoption for the EHR as appropriate for the specific setting type (see Table 7.2). These terminologies can facilitate the exchange of data with other settings for problems and care plans.

The Logical Observation Identifiers Names and Codes (LOINC®) is used for coding nursing assessments and outcomes while the Systematized Nomenclature of Medicine–Clinical Terms (SNOMED CT®) is more commonly used for problems, interventions, and observation findings. NANDA-I Nursing Diagnoses, NIC Interventions, NOC Outcomes, and NNN Linkages have been widely studied, and the evidence base supporting them will continue to evolve with an eye to consensus building about integration into the EHR (Macieira et al., 2018; Marcotullio et al., 2020; Moorhead et al., 2021; Swanson et al., 2021).

EHRs also provided the stimulus for institutions and practitioners to create greater access and transparency for patients so they can better understand their health status and engage in care (Tapuria et al., 2021). The development of patient portals has evolved to allow patients timely access to test results, appointment access, and direct communication with their care providers. OpenNotes evolved as the result of an international movement that urges healthcare providers to make notes that are written during visits, available to

TABLE 7.1 Definition of Functional Health Patterns

The following patterns were described by Gordon in the original text (1982). Patterns represent the patient's perception of typical daily living habits and routines that have been or can be affected by changes in health. The nurse obtains this health history as a basis for patient-centered care planning that considers the following: 1) each existing pattern, 2) factors affecting the patterns, and 3) the ways in which these patterns of living are managed to assure optimal health outcomes.

PATTERN	DEFINITION
Health status perception and management	View of one's health/well-being and how health is managed
Nutrition	Food and fluid consumption relative to metabolic need and local nutrient supply
Elimination	Regularity of excretory function including strategies and devices used to assist/control
Exercise/activity	Activities of daily living, leisure, and recreation
Sleep/rest	Sleep, rest, and relaxation practices
Sexuality/reproductive	Sexual preferences and satisfaction Reproductive patterns
Cognitive/perceptual	Cognitive and functional abilities including adequacy of sensory modes, experience of pain
Self-concept/self-perception	View of oneself as an individual and one's presentation
Coping–stress tolerance	Threshold and triggers for stress and effectiveness of coping strategies
Roles/relationships	Role engagements and responsibilities within the family and society
Values/beliefs	Life value, goals, or beliefs that guide choices or decisions

Source: Gordon, M. (1982). Nursing diagnosis: Process and application. McGraw-Hill Companies.

patients to read. OpenNotes is not a software program but rather a process that supports transparent communication between providers and patients (OpenNotes, 2019). Making such communication available directly to patients has the potential to improve safety by reinforcing therapeutic instructions, increasing patient engagement in self-care, and ultimately, improving the patient's health outcomes. Evidence suggests that there are strong preferences for "how to" learning through video demonstrations which can be streamed through portals rather than simply relying on printed text instructions (Smith et al., 2018).

USING TECHNOLOGY TO IMPROVE CARE DELIVERY PROCESSES

Shifts in population demographics and health demands have prompted considerable innovation in the use of technology to deliver care. The global response to the coronavirus disease 2019 (COVID-19) pandemic stimulated a significant expansion of this technology to address proximity and contact tracing, symptom monitoring, and quarantine control (Golinelli et al. 2020; Whitelaw et al., 2020). This experience has expanded our understanding of how care and

TABLE 7.2 ANA-Recognized Terminology and Data Set

ANA-RECOGNIZED TERMINOLOGY/DATASET	YEAR DEVELOPED	YEAR RECOGNIZED	NURSING CONTENT
NANDA-Nursing Diagnoses, Definitions, and Classification	1973	1992	Diagnoses
Omaha System	1975	1992	Diagnoses, interventions, outcome ratings
NMDS	1985	1999	Clinical data elements
NIC	1987	1992	Interventions
PNDS	1988	1999	Diagnoses, interventions, outcomes
CCC System	1988	1992	Diagnoses, interventions, outcome ratings
NMMDS	1989	1998	Management data elements
ICNP®	1989	2000	Diagnoses, interventions, outcomes
NOC	1991	1997	Outcomes
LOINC®	1994	2002	Assessments, outcomes
ABC Codes	1996	2000	Billing codes
SNOMED CT®	2000	1999	Diagnoses, interventions, outcomes, findings

ANA, American Nurses Association; CCC, Clinical Care Classification; ICNP®, International Classification for Nursing Practice; LOINC®, Logical Observation Identifiers Name and Codes; NANDA, North American Nursing Diagnosis Association; NIC, Nursing Interventions Classification; NMDS, Nursing Minimum Data Set; NMMDS, Nursing Management Minimum Data Set; NOC, Nursing Outcomes Classification; PNDS, Perioperative Nursing Data Set; SNOMED CT®, Systematized Nomenclature of Medicine-Clinical Terms.

Source: American Nurses Association. (2018). *Inclusion of recognized terminologies supporting nursing practice within electronic health records and other health information technology solutions.* www.nursingworld.org/practice-policy/nursing-excellence/official-position-statements/id/Inclusion-of-Recognized-Terminologies-Supporting-Nursing-Practice-within-Electronic-Health-Records/

important health messages can be delivered to support remote surveillance of disease symptoms and treatment adherence. In 2022, Internet penetration is estimated to be as high as 68% across the globe, with 93% penetration in North America (Internet World Stats, 2023). About three-quarters of U.S. adults own a desktop or laptop computer, and about half own a tablet computer. While ownership varies with age, education, and household income, technology has become a part of daily processes for care delivery (Pew Research Center, 2021a). In this section, we outline some of the ways in which technology can be used to improve care delivery processes and assure continuity of care outside the traditional hospital and clinical settings.

TELEMEDICINE STRATEGIES

Telemedicine is the diagnosis and treatment of patients by means of remote communication technology. Historically, it has been considered a reliable and promising method to increase access to populations particularly in rural and underserved areas where staff shortages and significant distances from healthcare facilities have prompted the use of innovative technology (Barbosa et al., 2021). Investigators have also shown that this technology has the potential to improve care for those who are socially isolated due to physical or financial limitations (Banbury et al., 2018).

Healthcare providers working with various populations have reported excellent results when using telemedicine in their practices for professional consultation and direct patient care. Indeed, specialty consultations and follow-up care have been associated with reduced costs and improvements in continuity and overall quality of care. Studies of newer rehabilitation models demonstrated the benefits of technology-based models (Gallagher et al., 2017; Oseran & Wasfy, 2019; Quanjel et al., 2019). Bellomo et al. (2020) reported that tele-rehabilitative therapy with home exercises in the form of interactive games for chronic stroke patients produced similar improvements in functional status, particularly in balance, motor and sensory function, and activities of daily living. In a scoping review, Alipour and Hayavi-Haghighi (2021) identified a variety of opportunities such as attention to improvements in clinical care delivery, organizational functioning (e.g., healthcare financing), application of technology, and assurance of equity. They also identified challenges in each of these categories, including the requirements for documentation and regulation.

Designing and implementing technology to provide care requires considerable insight into the patient experience, as well as technical expertise. Telemedicine workflows do not easily mimic in-person clinic visits, so determining the essential components of ambulatory care and how they can be adapted to the online environment is key. For example, how are vital signs and physical exams performed? How is medication reconciliation conducted? APRNs must be aware of both the benefits and the barriers as they plan for new services using advanced technologies. Patients and experts in the use of technology are key stakeholders in designing new interventions and care delivery programs that incorporate the use of technology. Implementing effective care delivery using telemedicine also requires appropriate training for patients and providers to maintain quality connections without interruption and assure patient confidentiality (see Chapter 8, "Concepts in Program Design and Development").

CASE STUDY

As the coordinator for the organ transplant program, an APRN is responsible to assure that patients receive information before they agree to a transplant and once they consent to a transplant. Upon evaluating the current materials, the APRN recognizes that some of the information patients and families receive does not address important issues that they need to know at the time of admission for their transplant. Further, they recognize that a long time can elapse while the patient is waiting. How can technology keep the APRN in touch with patients and families during this time so they have the necessary information when they need it?

MOBILE TELEPHONY AND MOBILE HEALTH

The general public is increasingly reliant on smartphones and other mobile devices. Estimates suggest that 97% of Americans own a cell phone and as many as 85% own a smartphone, usage which has more than doubled over the last decade (Pew Research Center, 2021b). With this trend, the use of remote technology to manage one's health has now been extended beyond clinical encounters in the hospital or outpatient visits. Mobile telephony (m-Health) allows for the transmission of health information using video and audio technologies, digital photography, and remote patient monitoring and services using cell phone technology (NEJM Catalyst, 2018).

Innovative technology demonstrated success as an enhancement for traditional cardiac rehabilitation (CR) with randomized trials using smartphone-based CR and avatars on social media platforms that demonstrated improvements in physical functioning (Dorje et al., 2019; Varnfield et al., 2014). While this work has typically focused on improving adherence and self-care behaviors, other benefits such as improved access and convenience for patients, as well as clinician efficiency in managing their caseloads, have also been identified. Payers and employers are also important stakeholders in the process and generally support the expanded use of telehealth strategies for their potential to reduce healthcare costs.

Texting has long been considered an effective strategy regardless of age or socioeconomic status and allows for individualization of the delivered message (Willcox et al., 2019). Reviews related to the use of mobile telephony and short message service (SMS) for patients with various chronic health conditions have been shown to facilitate behavior change and improved adherence to scheduled appointments and prescribed treatments. Although the use of text messaging and mobile phone applications to improve medication adherence has also shown promise in terms of feasibility and acceptability among adolescents with chronic illness, the approaches used to date have been varied with mixed results (Badawy et al., 2017).

Hilty et al. (2017) also reviewed opportunities for integrating mobile technology into mental healthcare and identified the need for clinicians to develop skills in using this technology and evaluate its effectiveness in care.

These examples illustrate the potential for improved outcomes from effective technology use and underscore the need for nurses to broaden their perspective as they design new interventions for specific populations. While pandemic experiences have informed the opportunities to gather data and plan interventions for improved public health, it has also raised many ethical and legal concerns about how policymakers and other decision-makers can and should use these tools in practice (Gasser et al., 2020). Snoswell et al. (2023) have also cautioned that while telehealth has not demonstrated any increase in mortality rates, we must be attentive to the potential for drift into a care delivery pattern that may be sub-optimal to in-person care.

USING TECHNOLOGY TO OBTAIN HEALTH INFORMATION

Technology is revolutionizing the way that health professionals and consumers worldwide access information and communicate with each other. Hitlin (2018) suggested that the United States had reached a plateau in the number of people who access the Internet.

A marked shift occurred in the number of people who relied solely on a smartphone to access the Internet, with more than 90% of adults younger than 50 years regularly online. Here, we summarize the different ways in which technology is being used to share and use health information.

INFORMATION AND INSTRUCTION

The use of technology in healthcare, education, and work settings became more commonplace due to the worldwide COVID-19 pandemic. Many sources of health information are now universally and readily accessible via the Internet. Population surveys indicate that approximately one in 10 people in the United States go online for health information (Gordon, 2021, pp. 1–5). While valuable and high-quality information is online, individuals can often be confused by the amount of data and unprepared to reconcile different facts in relation to the clinical scenarios at hand.

Although nurses and physicians are considered trusted sources of health information, many people, irrespective of gender, race, ethnicity, or political affiliation, will turn to the Internet first to gain some understanding about their condition, medications, and treatment options. In addition, quality ratings about providers and healthcare settings are now publicly available to inform decisions about where and how they can obtain care. Thapa et al. (2021) suggested that consumers use the information they find online to support the information they receive from their providers, although they identified the patient's relationship with their provider as an important factor in moderating potentially negative outcomes from online health information. This underscores the imperative for APRNs to use discretion in routinely evaluating patients' reliance and beliefs in online information, as well as providing guidance about valid and reliable sources of information. Timely access to information can be beneficial, but many organizations are challenged to update their websites and provide sufficient information that is applicable in individual situations.

PEER SUPPORT INTERVENTIONS

Over the last 20 years, web-based applications have been increasingly used to provide peer support to patients and caregivers with various conditions (Banbury et al., 2018; Vaughan et al., 2018). Peer support is generally intended to provide communication to groups of people with similar conditions using discussion forums, chat messaging, and video conferencing to deal with different circumstances related to diagnostic and treatment processes, as well as needs for caregiving by friends and loved ones. Varying degrees of benefit have been reported as people seek information and emotional support, and it is unclear the extent to which the presence of mediation by health professionals and trained peers has an impact (Berkanish et al., 2022). PatientsLikeMe (www.patientslikeme.com) is a unique digital health platform designed to facilitate patient access to health information through online communities with people with similar conditions. Blogs and other information resources to address self-monitoring and self-care strategies with personal agency establish PatientsLikeMe as a clinically robust resource with demonstrated impact, validated by more than 100 studies in peer-reviewed medical and scientific journals.

SELF-CARE AND BEHAVIOR CHANGE

Online education and coaching for groups and individuals to promote lifestyle changes such as smoking cessation, healthy eating, and weight control show successful results as well. Nothwehr (2013) demonstrated the feasibility of using remote coaching and a handheld electronic device with adults to increase the consumption of fruits and vegetables and decrease television viewing. Choi et al. (2014) described the effectiveness of a 16-week web-based nutrition program to assist patients with metabolic syndrome in decreasing overall body weight, waist circumference, body fat, and body mass index (BMI). Many commercial vendors have successfully adopted similar approaches and reported benefits, although there are inconsistencies in how program quality is measured. Cheung et al. (2017) suggested the need for greater transparency about the program offerings and related outcomes that can be achieved to avoid disappointment and frustration among participants about failed attempts at behavior change. Similarly, the requirements for one's digital literacy and threshold for computer use is another factor affecting positive outcome achievement.

Many studies have been conducted to determine how the use of technology can improve specific population outcomes and self-care behaviors alone and in combination with other interventions. Barnason et al. (2017) conducted a literature review of studies related to cardiovascular patient self-management. Based on this review, the authors recommend bundled strategies as the most beneficial method in optimizing self-care. Ultimately, caution must be exercised to determine the long-term effectiveness of these strategies in engaging patients in healthy behaviors. The novelty of technology use may impact use for different individuals initially but may not be sustained or necessary over time.

The Pew Internet Project tracks Internet use in many fields and reports that social determinants influence access to and use of online searches for health information. The *digital divide* is a term used to describe disparities in the use of the Internet and other forms of technology. It is often defined by age (younger people are more likely to use the Internet than older people), income (wealthier people are more likely to use the Internet than less wealthy people), geography (people living in urban or suburban areas are more likely to use the Internet than people in rural areas), and education (people who use the Internet tend to have attained higher degrees than people who do not). Some have predicted this divide will worsen in the coming years with the increasing emphasis on technology options for communication and care delivery (Pew Research Center, 2021c). Many individuals reported that the Internet served as a lifeline for them during the pandemic, prompting them to expand their use in ways they had not previously considered. On the other hand, many others have struggled with the fatigue and cost of increased reliance on the Internet (Pew Research Center, 2021b). APRNs must be attentive to not only the disparities in access to technology but also the patient's abilities and motivation to use available technology.

OPPORTUNITIES AND BARRIERS TO USING NEW TECHNOLOGY

The explosion of technologies is evolving to provide information that is timely and accessible to both clinicians and consumers to make decisions about treatment and care delivery. The proliferation of websites has also generated increasing concern about the reliability and trustworthiness of information for healthcare professionals as well as the general public. Indeed, online disinformation has been cited as a global risk due to individuals' limited ability to discern the credibility of online information (Ye, 2020). APRNs need to be mindful of both the usefulness and the limitations of technology.

Before making a decision about using online resources to supplement patient care, APRNs must conduct a comprehensive assessment about the patient's capacity and receptivity to using online communication. The prevalence of limited health literacy in the population suggests that routine screening, including an individual's reading ability, presence of any sensory deficits, and learning styles, must be integrated into routine practice. Consistent structures for documenting these assessments will facilitate data collection that supports aggregate analyses to better understand the population's needs and the profile of patients who may be disadvantaged. In this section, we summarize the opportunities for the future and the barriers to technology that nurse leaders must be aware of.

OPPORTUNITIES

Improved Clinical Decisions by Healthcare Providers

Researchers are now publishing at an exponential rate, often making it difficult for clinicians and patients to process and synthesize how the latest evidence is best applied in a particular situation. Similarly, no standard metric is adopted to capture the degree to which quality standards are achieved in various settings. This variety of metrics are publicly reported and impact healthcare system financing, as well as individual patient decisions about the choice of care providers. While these data are intended to improve decision-making about health, the plethora of available data can be confusing, making it difficult for providers as well as patients and families to make decisions. This underscores the need for a better understanding of the human-technology interface and the critical links between clinical data, essential interventions, and patient outcomes. Artificial intelligence and machine learning techniques are expected to contribute to the development of more valid and reliable alerts in the EHR to identify at-risk conditions and early signs of deterioration. For nursing, it will depend on the extent to which evidence evolves and supports a clearer and more standardized approach to documentation.

Tailored Patient Care and Shared Decision-Making

Many patients report that they use online health information to complement the information provided by their physicians. The patient–provider relationship is key to reducing the risk of potentially negative consequences occurring when information from various sources is not well synthesized or understood to one's specific circumstances (Thapa et al., 2021). APRNs have a unique opportunity to create trusting relationships with patients and families in terms of their life context and values related to health. It is critical that APRNs confirm a patient's ability, motivation, and preferences for health information to guide the appropriate selection of credible websites that can facilitate an accurate interpretation of this content in relation to their unique circumstances. Diviani et al. (2015) examined health literacy and its effect on the ability of persons to evaluate the effectiveness and accuracy of online information. Not unexpectedly, they determined that effective and informed evaluation of online health information is negatively impacted by low health literacy. Routinely encouraging patients and families to openly share any insights or concerns arising from online information with their healthcare providers will likely lead to earlier clarification and reduction in misunderstandings.

Improved Adherence to Self-Care

The Internet can also be a very helpful tool for APRNs and their patients to use for monitoring and tracking progress, as well as to explore alternative practices for the common goal of improving overall health. In recent years, there has been a proliferation of Internet applications ("apps") intended to help patients with a variety of self-care tasks. While similar concerns about the accuracy of the evidence base and the lack of regulation exist, apps also require attention to usability, privacy, security, and functionality. Boudreaux et al. (2014) recommend several strategies to guide their evaluation and selection. Searching the scientific literature, clearinghouses, and stores related to the use of a particular app can be useful in understanding a complete description of the app, any comparable products to address the specific self-care behavior, and user ratings and reviews. These search strategies are often limited by the lack of formal trials and standards and the difficulties in finding current information, as new technology is almost continuously evolving. Using social media to query professionals and patient groups can provide additional guidance in the process of selecting an app for a particular population.

Patients, consumers, and healthcare professionals also need to be educated on good practices of data sharing and access when they go online or use an app. Staccini and Lau (2018) suggested there is a need for more emphasis on considering the privacy features in the app's design, specific approaches to consent and data sharing mechanisms for users, and any sociodemographic characteristics that may influence access to personal health information. Perhaps the most effective techniques to guide selection of an app are in piloting its use and soliciting feedback from the patient population for whom the app is being selected. This will provide essential insights into the factors affecting the usefulness of the app for the targeted disease or health behavior and what might be required for successful implementation in the practice setting. More primary research is needed to determine the efficacy of health apps and their impact on health outcomes.

BARRIERS

Use of Social Media

Various social networking sites and communication methods, such as Facebook, LinkedIn, Pinterest, Tumblr, X (formerly Twitter), Instagram, TikTok, email, chat rooms, and texting, are widely used to exchange information. These communication channels are not well controlled and can often serve as a distraction for healthcare providers, patients, and families. The quality and accuracy of the available information and the privacy on such sites are often not well controlled. Some have suggested that the "new normal" of relying on technology may widen the digital divide and resulting healthcare disparities (Pew Research Center, 2021c).

Professional organizations have written guidelines for the use of social media, emphasizing patient confidentiality as a legal and ethical responsibility. Complaints to the

State Boards of Nursing against nurses who use social media have included patient privacy breaches as well as negative communication toward colleagues and/or employers (Balestra, 2018; Vukušić Rukavina et al., 2021). The Internet can be a valuable tool for patient care, communication, and social interaction and for boosting one's career, but nurses have also been fired, lost their licenses, and experienced bullying, all within the context of social media. The National Council of State Boards of Nursing (NCSBN) has produced social media guidelines for nurses. A video is available at www.ncsbn.org/347.htm, and *A Nurse's Guide to Professional Boundaries* (*NCSBN*) is located at www.ncsbn.org/ProfessionalBoundaries_Complete.pdf. Among the most important facts for people who use social media to remember is that once information is posted on the Internet, it is posted permanently, and that privacy settings are not 100% effective.

Patient Factors

Healthcare providers must also be attentive to patients' use of and vulnerability to social media messages. Many patients and family members will find online posts from others with similar health concerns, such as childhood illnesses and weight loss or conditions such as cancer or diabetes, helpful for information or a source of social support (Farrell, 2018; Vaughan et al., 2018). While the majority of information on these sites may be accurate, one must remain cautious about the misinformation arising from opinion and hearsay, without scientific evidence, that may be shared and interpreted incorrectly. Various investigators have also suggested that the browsers used can influence the sites that are accessed (Modave et al., 2014; Narasimhulu et al., 2016).

An individual's level of trust in online information varies and may be influenced by their interest in the specific piece of information, their level of stress, their sense of urgency, and how engaged they are in their plan of care (Horrigan, 2017). Reading level and comprehension are other major factors affecting an individual's understanding acceptance of online information. Social isolation and Internet dependency may also make the public more vulnerable to misinformation. Frequently, people are unaware of an organization or a company's influence through advertising. The world witnessed the most dramatic example of how social media influenced health behavior during the COVID-19 pandemic. Concerns about how politics, trust in government, and personal beliefs in conspiracy fueled social media postings spreading vaccine misinformation, influencing the global adoption of available COVID-19 vaccines (Jennings et al., 2021; Puri et al., 2020; Rathje et al., 2022).

Technical Issues

Technical issues can also lead to substantial barriers when one is seeking information or involved in a clinical encounter. Equipment updates and system downtimes create inconvenient delays and frustration for patients and providers. Local bandwidth can be an issue in remote areas and requires attention to the potential disparities in access. Assessing populations for their patterns of technology use is an important part of the APRN's role. Equally important are the privacy issues that often create a reluctance in adopting technology. Research and program evaluations are needed to fully evaluate the advantages and disadvantages of using technology in populations to improve health while maintaining privacy and sustainability.

The increased reliance on technology to engage patients in care raises concern for people who may face barriers to access or difficulties during their healthcare experiences. While 90% of Americans report that Internet technology has been essential or important to them following the pandemic, many people still struggle with the cost and fatigue of online communication (Pew Research Center, 2021a). APRNs must understand the patterns and preferences of technology use among different individuals and groups to effectively plan for its implementation in direct care or healthcare program planning. There must be a realistic appraisal of how technology can and should be used for self-care skill development in different populations. Limitations at the individual level require appropriate assistance for adoption or alternative sources of information, as systems increasingly shift to online materials and processes that require reading comprehension. Aggregating such utilization data (e.g., who uses the Internet, what types of information they are looking for, and what types of devices and methods they use to search for information) can provide insights into the needs for program development as discussed in Chapter 8, "Concepts in Program Design and Development."

EVALUATING THE QUALITY OF ONLINE INFORMATION

While online information provides many opportunities for advancing healthcare, caution is required to evaluate the accuracy of various sources of information and consider the ways in which Internet sources can be used effectively. APRNs have an opportunity to better serve their population by helping consumers use the Internet wisely and directing them to sites that provide evidence-based information and privacy protection. It is critical that they be prepared to evaluate websites for current and accurate information, given the evidence that many Internet consumers do not confirm the validity of the Internet resources that they use.

The Medical Library Association (MLA, 2019) and the U.S. National Library of Medicine (NLM) provide guidelines for evaluating online information. Links to these sites can be found in Table 7.3. The NLM has partnered with MedlinePlus (MedlinePlus, 2016) to create a useful tutorial for all audiences entitled *Evaluating Internet Health Information: A Tutorial from the National Library of Medicine*, which is accessible

TABLE 7.3 Links for Evaluating Online Information

RESOURCE	INFORMATION AVAILABLE
Medical Library Association: www.mlanet.org/p/cm/ld/fid=1717	Use the "For Health Consumers and Patients" link to find the MLA user's guide to finding and evaluating health information on the web, MLA's top health websites, and Deciphering Medspeak (What Did My Doctor Say?).
U.S. National Library of Medicine: www.nnlm.gov/public-libraries/evaluating-health-information	Use the health information site to find the guide to healthy web surfing, medical information on the Internet tutorial (from Medlineplus), Health Library Directory, and dozens of links for safe health resources for consumers.

at Evaluating Internet Health Information: A Tutorial from the National Library of Medicine (medlineplus.gov).

In the context of growing concerns about misinformation, various tools have been developed to evaluate online sources and cited as the criteria for evaluating the trustworthiness and usefulness of online health information. The SIFT guide suggests one should stop; investigate a source; find a trusted resource to corroborate; and trace claims, quotes, and media to some original source. The CRAAP is an acronym that reflects key indicators for currency, relevance, authority, accuracy, and purpose. DISCERN is another instrument that was developed by a team in the United Kingdom to evaluate and produce online information (www.discern.org.uk/background_to_discern.php). Portillo et al. (2021) reported on an evaluation of information on frequently used consumer health information websites related to COVID-19 pandemic. These investigators reported the five most frequently appearing websites included WebMD, Mayo Clinic, Healthline, MedlinePlus, and Medical News Today, respectively. DISCERN and CRAAP scores indicated that MedlinePlus was the most reliable health website.

- Who runs the site?

    Check the address (uniform resource locator or URL) of the website. Government sites have *.gov* in the address, educational institutions have *.edu*, and professional sites have *.org* suffixes. Commercial sites have *.com* in the address. Commercial sites may exist for commercial reasons—to sell products—but many provide useful and balanced information. Go to the "About Us" page. The sponsor and the credentials of the people who run the site should be clearly identified. The site should also include a method for contacting the webmaster or the people responsible for maintaining the site.

- Why have they created the site?

    The site should identify its intended audience. Some sites have separate sections for consumers and for health professionals, whereas other sites are designed exclusively for either health professionals or consumers.

- Who is sponsoring the site? Does the information favor the sponsor?

    The website should disclose all financial relationships such as the source of funding for the site. Advertisements should be clearly labeled as such. Users should examine sites for balanced information that does not favor a sponsor.

- Where did the information come from? Is the information reviewed by experts?

    Websites should provide the credentials of contributors and the process for selecting information that is posted. Look for information on an editorial board; this can usually be found on the "About Us" page. Look for a statement that indicates that it is a peer-reviewed site. The information on the site should be presented clearly and should be factual, not opinion.

- Is it up to date?

    Websites, especially those that provide health-related information, should be current and updated on a regular basis. Dates should be clearly posted.

- Is it readable?

    The website should present material that is visible for those with limited vision. The written word should be accessible for the intended audience and consider developmental stage, language, and literacy level. Illustrations should be used effectively to address complex topics.

- What is the privacy policy?

    There should be a privacy policy posted on the site. Check the policy to see whether information is shared. Do not provide personal information unless the privacy policy clearly states what information is and is not shared.

    In general, patients and the general public should be vigilant when using and interpreting information obtained on the World Wide Web.

ELECTRONIC RESOURCES THAT SUPPORT POPULATION-BASED NURSING

There are many Internet resources identified throughout this text that can be used to support population-based nursing. Table 7.4 provides many reputable online sites. The list and the descriptions of the sites are not meant to be exhaustive but can be used as a guide by APRNs to find sources of reliable health information.

The preeminent international source of health information is the World Health Organization (WHO). The U.S. Department of Health and Human Services (DHHS) is the U.S. government's principal agency for protecting the health of all Americans. It provides essential services (such as Medicare) and administers more grant dollars than all other federal agencies combined. Government sites (which have .gov in the URL) are a rich source of information and offer a variety of resources for both consumers and healthcare providers. Nongovernmental websites are also a source of excellent information for healthcare providers and consumers. Sites with .edu, owned by educational institutions, have extensive resources available for people who are looking for information on health-related topics, particularly universities that offer health-related degrees. Many professional organizations are operated as not-for-profits and work to further the interests of a profession and to protect the public. They are generally a rich source of information about healthcare professions and usually have .org in the address. APRNs should search their specialty organizations for resources and information.

Nonprofit organizations use their earnings to pursue their goals by providing resources to support and disseminate new knowledge to professionals and the general public. Well-known examples are the American Heart Association (AHA), the American Cancer Society (ACS), and the Asthma and Allergy Foundation of America (AAFA). Many of these sites have an impressive amount of information and resources available, often free of charge. Most of these groups have .org in their URLs. Many commercial (.com) sites can also be useful but should be evaluated carefully to ensure balance and accuracy in the information provided.

TABLE 7.4 Internet Resources That Support Population-Based Nursing

GOVERNMENT	LINK	DESCRIPTION
Agency for Healthcare Research and Quality	www.ahrq.gov	Information to guide consumers, employers, policymakers, and healthcare providers in decision-making, including health IT tools, recent research findings, available databases, and funding opportunities for research
Centers for Disease Control and Prevention	www.cdc.gov	Preeminent source of information for consumers, health professionals, policymakers, researchers, and educators including a large range of topics, including U.S. trend data and available clinical and educational tools (BMI calculator and educational slides), as well as professional reports (EID, MMWR, PCD, etc.)
Healthfinder.gov	healthfinder.gov	Easy-to-understand information about preventive health and how to access services. Health facilities and providers. A Guide to Everyday Healthy Living is available on various topics.
National Center for Complementary and Integrative Health	nccih.nih.gov/health/webresources	Source of information about research and application of complementary health products and practices
National Center for Health Statistics	www.cdc.gov/nchs	Full range of statistical data produced by the federal government linking to more than 100 agencies that provide data and trend information on such topics as diseases, demographics, education, healthcare, and crime
StopBullying.gov	www.stopbullying.gov	Information for all ages about the recognition, prevention, and termination of bullying and available services
The National Guideline Clearinghouse	www.guideline.gov	Public resource within AHRQ site for evidence-based practice guidelines This site is no longer funded. Guideline acceptance ended in March 2018.
The National Institutes of Health	www.nih.gov	Information about research funding and many science and health topics including slides and print material
U.S. Department of Health and Human Services	www.hhs.gov	Broad range of information related to healthcare including programs, insurance, laws, and regulations Project funding announcements are also available.

(continued)

7 USING INFORMATION TECHNOLOGY TO IMPROVE POPULATION OUTCOMES

TABLE 7.4 Internet Resources That Support Population-Based Nursing (*continued*)

GOVERNMENT	LINK	DESCRIPTION
Education		
American Nurses Association	www.nursingworld.org	Official source of information for professional registered nurses in the United States with 54 constituent member nurses associations and affiliations with 35 specialty nursing and workforce advocacy affiliate organizations; outlines standards of practice, lobbies regulatory agencies affective nurses and the general public, including an online consumer health resource developed and launched in 2011
American Public Health Association	www.apha.org	Professional source of information for public health professionals whose goals are to increase access to healthcare, protect funding for core public health services, and eliminate health disparities
HealthCareandYou.org	www.healthcareandyou.org	Explanation of the provisions and benefits in the Affordable Care Act by state, in language and format accessible to consumers
Howard Gotlieb Archival Research Center, Boston University	hgar-srv3.bu.edu/collections/nursing	Widely respected source of nursing history addressing the early years of nursing and public health including a collection of personal and professional papers, including 250 of Florence Nightingale's letters and records of schools and organizations within this country and internationally
National Academy of Medicine (formerly the Institute of Medicine)	nam.edu	Independent, nonprofit, nongovernmental source (within the National Academy of Sciences), with "unbiased and authoritative advice to decision-makers and the public" responsive to mandates from Congress, federal agencies, and independent organizations; list of available reports published after 1998
The American Nurses Credentialing Center, a subsidiary of ANA	www.nursingworld.org/ancc	Source of standards for professional nursing certification, continuing nursing education accreditation, and oversight for the Magnet Recognition Program

(*continued*)

TABLE 7.4 Internet Resources That Support Population-Based Nursing (*continued*)

GOVERNMENT	LINK	DESCRIPTION
Nonprofit		
American Cancer Society	www.cancer.org	Independent, nonprofit source of science, practice guidelines, and related health information for cancer prevention and treatment, including resources and software applications for educators, consumers, and healthcare professionals at all levels
American Heart Association	www.heart.org	Independent, nonprofit source of science, practice guidelines, and related health information for prevention and treatment of cardiovascular disease and stroke, including resources and software applications for educators, consumers, and healthcare professionals at all levels
Asthma and Allergy Foundation of America	www.aafa.org	Independent, nonprofit source of science, practice guidelines, and related health information for the prevention and treatment of asthma and allergies, including resources and software applications for educators, consumers, and healthcare professionals at all levels
The Pew Research Center, a subsidiary of the Pew Charitable Trusts	www.pewresearch.org	Respected source of public information from polls, demographic research, media content analysis, and other empirical social science research reflecting the issues, attitudes, and trends shaping America and the world
International		
World Health Organization (arm of the United Nations)	www.who.int	Source of global health matters and technical support for different countries related to health trends, including publications and resources in many languages on disease outbreaks, various health topics, and evidence-based clinical guidelines; multimedia site with information via podcasts and videos on various health topics for international travelers
Commercial		
Medscape	www.medscape.com	Online, peer-reviewed, free resource for health professionals, including peer-reviewed original articles and continuing medical and nursing education; offers a customized version of the NLM's MEDLINE database, a drug interaction checker, and a drug reference, with free downloadable apps for health professionals; copyright restrictions and privacy protection apply

(*continued*)

TABLE 7.4 Internet Resources That Support Population-Based Nursing (*continued*)

GOVERNMENT	LINK	DESCRIPTION
Analytic		
Epi Info	www.cdc.gov/epiinfo	A collection of free software tools available through the CDC website that can be used to create questionnaires, download data, and perform advanced statistical analyses and GIS mapping that allows users to map trends in disease or outcomes of interest using zip codes or city boundaries and integrate data into a geographical map to summarize health services utilization data based on geographical location
The ViSta	www.uv.es/visualstats/Book	Free, downloadable statistical system that can be used for both descriptive and inferential analytic analyses (copyright restrictions apply)

AHRQ, Agency for Healthcare Research and Quality; ANA, American Nurses Association; BMI, body mass index; CDC, Centers for Disease Control and Prevention; EID, Emerging Infectious Diseases; GIS, geographic information system; IT, information technology; MMWR, Morbidity and Mortality Weekly Report; NLM, National Library of Medicine; PCD, Preventing Chronic Disease; ViSta, Visual Statistics System.

CASE STUDY

A nurse specialist for cardiology patients was asked to develop educational materials to support self-care for patients after an acute event. This is an ideal time to engage patients in risk reduction efforts, but there is little time in the hospital to cover the many topics related to medications, lifestyle modifications, and follow-up. Knowing that patients and families can only absorb so much new knowledge for self-care at one time, how might the APRN design the information so patients' priorities and preferences are considered? Which patients will benefit from self-guided online instructions? What information will be best communicated directly with in person visits versus telehealth strategies? Take some time to think about how the APRN might design the current technology in a health system to make this information available to patients and families at their convenience.

SUMMARY

Technological innovation has become an important part of daily life in the form of smart TVs, wearable devices, household thermostats, and security systems. In the fast-moving world of healthcare, it has generated a whole new lexicon for healthcare providers and provided new opportunities for improving population outcomes. Software apps that can be downloaded to mobile devices and updated on a regular basis make important clinical information immediately available for clinicians and patients alike. Electronic alerts, really simple syndication (RSS), podcasts, videoconferencing, and social media are efficient and cost-effective ways to deliver healthcare information to both consumers and healthcare professionals. E-health also provides a means to enhance continuity of care and bridge the gap between patients and healthcare providers. Evidence is continuing to accumulate about how technology can be implemented and its long-term effectiveness on patient outcomes.

The examples cited in this chapter offer a mere glimpse into the opportunities for APRN creativity in improving patient outcomes. APRNs need to be technologically literate and willing to explore new ways to deliver healthcare. They must stay abreast of this evolving field, carefully evaluating the available resources for their potential application in practice. This is essential as APRNs lead care improvement activities and address future health demands. Of primary concern are the legal and ethical responsibilities related to patient preferences and privacy. Regardless of these challenges, technology is here to stay, and it is the responsibility of APRNs to educate themselves and their patients to use discretion in their use of technology.

END-OF-CHAPTER RESOURCES

EXERCISES AND DISCUSSION QUESTIONS

EXERCISE 7.1 Online databases are a rich source of information for healthcare professionals. Use the following CDC database to research the state that you live or work in: www.cdc.gov/nchs/data-visualization/mortality-leading-causes/index.htm.

- How do the leading causes of death in your state compare to national figures?
- Identify five important risk factors that need to be targeted in your state.
- Identify vulnerable groups for whom targeted services need to be provided.

EXERCISE 7.2 Using the criteria and guidelines provided in this chapter, identify two credible websites for patients with a chronic illness who manage their own care at home. Consider sources that address self-management practices such as diet, activity, and medication management. What are the strengths and weaknesses of the sites that you found?

EXERCISE 7.3 Identify at least two technological innovations that are used to manage the care of the population that you serve. What factors influenced the choice of these particular innovations? How do you (or how do you plan to) evaluate their effectiveness? What outcomes do you hope to achieve through their use?

A robust set of instructor resources designed to supplement this text is located at http://connect.springerpub.com/content/book/978-0-8261-4377-8. Qualifying instructors may request access by emailing textbook@springerpub.com.

REFERENCES

Alipour, J. & Hayavi-Haghighi, M.H. (2021). Opportunities and challenges of telehealth in disease management during COVID-19 pandemic: A scoping review. *Applied Clinical Informatics, 12*(4), 864–876. https://doi.org/10.1055/s-0041-1735181

American Association of Colleges of Nursing. (2021). *The essentials: Core competencies for professional nursing education*. https://www.aacnnursing.org/Portals/42/AcademicNursing/pdf/Essentials-2021.pdf

American Nurses Association. (2018). *Inclusion of recognized terminologies supporting nursing practice within electronic health records and other health information technology solutions*. https://www.nursingworld.org/practice-policy/nursing-excellence/official-position-statements/id/Inclusion-of-Recognized-Terminologies-Supporting-Nursing-Practice-within-Electronic-Health-Records/

Badawy, S., Barrera, L., Sinno, M., Kaviany, S., O'Dwyer, L., & Kuhns, L. (2017). Text messaging and mobile phone apps as interventions to improve adherence in adolescents with chronic health conditions: A systematic review. *JMIR Mhealth Uhealth, 5*(4), e66. https://doi.org/10.2196/mhealth.7798

Balestra, M. (2018). Social media missteps could put your nursing license at risk. *American Nurse Today, 13*(3), 21–22.

Banbury, A., Nancarrow, S., Dart, J., Gray, L., & Parkinson, L. (2018). Telehealth interventions delivering home-based support group videoconferencing: Systematic review. *Journal of Medical Internet Research, 20*(2), e25. https://doi.org/10.2196/jmir.8090

Banister, G., Carroll, D. L., Dickins, K., Flanagan, J., Jones, D., Looby, S. E., & Cahill, J. E. (2022). Nurse-sensitive indicators during COVID-19. *International Journal of Nursing Knowledge, 33*(3), 234–244. https://doi.org/10.1111/2047-3095.12372

Barbosa, W., Zhou, K., Waddell, E., Myers, T., & Dorsey, E. R. (2021). Improving access to care: Telemedicine across medical domains. *Annual Review Public Health, 42*, 463–481. https://doi.org/10.1146/annurev-publhealth-090519-093711

Barnason, S., White-Williams, C., Rossi, L. P., Centeno, M., Crabbe, D. L., Lee, K. S., McCabe, N., Nauser, J., Schulz, P., Stamp, K., & Wood, K. (2017). Evidence for therapeutic patient education interventions to promote cardiovascular patient self-management: A scientific statement for healthcare professionals from the American Heart Association. *Circulation: Cardiovascular Quality and Outcomes, 10*(6), 1–6. https://doi.org/10.1161/HCQ.0000000000000025

Bellomo, R. G., Paolucci T., Saggino, A., Pezzi, L., Bramanti, A., Cimino, V., Tommasi, M., & Saggini, R. (2020). The WeReha project for an innovative home-based exercise training in chronic stroke patients: A clinical study. *Journal of Central Nervous System Disease, 12*. https://doi.org/10.1177/1179573520979866

Berkanish, P., Pan, S., & Viola, A., Rademaker, Q., & Devine, K. A. (2022). Technology-based peer support interventions for adolescents with chronic illness: A systematic review. *Journal of Clinical Psychology in Medical Settings, 29*(4), 911–942. https://doi.org/10.1007/s10880-022-09853-0

Boudreaux, E. D., Waring, M. E., Hayes, R. B., Sadasivam, R. S., Mullen, S., & Pagoto, S. (2014). Evaluating and selecting mobile health apps: Strategies for healthcare providers and healthcare organizations. *Society of Behavioral Medicine, 4*(4), 363–371. https://doi.org/10.1007/s13142-014-0293-9

Castellan, C., Sluga, S., Spina, E., & Sanson, G. (2016). Nursing diagnoses, outcomes and interventions as measures of patient complexity and nursing care requirement in intensive care unit. *Journal of Advanced Nursing, 72*(6), 1273–1286. https://doi.org/10.1111/jan.12913

Cheung, K. L., Wijnen, B., & de Vries, H. (2017). A review of the theoretical basis, effects, and cost effectiveness of online smoking cessation interventions in the Netherlands: A mixed-methods approach. *Journal of Medical Internet Research, 19*(6), e230. https://doi.org/10.2196/jmir.7209

Choi, Y., Lee, M. J., Kang, H. C., Lee, M. S., & Yoon, S. (2014). Development and application of a web-based nutritional management program to improve dietary behaviors for the prevention of metabolic syndrome. *Computers, informatics, nursing: CIN, 32*(5), 232–241. https://doi.org/10.1097/CIN.0000000000000054

D'Agostino, F., Vellone, E., Cocchieri, A., Welton, J., Maurici, M., Polistena, B., Spandanaro, F., Zega, M., Alvaro, R., & Sanson, G. (2019). Nursing diagnoses as predictors of hospital length of stay: A prospective observational study. *Journal of Nursing Scholarship, 51*(1), 96–105. https://doi.org/10.1111/jnu.12444

DISCERN retrieved from http://www.discern.org.uk/good_practice.php

Diviani, N., van den Putte, B., Giani, S., & van Weert, J. C. (2015). Low health literacy and evaluation of online health information: A systematic review of the literature. *Journal of Medical Internet Research, 17*(5), e112. https://doi.org/10.2196/jmir.4018

Dorje, T., Zhao, G., Tso, K., Wang, J., Chen, Y., Tsokey, L., Tan, B. K., Scheer, A., Jacques, A., Li, Z., Wang, R., Chow, C. K., Ge, J., & Maiorana, A. (2019). Smartphone and social media-based cardiac rehabilitation and secondary prevention in China (SMART-CR/SP): A parallel-group, single-blind, randomised controlled trial. *Lancet Digital Health, 1*(7), e363–e374. https://doi.org/10.1016/S2589-7500(19)30151-7

Elenko, E., Underwood, L., & Zohar, D. (2015). Defining digital medicine. *Nature Biotechnology, 33*(5), 456. https://doi.org/10.1038/nbt.3222

Farrell, A. (2018). Accuracy of online discussion forums on common childhood ailments. *Journal of the Medical Library Association, 106*(4), 455–463. https://doi.org/10.5195/jmla.2018.355

Gallagher, J., James, S., Keane, C., Fitzgerald, A., Travers, B., Quigley, E., Hecht, C., Zhou, S., Watson, C., Ledwidge, M., & McDonald, K. (2017). Heart failure virtual consultation: bridging the gap of heart failure care in the community: A mixed-methods evaluation. *ESC Heart Failure, 4*(3), 252–258. https://doi.org/10.1002/ehf2.12163

Gasser, U., Ienca, M., Scheibner, J., Sleigh, J., & Vayena, E. (2020). Digital tools against COVID-19: Taxonomy, ethical challenges, and navigation aid. *Lancet Digital Health, 2*(8), e425–e434. https://doi.org/10.1016/S2589-7500(20)30137-0

Golinelli, D., Boetto, E., Carullo, G., Nuzzolese, A., Landini, M., & Fantini, M. (2020). Adoption of digital technologies in health care during the COVID-19 pandemic: Systematic review of early scientific literature. *Journal of Medical Internet Research, 22*(11), e22280. https://doi.org/10.2196/22280

Gordon, D. (2021). *1 in 10 Americans turn to social media for health information, new survey shows.* Retrieved from https://www.forbes.com/sites/debgordon/2021/10/06/1-in-10-americans-turn-to-social-media-for-health-information-new-survey-shows/?sh=2b5d893b3

Gordon, M. (1982). *Nursing diagnosis: Process and application.* McGraw-Hill Companies.

Hilty, D. M., Chan, S., Hwang, T., Wong, A., & Bauer, A. M. (2017). Advances in mobile mental health: Opportunities and implications for the spectrum of e-mental health services. *mHealth, 3*(34). https://doi.org/10.21037/mhealth.2017.06.02

Hitlin, P. (2018). *Internet, social media use and device ownership in the U.S. have plateaued after years of growth.* http://www.pewresearch.org/fact-tank/2018/09/28/internet-social-media-use-and-device-ownership-in-u-s-have-plateaued-after-years-of-growth

Honavar, S. G. (2020). Electronic medical records—The good, the bad and the ugly. *Indian Journal of Ophthalmology, 68*(3), 417–418. https://doi.org/10.4103/ijo.IJO_278_20

Horrigan, J. B. (2017). *How people approach facts and information.* http://www.pewinternet.org/2017/09/11/how-people-approach-facts-and-information

Internet World Stats. (2023). *Usage and population statistics.* Retrieved May 15, 2023 from https://www.internetworldstats.com

Jennings, W., Stoker, G., Bunting, H., ValgarÐsson, V. O., Gaskell, J., Devine, D., McKay, L., & Mills, M. C. (2021). Lack of trust, conspiracy beliefs, and social media use predict COVID-19 vaccine hesitancy. *Vaccines, 9*(6), 593. https://doi.org/10.3390/vaccines9060593

Jones, D. J., Lunney, M., Keenan, G., & Moorhead, S. (2010). Standardized nursing languages: Essential for the nursing workforce. *Annual Review of Nursing Research, 28*, 253–294. https://doi.org/10.1891/0739-6686.28.253

Macieira, T. G. R., Smith, M. B., Davis, N., Yao, Y., Wilkie, D. J., Lopez, K. D., & Keenan, G. (2018). Evidence of progress in making nursing practice visible using standardized nursing data: A systematic review. *AMIA Annual Symposium Proceedings, 2017*, 1205–1214.

Marcotullio, A., Caponnetto, V., La Cerra, C., Toccaceli, A., & Lancia, L. (2020). NANDA-I, NIC, and NOC taxonomies, patients' satisfaction, and nurses' perception of the work environment: An Italian cross-sectional pilot study. *Acta Biomedica, 20*(91), 85–91. https://doi.org/10.23750/abm.v91i6-S.8951

Medical Library Association. (2019). For health consumers and patients: Find good health information. https://www.mlanet.org/page/find-good-health-information

MedlinePlus. (2016). *Evaluating Internet health information: A tutorial from the National Library of Medicine.* http://www.nlm.nih.gov/medlineplus/webeval/webeval.html

Modave, F., Shokar, N., Penaranda, E., & Nguyen, N. (2014). Analysis of the accuracy of weight loss information search engine results on the Internet. *American Journal of Public Health, 104*(10), 1971–1978. https://doi.org/10.2105/AJPH.2014.302070

Moorhead, S., Macieira, T. G. R., Lopez, K. D., Mantovani, V. M., Swanson, E., Wagner, C., & Abe, N. (2021). NANDA-I, NOC, and NIC linkages to SARS-CoV-2 (COVID-19). Part 1. Community response. *International Journal of Nursing Knowledge, 32*(1), 59–67. https://doi.org/10.1111/2047-3095.12291

Narasimhulu, D. M., Karakash, S., Weedon, J., & Minkoff, H. (2016). Patterns of Internet use by pregnant women, and reliability of pregnancy-related searches. *Journal of Maternal Child Health, 20*, 2502–2509. https://doi.org/10.1007/s10995-016-2075-0

NEJM Catalyst. (2018). *What is telehealth?* https://catalyst.nejm.org/doi/full/10.1056/CAT.18.0268

Nothwehr, F. (2013). People with unhealthy lifestyle behaviors benefit from remote coaching via mobile technology. *Evidence Based Nursing, 16*(1), 22–23. http://dx.doi.org/10.1136/eb-2012-100953

Open Library. Advanced Professional Communication. Chapter 10.9: Evaluating Professional Sources. https://ecampusontario.pressbooks.pub/llsadvcomm/chapter/10-9-evaluating-sources

OpenNotes. (2019). *Everyone on the same page.* https://www.opennotes.org

Oseran, A. S., & Wasfy, J. H. (2019). Early experiences with cardiology electronic consults: A systematic review. *American Heart Journal, 215*, 139–146. https://doi.org/10.1016/j.ahj.2019.06.013

Pew Research Center. (2021a). *The Internet and the pandemic.* https://www.pewresearch.org/internet/2021/09/01/the-internet-and-the-pandemic/

Pew Research Center. (2021b). *Experts say the 'new normal' in 2025 will be far more tech-driven, presenting more big challenges.* https://www.pewresearch.org/internet/2021/02/18/experts-say-the-new-normal-in-2025-will-be-far-more-tech-driven-presenting-more-big-challenges/

Pew Research Center. (2021c). *Mobile fact sheet.* Retrieved from: https://www.pewresearch.org/internet/fact-sheet/mobile/

Portillo, I. A., Johnson, C. V., & Johnson, S. Y. (2021). Quality evaluation of consumer health information websites found on Google using DISCERN, CRAAP, and HONcode, *Medical Reference Services Quarterly, 40*(4), 396–407. https://doi.org/10.1080/02763869.2021.1987799

Puri, N., Coomes, E. A., Haghbayan, H., & Gunaratne, K. (2020). Social media and vaccine hesitancy: New updates for the era of COVID-19 and globalized infectious diseases. *Human Vaccines & Immunotherapeutics, 16*(11), 2586–2593. https://doi.org/10.1080/21645515.2020.1780846

Quanjel, T. C. C., Spreeuwenberg, M. D., Struijs, J. N., Baan, C. A., & Ruwaard, D. (2019). Substituting hospital-based outpatient cardiology care: The impact on quality, health and costs. *PLoS One, 14*, e0217923. https://doi.org/10.1371/journal.pone.0217923

Rathje, S., He, J. K., Roozenbeek, J., Van Bavel, J. J., & van der Linden, S. (2022). Social media behavior is associated with vaccine hesitancy. *PNAS Nexus, 1*, 1–11. https://doi.org/10.1093/pnasnexus/pgac207

Rossi, L., Butler, S., Coakley, A., & Flanagan, J. (2023). Nursing knowledge captured in electronic health records. *International Journal of Nursing Knowledge, 34*(1), 72–84. https://doi.org/10.1111/2047-3095.12365

Sanson, G., Vellone, E., Kangasniemi, M., Alvaro, R., & D'Agostino, F. (2017). Impact of nursing diagnoses on patient and organisational outcomes: a systematic literature review. *Journal of Clinical Nursing. 26*, 3764-3783. doi: 10.1111/jocn.13717

Smith, A., Toor, S., & Van Kessel, P. (2018). Many turn to YouTube for children's content, news, how-to lessons. Retrieved from Pew Research Center Internet and Technology website www.pewinternet.org/2018/11/07/many-turn-to-youtube-for-childrens-content-news-how-to-lessons

Snoswell, C. L., Stringer, H., Taylor, M. L., Caffery, L. J., & Smith, A. C. (2023). An overview of the effect of telehealth on mortality: A systematic review of meta-analyses. *Journal of Telemedicine and Telecare, 29*(9), 659–668. https://doi.org/10.1177/1357633X211023700

Staccini, P., & Lau, A. Y. S. (2018). Findings from 2017 on consumer health informatics and education: Health data access and sharing. *Yearbook of Medical Informatics, 27*(1), 163–169. https://doi.org/10.1055/s-0038-1641218

Swanson, E., Mantovani, V. M., Wagner, C., Moorhead, S., Lopez, K. D., Macieira, T. G. R., & Abe, N. (2021). NANDA-I, NOC, and NIC linkages to SARS-CoV-2 (COVID-19): Part 2. Individual response. *International Journal of Nursing Knowledge, 32*(1), 68–83. https://doi.org/10.1111/2047-3095.12307

Tapuria, A., Poratb, T., Kalrac, D., Dsouzac, G., Xiaohui, S., & Curcina, V. (2021). Impact of patient access to their electronic health record: Systematic review. *Informatics for Health and Social Care, 46*(2), 194–206. https://doi.org/10.1080/17538157.2021.1879810

Tastan, S., Linch, G. C. F., Keenan, G. M., Stifter, J., McKinney, D., Fahey, L., Lopez, K. D., Yao, Y., & Wilkie, D. J. (2014). Evidence for the existing American Nurses Association-recognized standardized nursing terminologies: A systematic review *International Journal of Nursing Studies, 51*, 1160–1170. https://doi.org/10.1016/j.ijnurstu.2013.12.004

Thapa, D. K., Visentin, D. C., Kornhaber, R., West, S., & Cleary, M. (2021). The influence of online health information on health decisions: A systematic review. *Patient Education and Counseling, 104*(4), 770–784. https://doi.org/10.1016/j.pec.2020.11.016

Varnfield, M., Karunanithi, M., Lee, C. K., Honeyman, E., Arnold, D., Ding, H., Smith, C., & Walters, D. L. (2014). Smartphone-based home care model improved use of cardiac rehabilitation in postmyocardial infarction patients: Results from a randomised controlled trial. *Heart, 100*(22), 1770–1779. https://doi.org/10.1136/heartjnl-2014-305783

Vaughan, C., Trail, T. E., Mahmud, A., Dellva, S., Tanielian, T., & Friedman, E. (2018). Informal caregivers' experiences and perceptions of a web-based peer support network: Mixed-methods study. *Journal of Medical Internet Research, 20*(8), e257. https://doi.org/10.2196/jmir.9895

Vukušić Rukavina, T., Viskić, J., Machala Poplašen, L., Relić, D., Marelić, M., Jokic, D., & Sedak, K. (2021). Dangers and benefits of social media on E-professionalism of health care professionals: Scoping review. *Journal of Medical Internet Research, 23*(11), e25770. https://doi.org/10.2196/25770

Whitelaw, S., Mamas, M. A., Topol, E., & Van Spall, H. G. C. (2020). Applications of digital technology in COVID-19 pandemic planning and response. *Lancet Digital Health, 2*, e435–e440. https://doi.org/10.1016/S2589-7500(20)30142-4

Willcox, J., Dobson, R., & Whittaker, R. (2019). Old-Fashioned technology in the era of "bling": Is there a future for text messaging in health care? *Journal of Medical Internet Research, 21*(12), e16630. https://doi.org/10.2196/16630

Ye, J. (2020). The role of health technology and informatics in a global public health emergency: Practices and implications from the COVID-19 pandemic. *JMIR Medical Informatics, 8*(7), e19866. https://doi.org/10.2196/19866

CHAPTER 8

CONCEPTS IN PROGRAM DESIGN AND DEVELOPMENT

LAURA P. ROSSI

INTRODUCTION

Advanced practice registered nurses (APRNs) are expected to integrate nursing science with knowledge from other fields in order to provide the highest level of nursing care. They are also expected to "[p]articipate in system-wide initiatives that improve care delivery and/or outcomes" (American Association of Colleges of Nursing, 2021, p. 44). In this chapter, the APRN will learn how to design new programs by addressing factors related to planning and organizational decision-making.

Effective program development requires the use of information that is accurate, pertinent, and timely. It is critical that programs be constructed in a way that takes into consideration factors that reflect the numerous internal and external forces that have the potential to impact the implementation and overall success of a program. Measures of success and desired outcomes should be defined early in the program design process so as to provide continuous checkpoints during the implementation and ongoing evaluation process. Program development, implementation, and evaluation will vary across geographical and practice settings because of the unique and varied characteristics of populations, communities, and healthcare professionals. To be successful, APRNs must demonstrate competency in conducting environmental assessments and building effective project teams to effectively develop analyses and reports that will guide the process.

MODELS FOR PROGRAM DESIGN AND IMPLEMENTATION

Selecting a model as an organizing framework for developing a program from beginning to end is often a helpful first step. Various models can be used as a guide to facilitate the process of program development, planning, implementation, and evaluation.

Some programs can take many years to implement depending on their focus and scope. Programs may be focused on individuals (patients or staff members), interpersonal processes (team communications), organizations (policy or practice development), communities (developing community resources), or environmental concerns (social determinants such as education and employment).

Different organizations and health systems may have preferences about the specific approach to new program development. The following approaches share many common characteristics. APRNs should be familiar with these models and select a model according to the environment they are working in, the characteristics of the target population, and/or the type of program to be developed.

QUALITY IMPROVEMENT MODELS

Hospitals and health systems routinely incorporate principles of quality improvement into their routine operations. Quality improvement (QI) models provide a framework to assist APRNs in introducing and evaluating specific program components and/or pilot programs before attempting to scale implementation with a broader reach. Frequently, these begin as carefully scoped projects to evaluate specific interventions that have the potential to become effective components of a more comprehensive care delivery program. Various QI models, such as Lean and Six Sigma, evolved from the work of Shewhart (1939) who identified the PDSA (also referred to as PDCA) cycle for improvement. The PDSA steps include the following:

- **Plan:** Plan the change.
- **Do:** Do it.
- **Study (Check):** Study the actual results, then tailor next steps based on the results.
- **Act:** Act to stabilize the change or begin to improve on the change with new information.

The PDSA model is an iterative process and reinforces the goal of continuous quality improvement through ongoing assessment and improvement of structure, process, and outcomes. While many industries outside of healthcare have adopted different models for their improvement activities based on these basic steps, the Institute for Healthcare Improvement (IHI) has become the preeminent organization committed to the global improvement of health and healthcare. The IHI recommends the PDSA cycle for improvement projects. The IHI project charter can be very useful as a guide to creating an improvement project. It also provides numerous resources for educating professionals, disseminating information related to improvement processes, and developing the science of improvement. The IHI website can be accessed at www.ihi.org/about/Pages/default.aspx.

The successful use of the PDSA model has been demonstrated widely in both inpatient and outpatient areas (Rosenthal et al., 2018; Saunders et al., 2022). An early example involved a multidisciplinary team that was convened in an acute care hospital and charged with improving the safety of blood administration practices. In this project, the team examined the extent to which existing policies and procedures were being followed. A training program was developed to assure consistency in carrying out the defined procedures, followed by direct observations to assure compliance with the process and reduction in transfusion errors (Saxena et al., 2004). Recent examples include efforts to advance improvements in patient care in different settings. Saunders et al. (2022) reported a successful project to improve care for hypertension patients in primary care. Rosenthal et al. (2018) developed a screening process in a general hospital to detect substance abuse in patients.

THE LOGIC MODEL

The *logic model*, developed by the W. K. Kellogg Foundation (2004), is commonly cited in the literature as a model for program planning, management, and evaluation. It is a tool used to help shape a program by identifying factors that may impact it and forecasting the resources necessary to achieve success. A logic model is a graphic display or "map" depicting the relationship among resources, activities, and intended short- and long-term results that identify underlying theory and assumptions. Further, it clarifies the specific proposed program interventions and their impact on individual behaviors, organizations, and communities. In this way, it helps key stakeholders and team members visualize their roles and accountabilities to the program development process so that collaboration and communication can be enhanced. Logic models identify goals, assign tasks and responsibilities, and communicate outcomes. The steps include the following:

- Describe the problem(s) and/or issue(s) your program is intended to solve/address.
- Specify the existing needs and/or assets that indicate this program will benefit the community.
- Explain the desired program and results, including both short- and long-term achievements.
- Identify the factors that will influence change in the population or community.
- Provide evidence of any successful strategies or "best practices" that demonstrate the effectiveness and potential benefits for the intended population.
- State assumptions underlying how and why the proposed program will work.

Logic models have been successfully utilized to mobilize community resources to address complex issues including breast health for rural, underserved women and school-based programs to address teenage pregnancy (Hutton, 2007; Lane & Martin, 2005). In 2018, efforts to develop more home-based, patient-centered care management prompted a large, urban academic medical center to partner with the local fire department to establish a Mobile Integrated Health Transitional Care program involving community paramedicine (Mobile Integrated Healthcare–Community Paramedicine [MIH-CP]). The logic model was employed to guide the development of this innovative program using community resources to provide support to patients and families as they transitioned home after discharge from inpatient settings (Seidl et al., 2021). A logic model was also used successfully in a nursing education setting to improve students' conceptualizations and clarity of project goals to assure program feasibility and success (Idzik et al., 2021).

The logic model provides a focus for leaders as they track and clarify program progress. The Community Tool Box, created as a public service and sponsored by the University of Kansas, is an online resource for individuals interested in promoting community health and development. This site incorporates many best practices and examples of how to promote change and improvement in the community (Community Toolbox, 2023). While logic models are helpful in visualizing the development of large-scale projects, the focus and linearity of steps without some theoretical perspective as a guide can affect the degree to which planning is flexible as when there are changes in the environment and new perspectives emerge (Dorsey et al., 2014; Kneale et al., 2015; Mills et al., 2019).

DEVELOPING A FRAMEWORK OR MODEL OF CHANGE

The model of change builds on the logic model and makes program planning more adaptable as new information emerges in the program planning process. Models of change can prompt thinking about process details and how changes will actually occur. The healthcare system is dynamic, and organizational willingness to proceed with new programs can quickly shift when contextual factors including cultural factors, system finances, and/or new regulations and population expectations surface. Similarly, flexibility is needed in program planning as evidence evolves about the effectiveness of new interventions, innovative technology, and other healthcare programs. Creating time points when program leaders will evaluate input and feedback from program participants, stakeholders, and representatives from the community assures that unanticipated barriers are limited and contingency plans can be implemented.

The framework or model of change is a detailed 12-step process to organize thinking and connect a sequence of events. It includes the following:

- Analyzing information about the problem or goal
- Establishing a vision or mission for the program
- Defining organizational structure and operating mechanisms
- Developing a framework for making change
- Developing and using action plans
- Arranging for community mobilizers
- Developing leadership
- Implementing effective interventions
- Ensuring technical assistance
- Documenting progress and using feedback
- Making outcomes matter
- Sustaining the work

These steps reinforce a focus on collective thinking to create a common understanding and ensure commitment to strategic action. Keeping abreast of comprehensive evidence-based interventions and known best practices will help clarify the rationale for programs, facilitate funding opportunities, and inform the need for ongoing data collection and outcome measurement. Several examples of how the model has been used to plan, develop, implement, and evaluate successful community programs are available on the Community Tool Box University of Kansas website (www.ctb.ku.edu).

THE PRECEDE–PROCEED MODEL

Another design model is the *PRECEDE–PROCEED model* of health program planning and evaluation which evolved at Johns Hopkins University and is grounded on the work by Green and Kreuter (1992). It is based on principles from epidemiology and health administration as well as the social, behavioral, and educational sciences. The two fundamental propositions underlying this model are the following: (a) health and health risks are caused by multiple factors, and (b) because of this, efforts to impact change must be multidimensional. Consequently, the model's goals are twofold: (a) to explain health-related behaviors and environments, and (b) to design and evaluate interventions that influence both behaviors and the environment.

The PRECEDE-PROCEED model has two distinct processes: one for planning and one for implementing and evaluating. The PRECEDE (predisposing, reinforcing, and enabling constructs in educational diagnosis and evaluation) process outlines the following program planning steps:

1. Determine population needs.
2. Identify health determinants of these needs.
3. Analyze behaviors and environmental determinants of health needs.
4. Outline factors that predispose, reinforce, or enable behaviors.
5. Ascertain interventions best suited to change behaviors.

The PROCEED (policy, regulatory, and organizational constructs in educational and environmental development) process defines four steps to program implementation and evaluation:

1. Implement interventions.
2. Evaluate interventions.
3. Evaluate the impact of interventions on the health behaviors and factors supporting the behaviors
4. Evaluate outcomes.

The model follows a continuous cycle, linking the information gathered in the PRECEDE steps with the actions in the PROCEED process. Experience in the PROCEED process in turn provides additional information to reinitiate the PRECEDE process for iterative changes. Systematic reviews provide supportive evidence about the effectiveness of the PRECEDE-PROCEED model in guiding health promotion programs especially in the context of screening and education to promote health-related behaviors in a variety of populations (Kim et al., 2022; Saulle et al., 2020). This work provides important insight into the contextual factors and the complexities affecting the likelihood of adopting new behaviors. Bammann et al. (2021) described a pilot program to promote physical activity among older adults and provided more detail in their use of the Precede-Proceed Model. In their article, they reinforced the need for involving individuals who will be participating in a program as key stakeholders in developing the program. The details of their plan are displayed in Table 8.1 as an example to follow.

EVALUATION FRAMEWORK FOR COMMUNITY HEALTH PROGRAMS

Produced by the Center for Advancement of Community-Based Public Health and based on work by the Centers for Disease Control and Prevention (CDC) (Framework for Program Development in Public Health) and the University of Kansas (Community Tool Box: A Framework for Program Evaluation), An Evaluation Framework for Community Health Programs (CDC, 2000) can be used for program development, implementation, and evaluation. This systematic approach involves procedures that are useful, feasible, ethical, applicable, and accurate. The framework emphasizes evaluation as the driving force for planning effective programs, improving existing programs, and demonstrating results to justify investment in resources. The framework comprises six interdependent steps that build on one another and facilitate understanding of the program context, including its history, setting, and organization. The recommended steps are as follows:

- Engage stakeholders (all who are impacted by the program in any way).
- Describe the program (the needs, expected outcomes, activities, resources, stages of development, operational chart).
- Focus on the evaluation design (program purpose, users, uses, questions, methods, agreements).
- Gather credible evidence (program indicators, sources, quality, quantity, logistics of data collection).
- Justify conclusions (program standards, analysis and synthesis, interpretation, judgments, recommendations).
- Ensure use and share lessons learned (program design, preparation, feedback, follow-up, dissemination, additional uses).

For more information on this model and a more detailed checklist, go to prevention.sph.sc.edu/Documents/CENTERED%20Eval_Framework.pdf.

Program design and implementation requires systematic and detailed planning with ongoing evaluation. There are no right or wrong answers about how to select a model to guide program design and development. Increasingly, hybrid designs are being considered to address the context and advance the science (Lynch et al., 2018).

Often, an intervention trial is implemented to evaluate for its effectiveness before it is implemented. Hybrid designs have two aims that are explored simultaneously to capture a real-world view with a process, formative, and summative focus. There may be some

TABLE 8.1 Adaptations and Application of the PRECEDE-PROCEED Model (PPM) in the OUTDOOR ACTIVE Pilot Study

CLASSICAL PPM	ADAPTED PPM	CHANGES	PRACTICAL APPROACH IN OUTDOOR ACTIVE PILOT STUDY
PRECEDE			
Phase 1: Social assessment	Phase 1: Outcome definition	More flexibility regarding the choice of an intervention outcome	Outcome (outdoor physical activity) was fixed in research proposal. • Literature research and empirical studies • Scientific literature • Community-specific documents (e.g., land use plans, meeting protocols, city traffic concept) • Small area statistics from the regional statistical office • Walkabouts and documentation of all streets in the district (walkability, bikeability, infrastructure) • Postal survey of all 110 registered clubs of the pilot district to collect already available offers and member statistics • Informal talks with key informants, including district parliaments • Population-based cross-sectional survey: physical activity (accelerometer), physical fitness (senior fitness test), blood pressure, basic anthropometry, self-administered questionnaire • Walking interviews and focus groups • Kick-off event: presentation of phase 2 results to the community • Initial participatory workshop: Choice of 3 broader determinants to be targeted and discussion on how to bring change to each of these determinants • Participatory workshops for action development • Participatory walkabouts to reassess situation and generate ideas for action (e.g., to a badly designated park)
Phase 2: Epidemiological assessment	Phase 2: Determinants research	Change of underlying model to a socio-ecological model	
Phase 3: Educational and ecological assessment	Phase 3: Model selection	Adaptation necessary due to change of underlying models in phases 2 and 4	
Phase 4: Administrative and policy assessment and intervention alignment	Phase 4: Actions development	Change of underlying model	

(continued)

TABLE 8.1 Adaptations and Application of the PRECEDE-PROCEED Model in the OUTDOOR ACTIVE PILOT STUDY (*continued*)

CLASSICAL PPM	ADAPTED PPM	CHANGES	PRACTICAL APPROACH IN OUTDOOR ACTIVE PILOT STUDY
PROCEED			
Phase 5: Implementation	Phase 5: Implementation	See phase 4	• Participatory workshops to generate ideas and gather information for implementation ideas • Community roundtables for networking and to generate and discuss implementation opportunities • Personal contacts to discuss implementation with actors (e.g., sports club to initiate a specific offer for older adults) • Documentation of all contacts with actors in the community (actor, initiator of contact, type of contact) • Evaluation of participatory actions (baseline statistics, short evaluation questionnaire) • Qualitative interviews with key informants • Follow-up survey • Follow-up survey
Phase 6: Process evaluation	Phase 6 Process evaluation	See phase 3	
Phase 7: Impact evaluation	Phase 7: Impact evaluation	See phase 2	
Phase 8: Outcome evaluation	Phase 8: Outcome evaluation	See phase 1	

PPM, PRECEDE-PROCEED model; PRECEDE, predisposing, reinforcing, and enabling constructs in educational diagnosis and evaluation; PROCEED, policy, regulatory, and organizational constructs in educational and environmental development.

Source: Bammann, K., Recke, C., Albrecht, B.M., Stalling, I., & Doerwald, F. (2021). Promoting physical activity among older adults using community-based participatory research with an adapted PRECEDE-PROCEED model approach: The AEQUIPA/OUTDOOR ACTIVE project. *American Journal of Health Promotion, 35*(3), 409–420.

variability in the extent to which one looks at the intervention effectiveness versus implementation issues. However, much insight can be gained from examining the system factors that enable a program to be carried out and achieve the desired outcomes. Consider the goals for achieving adherence to prescribed medication for hypertension. Nurses can be instrumental in this area and often focus on patient education. We can better understand the effectiveness of these efforts if we have more detail about the nurse's clinical reasoning and the contextual factors that affect the interaction between the patient and the nurse.

Combined design efforts to evaluate the process of implementing interventions and its relation to effectiveness can yield important insights into the contextual factors affecting a program's outcome. Programs may be easily integrated into one setting but not others. Understanding the factors that affect real world implementation can strengthen program designs and yield more reliable and valid evidence of a program's value (Bernet et al., 2013).

PROGRAM PLANNING: WHERE TO START

ESTABLISHING PROGRAM NEED

Designing new programs requires creative thinking and innovation by nurse leaders to improve the outcomes of care within a cost- and resource-constrained environment. Most organizations now have administrative structures that oversee efforts related to care redesign. New models or programs must operationalize the philosophy, values, and mission of the organization or health system. Programs must also consider the needs of diverse populations who are living longer with complex chronic conditions. The level of care needed and the skills and competencies of available staff are additional considerations that will ultimately affect operational costs.

Organizations place value on evidence-based practice, financial performance, program feasibility, and the achievement of improved outcomes of care. There are often structures that support accountability and operational processes to address regulatory and accreditation requirements. It is always important to be aware of the internal and external forces influencing organizational decision-making, that is, who is accountable for expected outcomes and who can assure that people will continue to work together even if there is a change in leadership.

A white paper commissioned by the Robert Wood Johnson Foundation (RWJF) outlined innovative care delivery models (2008). Eight common elements or themes were noted throughout the models (Joynt & Kimball, 2008):

1. Elevated roles for nurses: nurses as care integrators
2. Migration to interdisciplinary care: team approach
3. Bridging the continuum of care
4. Pushing the boundaries: home as setting of care
5. Targeting high users of healthcare: elderly plus
6. Sharpened focus on the patient
7. Leveraging technology in care delivery
8. Driven by results: improving satisfaction, quality, and costs

Following the publication of this white paper the American Academy of Nursing (AAN) created the Edge Runners Initiative. This program recognizes "nurse-designed models of care that reduce cost, improve health care quality, advance health equity, and enhance consumer satisfaction" (AAN, 2021).

As many as 50 Edge Runners models have been developed. The majority have demonstrated success in addressing the need for health promotion and wellness as well as acute and long-term care needs in various populations, including women, children, older adults, and those living in underserved communities. They demonstrate the potential for nurses to develop programs that can be scaled and sustained to address the nation's health (Martsolf et al., 2017). The process of care delivery in a specific program will vary with the population and service being provided. Edge Runners Initiatives reinforce the

RWJF white paper recommendations that nurse leaders involved in developing innovative models consider the following (Martsolf et al., 2017; Mason, et al., 2019):

- Focus on a specific population.
- Employ a team approach.
- Consider continuum of care, including the home environment.
- Implement strategies to engage the patient/client.
- Provide teaching or education.
- Focus on results or outcomes.

The delivery of healthcare is an ever-changing process. Changes in the healthcare needs of a population should be addressed and routinely reassessed to ensure the program's original goals are being realized and the patients' needs are being met. Iterative programmatic changes are often needed, but the end result must be well defined with measurable improvements in outcomes. In this next section, we address some key areas that require attention irrespective of the program objectives and the model selected to guide the process for design and development.

SOURCES OF DATA

There are many stakeholders both within and outside of organizations whose support of a new program will be influenced by programmatic-related data. Clinical performance and patient outcomes data are often very meaningful to clinicians, but that information must be assessed within the context of overall health outcomes and resource availability. Financial and health services utilization data are of critical importance to administrators who are challenged to support new program development while simultaneously managing the costs of care. Planners need to consider organizational goals to ensure a proper fit between an organization and a program. It is also important that they take into consideration the unique characteristics of the target population to ensure a proper fit between a program and a specific community. Data to guide program development are available from several sources.

POPULATION-LEVEL DATA

Population demographics guide APRNs in the development of population-based programs. For example, communities have their own unique identifying characteristics. These characteristics include age, socioeconomic status, and ethnicity, among others. A program targeting the administration of the influenza vaccine during influenza season may look different when implemented in an urban area such as New York City versus a rural community in Wisconsin. Information on population demographics as well as health service needs, utilization, and performance trends are publicly available from many government websites. The U.S. Department of Health and Human Services (HHS; HealthData.gov), the Agency for Healthcare Research and Quality (AHRQ; www.ahrq.gov/index.html), and the CDC (www.cdc.gov/datastatistics) are three excellent sources of information. Further, the Office of Minority Health (OMH) at the HHS (www.minorityhealth.hhs.gov) provides a wealth of information to address the health issues in racial and ethnic minority populations.

Existing data that can be used for benchmarking is available to program planners and is used to evaluate local health needs and program performance through registries that focus on the health status of a particular population, the care they receive, and their responses over a period of time. Blumenthal (2017) identified several registries in the United States that are designed to capture broad scope data from a mix of automated and manual data capture methods. Among the most common registry elements are comorbidities, adverse events, organization demographics, patient-reported outcomes, laboratory and test imaging results, quality of life, pharmaceuticals, functional status, and patient experience.

Databases that address specific needs can also be developed by program planners. A complete assessment of patient/consumer needs and characteristics and comparisons of population outcomes against standard benchmarks provide necessary information for the planning of new programs.

ORGANIZATION LEVEL DATA

APRNs are most likely to develop new programs in the organization or health system where they are employed. A major factor influencing the development and acceptance of new programs is the organization's mission and the population that is being served. Organizational data is increasingly available and publicly reported and accessible to guide the design of new programs or the restructuring of an existing program. Data related to length of stay, readmission, and emergency department use can often serve as proxy indicators for higher healthcare costs that must be addressed. Similarly, patient experience data can provide insights into the preferences of the population served and the degree to which care can be more patient centered. Developing programs to reduce lengths of stay and/or facilitate care transitions from hospital to home requires a comprehensive review of the data related to the number of hospital discharges, disposition (e.g., home, rehabilitation, skilled nursing facility), patient demographics, primary discharge diagnoses, rehospitalization rate and reason, and time from discharge to rehospitalization. A review of an organization's data might reveal a particular subset of patients with a specific need. For example, if a hospital's readmission rates for patients with heart failure trend above national benchmarks and the hospital has been penalized financially for this, the organization may place priority on developing a transitional care program. The APRN can approach program development to decrease readmission rates from several aspects, for example, by looking at discharge outcomes data, the reasons for readmission, and any specific social determinants suggesting which patients might benefit most from transitional care. The electronic health record provides an accessible source to evaluate patient populations and the impact of new programs within a specific organization or healthcare system.

Close examination of the characteristics of a patient population (e.g., age, education, absence of insurance, access to health services) and the processes involved in discharge (e.g., ability to fill discharge medications, clear discharge instructions, medical equipment available for home use) can help guide the development of program components to reduce readmission rates. Direct observation of patient movement through the system, along with an understanding of the typical disease course, may provide insight into the primary factors contributing to readmission as well as the most appropriate point of care for the introduction of a new program. At times, organizational metrics can provide information to compare program effectiveness across specific agencies or health systems. This is best facilitated when standard benchmarks are available in national databases. It is important to keep in mind that nationally reported data may not be consistently captured or risk adjusted across settings.

CONSUMER AND SOCIETAL TRENDS AND DEMANDS

Consumer and societal trends and demands provide information that drives the rationale for designing a specific program. It is not cost-effective to support a program that does not meet an identified consumer need. A simple dictionary definition of a trend is the general direction in which something tends to move. In what direction is healthcare technology moving? In what direction are consumer attitudes and beliefs about disease prevention moving? Consumer and societal trends and demands are constantly changing, making it difficult to know which trends or demands to pay attention to, if they will continue, and for how long. For example, in 2018, several information technology (IT) trends were identified by Health Data Management, including using IT to help achieve patient engagement and experience, protecting health information and data security, and the importance of population health management (Bazzoli, 2018). The coronavirus disease 2019 (COVID-19) pandemic produced many unanticipated and unprecedented changes in healthcare delivery and utilization. The use of telemedicine was expanded, but there were significant reductions in elective procedures and preventive care. While technology adoption was useful, it does not appear to have been sufficient to counter the reduction in face-to-face visits. The resulting health system capacity issues compound the concern about how these shifts have impacted disenfranchised populations. APRNs must continuously be aware of the changes within and outside their practice environment to confirm existing trends and demands and/or identify new ones. Efforts to reduce cost may improve efficiency but not consistently address patient-centered concerns.

Consumer attitudes and beliefs about how to access and manage healthcare are also changing. This creates a challenge in identifying which trends or demands to target in program development. As societal trends and demands shift, consumer needs and preferences also change, driving the demand for new programs. Consider the needs of an aging population in an era where hospital lengths of stay have declined and resources to provide care at home are limited. Changes in healthcare financing have resulted in higher copays for patients who may have multiple chronic conditions. It may not be cost-effective for health systems to develop or maintain programs that no longer meet an identified consumer or organizational need.

More than ever, consumers have access to information about the availability of healthcare services and programs. Quality and patient safety data related to institution and program performance are now publicly available on government, consumer, and institution websites. There is an expanding focus on transparency. The rapidly changing healthcare systems mandates that APRNs find ways to monitor and stay abreast of trends to confirm the viability of existing and/or new program opportunities in their practice environment. Involving consumers early in the program development process can be critical to developing a patient-centered process (see section on stakeholders). Hibbard and Greene (2013) emphasize the evidence on the importance of patient engagement in healthcare reform and its potential for improving patients' outcomes and perceptions of their experience with services. While it is unclear how costs are impacted, they suggest that programs are most successful when they consider patient activation and flexible opportunities for tailored interventions. Such measures of patient activation can be useful in evaluating the intermediate outcomes of a program.

It is difficult to predict how long a trend will persist or endure, so staying current on consumer preferences and available options for care and self-management is essential. Programs are often developed as a temporary bridge in anticipation of new technology becoming available. At other times, innovative programs can be nurtured and evolve as essential services that are available to a broader population. Careful consideration of the trends within and outside healthcare provides the basis for effective program development, sustainability, and growth.

IDENTIFYING KEY STAKEHOLDERS

Program development requires considerable buy in from many people. The term *stakeholders* refers to persons, groups, or organizations that have a direct or indirect stake in the program because they may be affected by the program and the related actions, objectives, and policies involved in implementation. Nurse leaders must be sensitive to the varied perspectives of stakeholders, internal and external to the program. It is important to know how and/or why some stakeholders may oppose the development of a program so that barriers can be anticipated and minimized. The following list of questions can guide the identification of key stakeholders who will provide constructive advice to facilitate successful program implementation:

- Who will be affected by the program?
- Who can influence the program in its development, implementation, evaluation, and ongoing operation, even if not directly involved?
- What groups are most committed to the program's success and outcomes?
- What is the impact of this program in the short term? Long term?

There are many stakeholders in healthcare, including patients/consumers, physicians and professional staff, board of directors, and administrators who assume responsibility for the financing and operations of a program or sponsoring organization. Think broadly about the range of potential stakeholders and their potential influence on the program. Regulatory bodies, government agencies, and professional associations will be concerned with the scope and standards of practice as well as service reimbursement. Local communities and the public at large will typically be concerned with issues of access and impact related to the influence of suppliers, competitors, and media. An APRN will also want to consider the views of frontline caregivers who will be responsible for delivering the service offered in the program during the initial and ongoing implementation. Regular and timely communication with stakeholders about the program development and implementation process is essential to ensure the engagement and commitment from those decision-makers who allocate resources and provide support.

There may be considerable variability and/or overlap in stakeholders' expectations, including healthcare quality, adequacy of resources, and costs and profitability. Publicly reported indicators may impact consumers' perception of a hospital's quality of care. The board of trustees will be very invested in the organization's image, which can directly impact a consumer's decision about where to seek care or a physician's decision about where to admit patients. Healthcare organizations have mission statements that reflect organizational values, and in many cases, these statements reflect the value placed on the development of various programs.

The power or influence of stakeholders can change with time as a result of their individual position, philosophy, and values. Changes in system and organizational leadership can also affect the identification and influence of stakeholders over time. This will have an important influence on the evolving culture and thereby impact expectations of a new program and the justification required to move it forward. Addressing the concerns and expectations of stakeholders when designing a program can improve the likelihood of ongoing support and program success. Focusing on the program outcomes that matter most to the stakeholders will help win their support.

ASSEMBLING A TEAM

Program development requires a team of people who are directly familiar with each aspect of the process that will be part of the program. The composition of the team will depend on its scope and generally should include individuals who will provide direct program services and those who will support direct providers at various stages of program implementation. Those closest to the process provide essential information and support for making changes. The type and number of staff members needed to provide direct program services depends on the nature of the services that will be provided and the number of program locations. The same is true for the type and number of support staff needed for program implementation and evaluation.

There are many specific roles and tasks that individuals can assume during the program development phase in order to encourage shared commitment and to ensure broad ownership for success. Involving an executive sponsor is often very helpful to ensure resources for development, such as protected staff time. The appointment of a process owner should also be considered. This team member could be an APRN with an administrative role in the program area who will ultimately be responsible for implementing the process and maintaining the program using resources appropriately to assure the outcomes required by the sponsoring group/organization. These individuals can provide essential advice about internal and external forces that should be considered when designing a program.

A lead player is the program administrator or manager who will drive the project and manage the associated changes. Regardless of industry or setting, this essential role requires an individual who can provide oversight and direct the work of the team members' performance as well as monitor and provide ongoing feedback about the team's performance. This role usually involves the following common responsibilities:

- Identifies, researches, and solves program issues effectively
- Identifies the resources required for a program's success
- Recognizes and manages unanticipated issues and opportunities for improvement
- Documents and communicates operation of the program
- Ensures that the program complies with standards, regulations, and procedures
- Plans and sets timelines for program goals, milestones, and deliverables

Regardless of the number and type of team members, the program manager or administrator plays a critical role in building and leading a successful team. A team that is effective and focused contributes to the success of the program. This requires attention to the charge to the team (sometimes referred to as the project charter), the expectations of individual team members, and the specific reasons/roles for the team's composition. A useful framework for building successful teams is described best by the acronym TEAM, which stands for "together everyone achieves more." The origins of the model are difficult to trace, but its concepts are sound and used by many. Successful teambuilding requires attention to the following:

- Commitment
- Competence
- Control or sense of ownership
- Collaboration
- Communication
- Awareness of positive and negative consequences
- Coordination

Stakeholders, team leaders, and team players all play a critical role in the success and/or failure of a program. Each member has a role and an expectation based on the anticipated outcome of a new program. Values influence a team's success, and it is important to share these values and address them early. Often, consideration of a new program requires creative thinking that could shift the culture and current thinking about how things are done. Engaging the team in consensus about this early on can be enabling and empowering as the program development process advances. Ultimately, commitment, communication, and collaboration are some of the most important characteristics a team requires for a successful program.

JUSTIFICATION

Justifying a program requires an articulation of scope and potential impact to engage stakeholders. Once the information from relevant data sources has been collected, a data-driven rationale must be developed to appeal to the various stakeholders and program participants. This is a critical step in establishing need and securing necessary resources for moving ahead with program development.

Producing a well-defined set of expectations and value propositions will make key stakeholders feel confident about approving and funding a program. The identification of a trend (such as increasing readmission rates for a particular population) is one possible justification for a program, especially when the trend leads to increasing costs or morbidity/mortality. Local and national trends may serve as a sign of competition or new demands. Newly published evidence may also be available that can stimulate interest in the development of new health programs.

A literature search can reveal compelling evidence to support the design and implementation of an effective transitional care program to reduce readmissions. Transitional programs that already exist may be expanded or adapted for another patient population. Prior programs can be enhanced or redesigned as an innovation, especially if those programs have been successfully implemented in comparable settings. Friedan (2014) suggests that innovations might emerge as a result of combining a reasonable number of evidence-based interventions as a "bundle." Often, a selected number of interventions can be integrated into a model of care delivery that has the potential to produce a more significant impact than introducing isolated interventions.

Once a program objective is conceived and a literature review is completed, it is important to consider whether the program is feasible. A pilot or feasibility study can help frame the program structure and identify potential risks and barriers associated with implementation. Basic questions need to be addressed and answered in the preparation of a program justification, such as the following:

- How is this program different from other programs in place to serve a similar purpose?
- Are there other alternatives and/or options to the proposed program?
- Is the program economically and technically feasible in the proposed practice setting?
- What are the potential costs and benefits with various program options? (Table 8.2)
- What operational issues must be addressed for successful implementation? (Table 8.3)
- How will the program be sustained?

Nurse leaders must be cognizant of the organization's current strategic goals and administrative directives to determine whether the climate and the timing are appropriate for the program's development. The healthcare environment and the political landscape are in constant flux, so it may be difficult to anticipate the number of external

TABLE 8.2 Potential Costs and Benefits of Proposed Program Worksheet

	POTENTIAL COSTS	POTENTIAL BENEFITS
Quantitative measures		
Qualitative themes		

forces that may affect a program's acceptability. Being prepared with contingencies and adaptations to a program can be essential to gaining support to move ahead.

Programs with the potential to save money and improve patient outcomes are often very appealing because the Centers for Medicare and Medicaid Services (CMS) ties reimbursement to certain key quality indicators. The Affordable Care Act (ACA) established the *Hospital Readmissions Reduction Program*, which requires the CMS to reduce payments to inpatient prospective payment system (IPPS) hospitals with excess readmissions. The ACA went into effect on October 1, 2012, and hospitals that are above the national average for 30-day readmission rates have seen decreased reimbursement rates (CMS, 2019). Improving readmission rates makes good financial sense. Increasingly, healthcare financing strategies apply the concept of value-based care. This approach to reimbursement calls for models in which healthcare providers are paid based on patient outcomes rather than the amount of service provided. "Value" is calculated by measuring the outcomes given the cost of producing these outcomes (Larsson, Clawson, & Howard, 2023). The APRN should assess the community to determine whether other similar programs exist that would compete with the proposed program or whether the proposed program could be built into an existing program. If a hospital has an existing community outreach department, the APRN could use the existing structure to house a new program.

In summary, justification of a program can be strengthened significantly by providing sound evidence such as a thorough review of the literature to establish the background of the problem and by examining current successful programs that may be applicable to the APRN's population of interest. Additionally, by following trends, APRNs can compare

TABLE 8.3 Operational and Support Issues for Designing New Programs

OPERATIONAL ISSUES	SUPPORT ISSUES
• What tools are needed to support the program (e.g., equipment and facilities)? Do we currently have these resources? • What skills training does the staff need? • What procedures or processes need to be created and/or updated? • What will be needed to maintain and support the program once it is implemented? • Is the program politically feasible considering strategic goals and administrative directives?	• What support staff will be needed? • What program materials will the staff use? • What and how will staff training be provided? • How will changes be introduced and managed? • Will the program be allowed to succeed?

outcome measures to national quality indicators and benchmarks and follow these performance measures over time with a goal toward improving patient outcomes and reducing costs. Finally, ascertaining the program's feasibility will further strengthen the justification. Feasibility studies provide a systematic framework in which a program can be assessed and thoughtfully implemented or integrated into current practice. Outlining a system of accountability for the program through ongoing monitoring, evaluation, and improvement is an essential component and inspires confidence in those who implement the program.

PROGRAM DESIGN AND IMPLEMENTATION

Designing a program is different from implementing it, although the steps are iterative. In the design process, nurse leaders must also consider how the program will be viewed, as well as how it can be effectively operated and supported. Critical issues such as image, funding, and infrastructure related to location, space, and equipment must be considered. During implementation, the nurse leader will be evaluating the sufficiency of these operational resources and staffing to achieve and sustain the program goals. Table 8.3 offers a non-exhaustive list of issues to consider.

STRUCTURE

As the team moves forward, APRNs must be focused and cautious about employing complex approaches to program structure. Complex designs can lead to failure if discrete outcomes are not easily measured or if too many measures or variables are involved. The structure of a new program can be as simple or detailed as desired if there is clarity about the goals, components, and specific outcome measures that will determine success. Funding sources may also dictate program structure. In general, a simple approach to outlining the structure of a program proposal is displayed in Table 8.4.

This structure is the "skeleton" with which a program can be designed and can serve as a reference when planning resources, budgets, staffing, and operational procedures. A program's structure consists of the program's goals and objectives, which follow directly from strategic planning. The plan should include a description of the resources needed to achieve the goals and objectives, including necessary funding. A major component of these resources may include human resources described in terms of required skills and scope of practice. Technical resources for data, including their analysis and storage, will need to be considered when designing a program budget. Initial budget proposals for new programs usually estimate costs in broad categories. Final program budgets require careful attention to all aspects of program planning, implementation, and evaluation and should estimate yearly costs as closely as possible. Funding is determined after a program budget is created. The source may be a state or federal grant, or it may be self-financed through health insurance held by consumers or a combination of funding sources. Whatever the source (or sources) for financing costs, a method of funding must be identified before the program can move forward.

TABLE 8.4 Structure of Program Proposal Outline

1. What	• What is the title of the program? • What is the focus of the program? • What are the goals of the program? • What are the objectives of the program? • What outcomes will be measured? • What is the budget for the program? • What is the timeline for program development, implementation, and evaluation?
2. Where	• Where will the program take place? • Where is the program's base location? • Where will staff be housed? • Where will supplies or resources for the program be stored?
3. Who	• Who are the stakeholders? • Who is in charge of the program? • Who are the staff members involved in program development, implementation, and/or evaluation? • Who is the program attempting to reach? • Who will fund this program?
4. When	• When will the program be implemented? • When will the program end?
5. Why	• Why is the program needed (justification)? • Why might the program succeed or fail?
6. How	• How will data be collected? • How often will data be collected? • How often will outcomes be examined? • How will the program be developed? Implemented? Evaluated? • How will the program sustain its funding or obtain future funding? • How will the program's success be determined?

OUTCOMES

Outcomes are the measurable results of the program objectives. They provide a method of evaluating the success of a program. Outcomes are often defined by regulatory, governmental, or certifying agencies such as The Joint Commission (TJC), the American Nurses Credentialing Center (ANCC), and the AHRQ. An outcome measure is often expressed as a rate or percentage and represents the result of some process in a patient population over a set period of time. TJC often looks for the results of improvement projects designed to meet standards for accreditation. The ANCC manages the Magnet® designation program that provides a prestigious distinction to healthcare organizations for nursing excellence and high-quality patient care. To receive Magnet designation, the ANCC looks for systematic data collection related to outcomes of care for specific groups of patients and a demonstration that most nursing units or practice arenas have outperformed the national benchmarks the majority of the time (ANCC, 2023). Performance on nurse-sensitive indicators is often the focus. The AHRQ also provides guidance for the identification of quality indicators that can be used as outcome measures. For a complete list, go to www.qualityindicators.ahrq.gov/Default.aspx.

Often, the data used to justify a program's development and implementation can provide insights into the outcome data that are readily available. What does the program do? Why does the program exist? State and national statistics can be used as benchmarks when examining outcomes. Comparisons to quality indicators can also serve as benchmarks to evaluate success or progress in a program. Measures can be defined in terms of structure, for example, equipment and personnel, processes (i.e., actions involved in evaluation and treatment), and/or outcomes (i.e., results). These measures should prompt consideration of how various aspects of a program work together. Several questions will emerge:

- How will you know the parts or steps in the system are performing as planned to affect the outcome?
- How will you know you have achieved the intended result?
- How can you tell you if you have unintended consequences?

Outcomes should be established for short-term, intermediate, and long-term objectives. The mnemonic SMART provides a template for writing such objectives (CDC, 2022).

- *Specific*: The outcome is well defined and unambiguous.
- *Measurable*: Concrete methods and criteria for assessing progress are used.
- *Achievable*: The goal can be a stretch but must be reasonable, given the program's resources and sphere of influence. Reasonable goals and objectives must be motivational; they should provide incentives for the program staff and stakeholders.
- *Relevant*: The outcome must be relevant to the program's vision, mission, and goals. Outcomes must also be relevant to all people affiliated with or impacted by the program.
- *Time*: The time period for accomplishing goals and evaluating outcomes is reasonable.

Outcomes can be incremental and subtle. Framing personal observations or subjective experiences as concrete, specific, observable measures can be a daunting task. Hence, both quantitative and qualitative outcomes can be both helpful and necessary.

The assessment of impact is viewed in broader terms and may be less specific than outcomes. Mindell et al. (2003) provide insight into the various definitions and areas of impact that can be considered in the evaluation of a program. Further, they emphasize the use of many different procedures, methods, and tools to evaluate a program's potential effects on the health of a population. Qualitative and quantitative data are needed to capture the effects of those directly involved in a program, as well as those who are not (Mindel et al., 2003). Impact evaluation is also intended to determine, in broad terms, whether a program has desirable or undesirable effects on individuals, households, and institutions and whether those effects are attributed to the interventions associated with the program. The following are examples of how the impact of a transitional program intended to reduce readmission rates for heart failure patients might be articulated in quantitative and qualitative terms:

- Within 1 year of the inception of the hypertension monitoring and self-care program, the community's rate of fatal strokes was reduced.

- In a recent 10-month tracking period, the rate of readmissions for pneumonia was reduced after 50 patients successfully completed the program.
- A patient's wife describes its value this way: "Thank you so much for your excellent program! I sincerely believe you and your team deserve an award for excellence in patient care. I don't know what we would have done without your support and guidance."
- The personal impact of the program and its professional staff is acknowledged by one participant: "[T]he staff helped me realize I was not eating as well as I should and got me moving in the right direction. Also, I noticed that when I eat so many fruits and vegetables, I don't have room for so much junk food. Before this program, I didn't realize how much salt was in the food I was eating."

On the other hand, program outcomes can illustrate whether the program is doing what it was intended to do. Outcomes should provide information that can be used for ongoing quality improvement. After defining program outcomes, consider using the SMART criteria to evaluate the program's stated outcomes. These questions may also be helpful:

- Is it clear what the program is assessing?
- Is the outcome measurable?
- Is the intended outcome measuring something useful and meaningful?
- How will the outcome be measured?
- Are the outcomes realistic for the time frame of the program?

Outcome data should be collected continuously at appropriately prescribed intervals (e.g., at specific milestones, quarterly) throughout the program implementation. Outcome data is collected at varying frequencies to monitor trends effectively. For example, ensuring that program activities are being carried out may require more frequent monitoring in the initial stages where volume and patient experience ratings will have more relevance than once the program is felt to be up and running.

In summary, the outcome measures selected should show the progress (or ineffectiveness) of a program and allow for objective evaluation. Outcome measures must be clear, concise, measurable, and easily compared to quality indicators when possible. They should be realistic and time delimited. Evaluation of the impact of a program can also be helpful when dealing with qualitative and quantitative measures.

IMPLEMENTATION

OPERATING POLICIES AND PROCEDURES

Once the program proposal has taken shape, well-designed policies and procedures are important to guide implementation. These policies and procedures should reflect the proposed structure, processes, and outcomes. Ensuring alignment with existing policies and compliance with regulatory mandates helps to ensure consistent performance and risk management while serving as a basis for evaluating process improvements. A program does not need a policy for every possible contingency. It should allow for flexibility in clinical decision-making and administrative operations. Similarly, policies and procedures require ongoing monitoring to evaluate their impact on daily operations and the means for assuring accountability in the context of new evidence and health system changes. Attention to the following tasks facilitate ongoing program implementation and alignment of logistics:

- Coordination of the writing and review of the policies and procedures
- Reviewing and discussing the policies and procedures with the program staff
- Ensuring policies and procedures are supported by evidence
- Interpreting and integrating the policies and procedures into program practices
- Providing administrative support and possible legal review
- Ensuring compliance with the policies and procedures

Using the earlier example, if a program was designed for transitioning patients with heart failure from hospital to home, it requires a review of the literature to determine evidence-based strategies that have been used by other organizations to prevent or delay readmissions. Program planners also need to review state and federal regulations related to important factors such as reimbursement for services and zoning requirements for program facilities. The synthesis of evidence provides a framework for the development of policies and procedures for clinical services and program implementation.

A carefully constructed policy and procedure manual is critical for program success. It can be modeled after evidence-based protocols and provide the framework for consistent training of staff and community outreach workers. Policies and procedures also serve as guidelines for staff to follow to ensure delivery of quality care and consistent practices in the program.

COMMUNICATIONS AND MARKETING

Clear and consistent communication is essential to keep team members and stakeholders engaged during program design and implementation. The following questions highlight a realistic problem that is faced when communicating about a program. You may have the best program in the world, but if you do not communicate the benefits and features of the program to the right audience, how are consumers going to find out about it? How are stakeholders and program team members going to buy into the program?

Marketing is an important component to consider in program design and development. Effective marketing of healthcare services requires in-depth knowledge of the patients' actual and potential needs and offering new services that patients may not be aware exist or explicitly request. It is also important to consider who the target market actually is. For example, is it the physician who must prescribe a referral? Is it the health plan that must authorize payment? Or is it the patient who must bear out-of-pocket costs? Profitability and sustainability of a program are additional considerations for a marketing plan (Purcarea, 2019).

The American Marketing Association (2013) defines *marketing* as "the activity, set of institutions, and processes for creating, communicating, delivering, and exchanging offerings that have value for customers, clients, partners, and society at large" ("Marketing" section, para 1). It is important to be aware of not only your competitors but also what will appeal to your audience (i.e., potential participants). A strong marketing campaign can lead to long-term successes not only for your program but also for future programs. Stakeholders will see the value in a well-constructed marketing plan, which ultimately is important for program sustainability. Marketing requires activity and is not passive. It is a group effort involving a variety of individuals and groups, internal and external to the program or organization.

Marketing is also process driven. Communication is essential to the process and can be delivered in many forms. The plan requires definition of the senders, receivers, and the media to be used. Use of various social media channels also provides new opportunities to reach patients and families of all ages as well as program referral sources. Consider the following basic questions when engaging in strategies to communicate about a program:

- Who will be responsible for communicating information about the program?
- What is the message being communicated?
- Who is the intended recipient of the communication?

A well-mapped-out process for communication and marketing is critical for success. For some programs, market research may be required to determine how interested patients/consumers and referring providers will get information about the program. The communication plan can include verbal and nonverbal communications. Verbal communication may include word of mouth, telephone voice messages, and presentations at meetings. Communication through nonverbal means includes ads in newspapers, information on an organization's website and social media accounts, newsletters, posters, text messages, and emails. Advertising is only one part of marketing. Without clearly defined and targeted processes, nurse leaders cannot launch an effective communication plan and will have difficulty determining which communication strategies are working and which are not.

Positioning is another marketing concept that nurse leaders must be aware of so as to differentiate a program from the competition. Positioning happens in one place, in the mind of the consumer, and occurs in a moment. Nurses must be prepared to present a "brand" of service in the healthcare marketplace to get the attention of the patients and/or the referring providers who are the customers you are reaching out to. Interested customers will spend time and energy evaluating one program in relation to others before making a choice about which program to participate in. The following questions related to the concept of positioning can be helpful throughout the design and development phase but are particularly important during implementation (McNamara, n.d.):

- Who is the target market?
- Who are the competitors for the program?

- What should be considered when determining the logistics of the program, including costs?
- What should be considered when naming the program?

Programs are successful only if they attract the participation of their identified target population. There must be buy-in by its members, and without effective communication by a variety of modalities, this message may never reach the intended audience. As noted earlier, there are both verbal and nonverbal forms of communication. Verbal communication is probably the most effective for some populations, as the value of face-to-face interaction and relationship building is difficult to replace with nonverbal methods. With that said, communication requires an investment of both time and money, and these costs need to be included in the program budget. Generally, marketing is 5% to 10% of a program's budget.

CASE STUDY

Consider this scenario:

Your hospital has been working to reduce the use of unnecessary health services by offering more access to the patients in the community they serve. There are more arthroplasty procedures being moved to the ambulatory center so patients are no longer hospitalized after surgery. The emergency department has been overcrowded and the overall length of hospital stay is over the national benchmark. Last year, the hospital incurred significant financial penalties for readmission. As a clinical leader, you have been asked to work with a team to identify opportunities for improving the delivery of care with attention to patient experience and health outcomes.

Think about how you will begin working with this team.
- What steps will you take?
- What data will you request?
- How will you help the group identify priorities for program planning?
- What is the rationale/justification for these priorities?
- What measures will you use to determine the achievement of program goals?
- What support will you request from your stakeholders and executive sponsors?

OVERCOMING BARRIERS AND CHALLENGES

New programs require continuous monitoring and surveillance to troubleshoot any barriers and challenges that arise during implementation. Leaders must remain close to the staff members on the front line as they will often be the first to identify obstacles. Their insights can pave the way toward developing action plans to overcome the barriers and challenges. This may require revisiting the overall design of the program or the unanticipated needs for staff time and other resources. Challenges may also relate to the lack of information about competition and/or lack of essential data about operational issues.

Gaglio et al. (2013) explain that areas that correspond to the structure, process, and outcome components of a program should guide program administrators during the quality improvement process. Structure and process measures established during program planning should be evaluated to determine if the program was implemented as intended or if sufficient time has been allotted to facilitate adoption. Adoption is the absolute number, proportion, and representativeness of settings and intervention agents who are willing to initiate and/or participate in the program. Initially, measures of adoption and staff engagement should be scrutinized to provide direction if additional communications, outreach, and training might be needed before program outcomes can be appreciated. Another important area is program maintenance which reflects the implementation process and the extent to which a program is assimilated into routine organizational practices and policies. Unanticipated issues often arise and provide an opportunity to tweak the implementation plan to assure program efficiency and/or effectiveness. Schell et al. (2013) suggest that a careful reflection of the program proposal elements, for example, a sound implementation plan, ongoing monitoring, stakeholder support, capacity constraints, and stability of funding, will guide the assessment of sustainability. Ultimately, ongoing assessment is key to assure a program's ability to sustain its activities and benefits over time.

SUMMARY

This chapter provides APRNs and nurse leaders with various tools and resources for detailed program design and development, including multiple components ranging from the identification of key stakeholders to marketing and communication strategies. Program designs that address consumer and societal trends are more likely to be successful and produce improved quality of care. Ultimately, the goal is to generate improved patient outcomes. Successful programs must incorporate knowledge from many fields to address issues related to the structure, process, and outcomes involved in program planning, development, implementation, and evaluation. Various program models provide a standard and tested method for helping nurse leaders throughout the process of program implementation.

END-OF-CHAPTER RESOURCES

EXERCISES AND DISCUSSION QUESTIONS

EXERCISE 8.1 Using data that can be found on the HHS or the CDC websites, identify trends in population demographics and health in an area that you serve.

- What are the implications for healthcare providers?
- What type of healthcare services and programs are needed right now?
- What type of services do you believe will be needed in 10 years?
- From a demographic point of view, in 10 years, what will be the important characteristics of the population that you serve if you continue to practice in this geographical region?

EXERCISE 8.2 You are interested in developing a program to reduce the rate of readmissions for patients with heart failure who have been hospitalized in an urban academic medical center. There have been many prior initiatives to address this issue, but you have identified many patients who have limited health literacy and cognitive impairments. Explain the process you will undertake to develop an effective program including consideration of established best practices and the outcomes of past initiatives.

- What are the important characteristics of the population you are serving in this geographical region?
- Consider the data you will need and how you will obtain it.
- How would you go about the analysis of the data?
- What steps would you take to identify the priority needs your program will be addressing?
- Using the "SMART" method, write short-term, intermediate, and long-term objectives for the program.
- How might you use the PRECEDE–PROCEED Model to plan, implement, and evaluate the program?
- How will you market the program?

A robust set of instructor resources designed to supplement this text is located at http://connect.springerpub.com/content/book/978-0-8261-4377-8. Qualifying instructors may request access by emailing textbook@springerpub.com.

REFERENCES

American Academy of Nursing. (2021). *Edge runners*. Retrieved from Edge Runners - American Academy of Nursing Main Site (aannet.org)

American Association of Colleges of Nursing. (2021). *The essentials: Core competencies for professional nursing education.* Author. Retrieved from https://www.aacnnursing.org/Essentials

American Marketing Association. (2013). *Definitions of marketing.* Retrieved from https://www.ama.org/AboutAMA/Pages/Definition-of-Marketing.aspx

American Nurses Credentialing Center. (2023). *2023 Magnet® application manual updates and FAQs.* Retrieved from 2023 Magnet Application Manual Updates and FAQs | ANCC | ANA (nursingworld.org)

Bammann, K., Recke, C., Albrecht, B.M., Stalling, I., & Doerwald, F. (2021). Promoting physical activity among older adults using community-based participatory research with an adapted PRECEDE-PROCEED model approach: The AEQUIPA/OUTDOOR ACTIVE project. *American Journal of Health Promotion, 35*(3), 409–420.

Bazzoli, F. (2018). *12 trends that will dominate healthcare IT in 2019.* Retrieved from https://www.healthdatamanagement.com/list/12-trends-that-will-dominate-healthcare-it-in-2019

Bernet, A. C., Willens, D. E., & Bauer, M. S. (2013). Effectiveness-implementation hybrid designs: Implications for quality improvement science. *Implementation Science, 8*(Suppl. 1), S2. Retrieved from http://www.implementationscience.com/content/8/S1/S2

Blumenthal, S. (2017). The use of clinical registries in the United States: A landscape survey. *EGEMS The Journal for Electronic Health Data and Methods, 5*(1), 26. http://dx.doi.org/10.5334/egems.248

Centers for Disease Control and Prevention. (2000). *An evaluation framework for community health programs.* Retrieved from An evaluation framework for community health programs (cdc.gov)

Centers for Disease Control and Prevention. (2022). *Develop SMART objectives.* Retrieved from: https://www.cdc.gov/publichealthgateway/phcommunities/resourcekit/evaluate/develop-smart-objectives.html

Centers for Medicare & Medicaid Services. (2019). *Hospital readmissions reduction program (HRRP).* Retrieved from http://www.cms.gov/Medicare/Medicare-Fee-for-Service-Payment/AcuteInpatientPPS/Readmissions-Reduction-Program.html

Community Toolbox. (2023). *Tools to change our world.* Retrieved from http://ctb.ku.edu/en

Dorsey, S. G., Schiffman, R., Redeker, N. S., Heitkemper, M., McCloskey, D. J., Weglicki, L. S., & Grady, P. A. (2014, December). National Institute of Nursing Research Centers of Excellence: A logic model for sustainability, leveraging resources, and collaboration to accelerate cross-disciplinary science. *Nursing Outlook, 62*(6), 384–393. http://dx.doi.org/10.1016/j.outlook.2014.06.003

Friedan, T. R. (2014). Six components necessary for effective public health program implementation. *American Journal of Public Health, 104,* 17–22. http://dx.doi.org/10.2105/ajph.2013.301608

Gaglio, B., Shoup, J. A., & Glasgow, R. E. (2013). The RE-AIM framework: A systematic review of use over time. *American Journal of Public Health, 103,* e38–e46. http://dx.doi.org/10.2105/ajph.2013.301299

Green, L. W., & Kreuter, M. W. (1992). CDC's planned approach to community health as an application of PRECEDE and an inspiration for PROCEED. *Journal of Health Education, 23*(3), 140–144. http://dx.doi.org/10.1080/10556699.1992.10616277

Hibbard, J. H., & Greene, J. (2013). What the evidence shows about patient activation: Better health outcomes and care experiences; Fewer data on costs. *Health Affairs, 32*(2), 207–214. http://dx.doi.org/10.1377/hlthaff.2012.1061

Hutton, L. (2007). An evaluation of a school-based teenage pregnancy prevention program using a logic model framework. *The Journal of School Nursing. 23*(2), 104–110. http://dx.doi.org/10.1622/1059-8405(2007)023[0104:AEOAST]2.0.CO;2

Idzik, S., Buckley, K., Bindon, S., Gorschboth, S., Hammersla, M., Windemuth, B., & Bingham, D. Lessons learned using logic models to design and guide DNP projects. *Nurse Educator, 46*(5), E127–E131. http://dx.doi.org/10.1097/NNE.0000000000001025

Joynt, J., & Kimball, B. (2008). *Innovative care delivery models: Identifying new models that effectively leverage nurses* (white paper). Robert Wood Johnson Foundation.

Kneale, D., Thomas, J., & Harris, K. (2015). Developing and optimising the use of logic models in systematic reviews: Exploring practice and good practice in the use of programme theory in reviews. *PLoS ONE, 10*(11), e0142187. http://dx.doi.org/10.1371/journal.pone.0142187

Kim, J., Jang, J., Kim, B., & Hee Lee, K. (2022). Effect of the PRECEDE-PROCEED model on health programs: A systematic review and meta-analysis. *Systematic Reviews, 11,* 213. https://doi.org/10.1186/s13643-022-02092-2

Lane, A., & Martin, M. (2005). Logic model use for breast health in rural communities. *Oncology Nursing Forum, 32*(1), 105–110. https://doi.org/10.1188/05.onf.105-110

Larsson, S., Clawson, J., & Howard, R. (2023). Value-based health care at an inflection point: a global agenda for the next decade. *NEJM Catalysts.* Retrieved from https://catalyst.nejm.org/doi/full/10.1056/CAT.22.0332

Lynch, E. A., Mudge, A., Knowles, S., Kitson, A. L., Hunter, S. C., & Harvey, G. (2018). There is nothing so practical as a good theory: A pragmatic guide for selecting theoretical approaches for implementation projects. *BMC Health Services Research, 18*, 857. https://doi.org/10.1186/s12913-018-3671-z

Martsolf, G. R., Mason, D. J., Sloan, J., Sullivan, C. G., & Villarruel, A. M. (2017). *Nurse-designed care models and culture of health: Review of three case studies*. RAND Corporation. Retrieved from https://www.rand.org/pubs/research_reports/RR1811.html

McNamara, C. (n.d.). *Designing and marketing your programs*. Retrieved from the Free Management Library website http://managementhelp.org/np_progs/mkt_mod/market.htm

Mills, T., Lawton, S., & Sheard, L. (2019). Advancing complexity science in healthcare research: The logic of logic models. *BMC Medical Research Methodology, 19*, 55. Retrieved from https://doi.org/10.1186/s12874-019-0701-4

Mindell, J., Ison, E., & Joffe, M. (2003). A glossary for health impact assessment. *Journal of Epidemiology and Community Health, 57*, 647–65. http://dx.doi.org/10.1136/jech.57.9.647

Purcarea, V. L. (2019). The impact of marketing strategies in healthcare systems. *Journal of Medicine and Life, 12*(2), 93–96. http://dx.doi.org/10.25122/jml-2019-1003

Rosenthal, L. D., Barnes, C., Aagaard, L., Cook, P., & Weber, M. (2018). Initiating SBIRT, alcohol, and opioid training for nurses employed on an inpatient medical-surgical unit: A quality improvement project. *MedSurg Nursing, 27*(4), 227–230.

Saulle, R., Sinopoli, A., De Paula Baer, A., Mannocci, A., Marino, M., de Belvis, A. G., Federici, A., & La Torre, G. (2020). The PRECEDE–PROCEED model as a tool in public health screening: A systematic review. *La Clinica Terapeutica, 171*(2), e167–e177. http://dx.doi.org/10.7417/CT.2020.2208

Saunders, E., Teall, A. M., Zurmehly, J., Bolen, S. D., Crane, D., Wright, J. Jr., Perzynski, A., & Lever, J. (2022). Coaching quality improvement in primary care to improve hypertension control. *Journal of the American Association of Nurse Practitioners, 34*(7), 932–940. http://dx.doi.org/10.1097/JXX.0000000000000731

Saxena, S., Ramer, L., & Shulman, I. (2004). A comprehensive assessment program to improve blood-administering practices using the FOCUS-PDCA model. *Transfusion, 44*, 1350–1356. http://dx.doi.org/10.1111/j.1537-2995.2004.03117.x

Schell, S. F., Luke, D. A., Schooley, M. W., Elliott, M. B., Herbers, S. H., Mueller, N. B., & Bunge, A. C. (2013). Public health program capacity for sustainability: A new framework. *Implementation Science, 8*, 15. http://www.implementationscience.com/content/8/1/15

Seidl, K. L., Gingold, D. B., Stryckman, B., Landi, C., Sokan, O., Fletcher, M., & Marcozzi, D. (2021). Development of a logic model to guide implementation and evaluation of a mobile integrated health transitional care program. *Population Health Management, 24*(2), 275–281. http://doi.org/10.1089/pop.2020.0038

Shewhart, W. A. (1939). *Statistical method from the viewpoint of quality control* (p. 45). Department of Agriculture. Dover.

W. K. Kellogg Foundation. (2004). *Logic model development guide*. Retrieved from W.K. Kellogg Foundation logic model guide | BetterEvaluation

CHAPTER 9

EVALUATION OF PRACTICE AT THE POPULATION LEVEL

BARBARA A. NIEDZ

INTRODUCTION

Early in their careers, nurses often have an enthusiasm and energy in caring for one patient at a time. Over the years, that focus broadens as the more experienced nurse embraces a role that is more expansive and addresses issues at a population level. As administrators, leaders, educators, and managers, the advanced practice registered nurse's (APRN's) scope of practice widens even further. Quality nurse professionals expand their view to the entire organization and across departments. Nurses have, over the years, moved in many diverse directions. They not only care for patients at the bedside but also in their homes, businesses, schools, prisons, rehabilitation settings, and in outpatient and mental health facilities. Nurses also serve in settings that may be considered more "nontraditional," for example, working for managed care organizations (MCOs) by providing utilization management (UM) and designing and implementing case and disease management (CM and DM) programs. Another critical responsibility of APRNs is the oversight of clinical outcomes at the population level.

The advancement of many educational opportunities for nurses has moved our profession into new and exciting places. The advent of the advanced practice licensure designation has opened doors for nurses that did not exist 20 years ago. Nursing is proactive and responsive to the needs of the healthcare environment and to the needs of patients. APRN status and licensure expand the nursing role to include status as primary care providers (PCPs), and APRNs are recognized in many preferred provider networks across the country, receiving appropriate reimbursement. Our potential to influence the health of patient populations has expanded accordingly.

This chapter describes ways to evaluate population outcomes; systems changes; and effectiveness, efficiency, and trends in care delivery across the continuum. Strategies to monitor healthcare quality are addressed, as well as factors that lead to success. Most importantly, these concepts are explored within the role and competencies of the APRN. Specifically, this chapter addresses at least three of the American Association of Colleges of Nursing (AACN) domain essentials (AACN, 2023). These are (a) population health, (b) quality and safety, and (c) systems-based practice.

MONITORING HEALTHCARE QUALITY

Nurses have been concerned about the quality of patient care for many years. Although our definitions of quality have varied, at the heart of this discussion is our collective desire to continuously improve patients' health and management of various disease states, regardless of where a given patient fits on the continuum.

DEFINITIONS OF QUALITY AND THEORETICAL MODELS

Just as nurses have cared for one patient at a time, initial models for quality dealt with individual patient reviews. Donabedian (1980, 2005) defines *quality* in broad terms: "Quality is a property that medical care can have in varying degrees" (p. 3). His definition holds that "attributes of good care… are so many and so varied that it is impossible to derive from them either a unifying concept or a single empirical measure of quality" (p. 74). This notwithstanding, Donabedian's model of structure, process, and outcome addresses how quality can be maximized in organizations and continues to be used today to structure research on quality methods throughout the globe (Tossaint-Schoenmakers et al., 2021).

In recent years, Donabedian's influence continues in the way organizations are required to demonstrate their quality endeavors. For example, most accrediting bodies, such as The Joint Commission (TJC), the National Committee for Quality Assurance (NCQA), and the Utilization Review Accreditation Commission (URAC), all require evidence of a quality structure. Trilogy documents (a program description for quality, the annual work plan, and an annual program evaluation) are developed and reported through a committee structure that provides insight into the structure of the quality program from frontline staff through governance. In addition, process indicators of quality, such as whether the patient presenting in the emergency department (ED) with chest pain had an EKG performed within 10 minutes is a mandate within TJC's chart abstracted measures for both primary and comprehensive heart attack centers seeking certification (Joint Commission Resources, 2023). Finally, the emphasis of outcomes in recent years also emerges from the Donabedian model. The model provides for a robust relationship between structures and processes, which, taken together, enhance the potential for maximizing outcomes, such as reducing the incidence of readmissions within 30 days for a patient who experienced an acute myocardial infarction (AMI) hospitalization (Core Quality Measures Collaborative, 2023).

Population health includes an integrated system of care across the continuum. Hummer and Hamilton (2019) identify significant healthcare disparities in the

United States and across the board. The population health model seeks to address and reduce those disparities. From a population health perspective, quality is defined in terms of clinical data and outcomes, both economic and patient centered. Guided by research evidence, population health models describe the relationship between quality of care and the cost of care and essentially purport that if the quality of care improves, the cost of care is reduced. Goldberg and Nash (2022) describe the importance of prevention, screening, and patient self-care management. Population health principles identify risk factors implicit in the development of chronic illness, incorporate the influence of the community, and design various programmatic elements. Taken together, these key model components can help manage and reduce the cost of care (Goldberg & Nash, 2022; Hummer & Hamilton, 2019; National Academies of Sciences et al., 2021).

For example, the incidence of diabetes mellitus could potentially be reduced by getting control of the rampant obesity problem across the United States. As an example of a prevention indicator of quality for health plans, monitoring the patient's body mass index (BMI) is an important Healthcare Effectiveness Data and Information Set (HEDIS) (NCQA, 2023c) measure and is also included in the Centers for Medicare and Medicaid Services Five-Star Quality Rating System (CMS STARs) measures (CMS, 2023a). Preventing the incidence of diabetes mellitus can potentially result in reducing its short- and long-term complications, which could subsequently save thousands, perhaps hundreds of thousands, of healthcare dollars. As an example, consider the impact of preventing the incidence of type 2 diabetes mellitus on end-stage renal disease (ESRD) and the cost of dialysis as well as the cost of kidney transplantation. In 2016, Medicare expenditures for 2016 dialysis costs were $28 billion and $35 billion for kidney failure patients (University of California San Francisco, 2023).

The Institute for Healthcare Improvement (IHI) puts population health ideas into action in the Triple Aim initiative. The goals of the Triple Aim are (a) better health, (b) better experience of care, and (c) lower cost. The Triple Aim framework serves as the model for many organizations and communities. The Triple Aim site can be accessed at www.ihi.org/Topics/TripleAim/Pages/default.aspx. Similarly, national healthcare reform has brought this issue front and center (IHI, 2023f). The IHI's Pathways to Population Health (P2PH) describes a collaboration between four organizations that provide practical tools and resources to improve population health (IHI, 2023b). Though no one present unit possesses all the features needed, the role of Accountable Care Organizations (ACOs) in total population health is explored. (See Chapter 10, "The Role of Accreditation and Certification in Validating Population-Based Practice/Programs," for more information on ACOs.)

Juran offers a definition of quality that is both parsimonious and applicable across disciplines (DeFeo, 2019). Within the Juran Trilogy, quality is defined in terms of the customer and holds that a product or service has quality if it is "fit for use" in the eyes of the customer, with three major components: (a) quality planning, (b) quality improvement, and (c) quality control (DeFeo, 2019). Patients, as consumers of healthcare products and services, fit the definition of customers, regardless of the payment source. Juran explains that for a product or service to meet the needs of the customer, it must have the right features (quality by design) and must be free from deficiencies (quality improvement using a Lean Six Sigma approach) (DeFeo, 2019).

In the Juran model, new features (such as new cardiac surgical equipment or the capacity to provide outpatient dialysis) may require capital and operating expenses. Deficiencies or defects in healthcare products or services always contribute to the cost of poor quality, and although there might not be an outlay of dollars, there are still financial consequences. In years past, hospitals were reimbursed for service provided regardless of the outcome. Today, hospitals are no longer reimbursed for the cost associated with the development of a stage III or IV pressure ulcer in a patient if that ulcer was hospital-acquired and not present on admission or other hospital-acquired conditions (HACs). The CMS, which functions under the aegis of the U.S. Department of Health and Human Services (DHHS), promulgated rules to this effect in 2008 (see www.cms.gov/medicare/payment/fee-for-service-providers/hospital-aquired-conditions-hac/hospital-aquired-conditions) (CMS, 2023). The development of a hospital-acquired stage III or IV pressure ulcer is also included in the National Quality Forum's (NQFs) list of "never events" defined as serious reportable events (SREs) (NQF, 2023b). In recent years, the CMS has dictated by law and regulation that hospitals will not be reimbursed for care related to several SREs that occur during an inpatient admission (CMS, 2023).

In the 14 years since the abovementioned reimbursement change, researchers have observed improvement in rates, demonstrating that by tying reimbursement to quality, improvements become noticeable (Centers for Disease Control and Prevention [CDC], 2017, 2021). Other preventable outcomes that contribute to the cost of poor quality have consequences that go beyond dollars and cents. Deficiencies that result in complications and even deaths arise from poor systems and human failures. These have gotten significant and appropriate attention through the patient safety movement (*Crossing the Quality Chasm*, 2003; Institute of Medicine, 2000). Through TJC and the National Patient Safety Goals, attention to hospitals and other healthcare organizations has resulted in significant strides toward reducing deficiencies. Improving quality by preventing the "never events" and reducing deficiencies have reinforced the necessity of accurate and thorough documentation and medical decision-making by all healthcare providers.

Improvements in measurement for both outcome and process indicators of quality have emerged. For example, research literature has shown that in order to decrease the incidence of central line-associated bloodstream infections (CLABSIs), an evidence-based *bundle* is needed. The bundle includes more than one strategy and requires a diligent implementation over time to see results (see also, Chapter 12 "Challenges in Program Implementation") (Agency for Healthcare Research and Quality [AHRQ], 2018; Buetti et al., 2022; IHI, 2012). Surveillance methods have improved, reducing the incidence of overreporting false positives (causing hospitals to lose additional revenue) and underreporting (false negatives), which compromises the integrity of the comparison, benchmark, and risk-adjusted data (Bagchi et al., 2018; Hampe et al., 2017). Thus, measurement mechanisms emerge from Juran's definition of quality (DeFeo, 2019), which also fit with the Donabedian (1980) framework of structure, process, and outcome and the IHI's population health model (IHI, 2023b).

ORGANIZATIONAL MODELS FOR EXCELLENCE

Nurses provide the backbone of healthcare organizations, regardless of venue, whether the setting is inpatient, outpatient, rehabilitation, home care, community health, or in an MCO. Services can be provided in person or sometimes via the telephone. In certain circumstances, nurses provide support by developing and monitoring telehealth programs. As such, understanding the organizational framework that can maximize positive outcomes and minimize deficiencies through the role of the nurse has value. The APRN adds value, particularly through oversight and development of these newly emerging models of care.

Both the Juran model (DeFeo, 2019) and Donabedian (1980) put the concept of quality into the framework of an organization. Care of a patient across the wellness–illness continuum requires consistent and cogent processes and systems. Accordingly, Donabedian's view is that healthcare organizations require appropriate structure and key processes. Taken together, the structure and processes assist the organization in producing desired outcomes for their patients (Donabedian, 1980, 2005). Juran characterizes organizations as high functioning and marked by positive outcomes if features are maximized and deficiencies are minimized (DeFeo, 2019). To accomplish this, organizations plan for, control, and continuously improve quality. Both clinical and service quality characteristics are defined in terms of customers' needs and expectations.

In 1987, the federal government instituted the Malcolm Baldrige Award, which recognizes those organizations that demonstrate principles characteristic of high performance and achieve significant business results through quality improvement techniques. This award is based on seven key guiding principles and embodies a theoretical model of quality consistent with Juran (DeFeo, 2019) and the IHI (IHI, 2023f). In the late 1990s, this award was opened to healthcare organizations. Between 2002 and 2020, there were 29 winners of the Baldrige Award in the healthcare division (National Institutes of Standards and Technology [NIST], 2023).

For organizations to maximize positive outcomes and minimize deficiencies, planning must take on a strategic focus. Leadership and governance have responsibility and oversight for quality and are essentially responsible for organizational planning (Drew & Pandit, 2020; Sfantou et al., 2017). Quality planning provides depth, breadth, and scope of how the product or service is designed, developed, and implemented. Key quality characteristics in the form of measurable goals and objectives for the organization and for patient outcomes are designed in the system or process before that product or service begins. Once that product or service is in operation, customers' needs and expectations (whether in the form of clinical quality, customer satisfaction, core business processes, or utilization of healthcare resources) can be understood, defined, and measured.

The advent of the electronic health record (EHR) in hospitals and other healthcare organizations changed the way that organizations capture documentation and evidence of the patient's history across the continuum of care, as well as contributing to overall patient safety and reduction of medical error. These complex operational processes in hospitals exemplify organizational processes and systems that can address the needs of key customer groups: patients and providers of care. The EHR has facilitated real-time data in the form of reports as well as alerts and patient safety provisions, making accurate and actionable reports on key indicators of quality.

Standardized data definitions for surveillance and payment models also facilitate collective organizational insight as to the level of compliance and excellence achieved. External benchmark comparison data, particularly with risk adjustment, can be helpful in goal setting and in evaluating the extent to which a product or service meets customers' expectations. High-performing organizations design processes and systems to meet customer needs consistently, reducing variation in outcomes and minimizing defects.

W. Edwards Deming developed a landmark theory of quality and consistently modeled the theme of reducing variation and building quality into a product or system so that there is less need to depend on inspection, after the fact (Deming, 2000; The Deming Institute, 2023). Deming's model was also influenced by the work of other quality giants like Shewhart and Feigenbaum. Ishikawa paved the way for Japan's economic turnaround after World War II, largely based on the work of both Juran and Deming, who were sent by the U.S. government to support Japan after the war ("Guru Guide: Six Thought Leaders who Changed the Quality World Forever," 2010). These models rely heavily on the theory that all of quality is measurable and that reducing variation in processes holds a vital role in reducing the incidence of defects and, ultimately, ensuring better outcomes. Thought leaders in healthcare, including many at the IHI, promulgate the use of Deming's ideas in healthcare (IHI, 2023a, 2023e; Sampath et al., 2021).

Berwick et al. (1990) were preeminent in applying these theoretical models to healthcare. Six leading healthcare organizations were armed with a national demonstration grant from the Robert Wood Johnson Foundation; within this seminal work, the authors cataloged the experiences of these organizations in applying this theoretical approach to quality. Their experiences clearly indicate that the models and tools had merit and value in reducing defects, improving processes, and maximizing outcomes. This landmark work demonstrated that what had been shown repeatedly in manufacturing and in service industries throughout the country (and, in fact, worldwide) could be repeated in healthcare and laid the groundwork for potential application throughout the healthcare industry.

Deming, Juran, Crosby, and others explain that reducing variation is a continuous task, even when a given product or service is exceeding the needs of customers and especially when a given product or service is not competitive in the marketplace ("Guru Guide: Six Thought Leaders who Changed the Quality World Forever," 2010; Juran, 2023; The Deming Institute, 2023). The Six Sigma movement emerged from a qualityimprovement initiative at General Electric in the 1980s and set out to reduce defects or deficiencies to fewer than 3.4 defects per 1,000,000 opportunities; a *lean* strategy was added, making a Six Sigma approach particularly attractive to healthcare (American Society for Quality [ASQ], 2023; Pyzdek & Keller, 2018). In essence, this model for quality improvement and planning is built on the work of Juran, Deming, Crosby, Ishikawa, Feigenbaum, and others. Donabedian's work is theoretically sound and resonates with this thinking.

Developing a Lean Six Sigma approach works best when it is done broadly, across the entire organization. When a Six Sigma approach is well defined for a given organization, the impetus and funding source for the program comes directly from governance and cascades from the senior leadership team to the frontline employees, who use the Lean Six Sigma tools on a day-to-day basis. Deciding which projects are convened and which are not is also a governance process and would likely emerge out of the quality infrastructure. Governance provides for an educational process to learn and apply the use of the many tools in the Lean Six Sigma tool chest, many of which have a heavy statistical process control overlay. Lean Six Sigma leadership uses an educational process in the form of various "belts" for certification. For example, a master black belt possesses the skills to oversee multiple Lean Six Sigma projects simultaneously. The black belt is typically the project facilitator; green belts are often process business owners and may serve as the team lead in a Lean Six Sigma team. The yellow belt is the team member who will be schooled in the use of many of the tools (Pyzdek & Keller, 2018).

The patient safety movement in healthcare has given rise to a wider application of the Lean Six Sigma model. In addition, the language of defects and deficiencies, though developed out of manufacturing and other types of product development, has resulted in consistent thinking that complications heretofore considered risks of procedure or hospitalization are now considered preventable (Courtney et al., 2006). The patient safety movement in the United States emerged largely due to TJC and their attention to sentinel events (TJC, 2020). The consensus report "To Err Is Human," published by the Institute of Medicine (IOM) over 20 years ago, provides a focus on the potential for preventable error. One of the most telling comments early in the report explains that at that time, there were between 44,000 and 98,000 preventable medical errors annually in the United States that lead to patient deaths (Institute of Medicine, 2000). The variability in the range is significant. Measurement mechanisms that would provide accurate descriptions of these sentinel events did not exist at that time. In the language of the process improvement gurus, these are defects and deficiencies. Applying these theoretical models to healthcare has tremendous potential in accurately describing quality of care by improving outcomes through attention to structure, process, and outcome. Though there was a time when the focus was on the individual patient, EHR systems, competitive data comparisons with or without risk adjustment, and improvement models that have been developed over the past 20 years have made inroads in the availability of tools and a system-wide approach (AHRQ, 2023b; IHI, 2023b, 2023f; Sampath et al., 2021)

The advent of the EHR in healthcare has facilitated data collection and the availability of data to drive decisions organizationally and dashboards abound. Introduced over 30 years ago, Kaplan and Norton (1992) take measurement in organizations a step further and link progress against the strategic planning cycle to organizational goals and objectives. Their *balanced scorecard* (BSC) model lends itself to healthcare well and has been applied internationally (Balanced Scorecard Institute, 2023; Carnut & Narvai, 2020; Heidary Dahooie et al., 2021). The Malcolm Baldrige Award has several specific criteria and one of the most important is the recognition of *results* (NIST, 2023). The results criteria require evidence of measurement and improvement of quality across organizations and systems. A well-defined scorecard at the enterprise level, which is balanced across several categories relating to the customer's experience, is a useful and important tool for senior leadership and governance. As we move into a discussion about planning, controlling for, and improving quality across the entire patient population, understanding theoretical models for process improvement and their application becomes not only useful and accepted but also necessary and, most important, leads to improved outcomes of care.

PROCESS IMPROVEMENT MODELS AND TOOLS

The literature provides applied evidence of various process improvement models that have many commonalities. Deliberate and thoughtful use of applied evidence and the use of process improvement models can result in reduction of defects and deficiencies to levels that meet and exceed customers' expectations, whether those expectations surround clinical quality, customer satisfaction, core business processes, or utilization of healthcare resource expectations. The "plan, do, check, act" (PDCA) process improvement model (IHI, 2023c) or Six Sigma's define, measure, analyze, improve, and control (DMAIC) model (Pyzdek & Keller, 2018) both have common features. They are problem-solving models that drive measurable improvement when used properly. They can facilitate a thought process and require a team initiative. They will work whether the problem is related to clinical quality, customer satisfaction, core business processes, or utilization of healthcare resources. They work inside and outside of healthcare, whether the problem is simple or complex and whether one is concerned about the care of patients or developing tangible products for retail sale. Box 9.1 describes characteristics that are commonly found in process improvement models.

Process improvement models have these common characteristics. In addition, a variety of tools support the quality professional along the process improvement path. Tools such as process flow charting, barriers and aids charts, cost–benefit analyses, data collection tools and statistical methods, SIPOC (suppliers, inputs, process, outputs, and customers) analyses, project planning tools, lean thinking, and many others provide useful insight and drill closer to improvement goals (IHI, 2023c, 2023d) (American Society for Quality [ASQ], 2023; Messinger et al., 2019).

POPULATION-BASED MODELS

On a continuum from health and wellness (H&W) products to complex care management, a variety of population-based models have emerged over recent years (Box 9.2). Patients move across a continuum from good health to the end of life and enter a variety of settings in doing so. Programs are designed to offer both telephone care and field-based approaches to prevention, DM, care coordination, CM, and care integration. Patients are identified through predictive models and other stratification methods. The extent of outreach is determined by various levels of acuity, and the frequency of patient contact may depend on clinical assessment and care planning. Motivational interviewing and health education are primary strategies to engage patients into modifying their behaviors, but a hallmark of all these programs is ultimately a change in health behaviors, which leads to desired outcomes. Preventive strategies, such as smoking cessation programs, and care

> **BOX 9.1**
>
> **CHARACTERISTICS AND COMMONALITIES OF PROCESS IMPROVEMENT MODELS**
>
> 1. The problem is defined in measurable terms.
> 2. The problem is stated in terms of the customer's needs and expectations.
> 3. External comparative benchmark data are sometimes drawn on to help set the goal for the project.
> 4. Members of the team have well-defined responsibilities.
> 5. Most teams should have six to 10 members. Larger teams may not be able to control the problem process and might need to break into smaller groups to be effective. Smaller teams may have inadequate representation to fully address all facets of the problem.
> 6. The team includes an executive sponsor to usher the project as a priority in the organization.
> 7. Other team roles include business process owner as team leader, internal or external consultant as facilitator, and clearly described roles for remaining team members.
> 8. There is an analysis phase. This phase employs both qualitative and quantitative methods to arrive at barriers, obstacles, and root causes of the problem.
> 9. The analysis phase should be well supported with qualitative data (like a cause–effect diagram) and quantitative "theory testing" data (like a diagnostic study of the root causes of the process problem).
> 10. Remedies that address both the qualitative and quantitative barriers are designed.
> 11. A plan for piloting or testing the remedies is well defined, engages the full team, considers the cost of implementation and decision-making therein, and defines whether or not they are sufficient to achieve the desired improvement.
> 12. A measurement mechanism is designed to evaluate the effectiveness of the change strategy and the degree to which an additional remedial plan is needed.
> 13. A mechanism for evaluating ongoing data collection, day to day and month to month, is put in place, to ensure that the gains are held constant.
> 14. In order to provide an effective use of a process improvement model, the focus must be clear and well defined. Teams must sometimes winnow down a larger project to its smaller component parts. At the end of a successful process improvement project, consider going back to revisit other improvement opportunities, which may have been set aside from the focal interest.

coordination strategies, such as identifying a medical home and ensuring medical transportation to an outpatient facility, combined with condition-specific strategies in the presence of various chronic disease states, to reduce the incidence of ED usage for primary care and reduce inpatient admissions are all examples of ways to improve access to care in the hopes of ensuring overall quality of care (Affentranger & Mulkey, 2023; Kalata et al., 2023; Mukherji et al., 2022). DM and CM programs are effective in reducing the trajectory of chronic disease by lessening utilization of healthcare resources and enhancing patient satisfaction by improving the patient's ability to perform activities

> **BOX 9.2**
>
> **POPULATION HEALTH MODELS**
>
> 1. Health and Wellness (H&W): These programs are primarily telephonic and may have a biometric screening component; program awareness and patient education materials are often part of a direct mail campaign. These programs aim at identifying patients with significant health risk and encourage patient participation in screening. Completion of a health risk assessment is often a key component of lifestyle management programs. Smoking cessation, weight reduction, and attendance at preventive care visits are examples of desired outcomes for this patient population. Although significant health risks may emerge here, this patient population is essentially healthy without the presence of diagnosed disease states; the focus of H&W programs is aimed at identifying risks, with prevention of chronic illness as the ultimate target.
>
> 2. Disease Management (DM): These programs are likely to be telephonic, field based, or a combination of both. Patients qualify for DM programs on the basis of identified disease states, singly or in combination. Most DM programs target at least five or six disease conditions: persistent asthma, COPD (chronic obstructive pulmonary disease), CAD (coronary artery disease), diabetes mellitus, CHF (congestive heart failure), and depression. Other programs are broader and capture superutilizers—high-risk patients with varied chronic disease states. DM programs often have a care coordination component, which can provide such things as assistance in placing patients in a medical home, medical transportation (to help reduce the overuse of emergency medical services and ED care), or help in finding funding sources for medication management (to avoid disease exacerbations due to medications not being filled), and so on. Examples of outcomes for this patient population include, but are not limited to, (a) ensuring that a diabetic patient gets HbA1C testing done at least annually, (b) ensuring that a patient with persistent asthma has a prescription for controller medications, and (c) confirming that a CHF patient knows the importance of measuring their daily weight and what to do if symptoms worsen. For example, when a patient who has CHF and an ejection fraction of less than 40% is being discharged from the inpatient setting with proper discharge plans and instructions, we ensure that the patient is appropriately prescribed an angiotensin-converting enzyme (ACE) inhibitor and knows the importance of weighing themselves daily. In summary, care coordination ensures that the patient has the ability to fill the prescription (has transportation to obtain and financial resources to buy), has a scale at home or the means to purchase one, and has transportation to the doctor's office for follow-up or preventive care.
>
> 3. Case Management (CM): These programs capture patients who have complex needs and multiple health conditions. These patients are often high risk and high cost and come to the surface in stratification and predictive models because of overutilization of EDs and multiple admissions due to poor outpatient management or lack of a medical home. These patients account for a very small percentage of the total population but account for more than 60% of the total healthcare dollar. Models that integrate care across various specialties for a given patient set (e.g., patients with severe mental illness who also have multiple medical disease conditions) are emerging.

of daily living and improving their ability to manage chronic diseases (self-efficacy) (Deutschbein et al., 2020; Dillon et al., 2021; Hansen et al., 2022).

One of the most interesting recent trends in population-based care management is care integration. Care integration is a concept that is well known to nurses but may not be as familiar to other health professionals. Here is an example: A patient is admitted to an inpatient acute care hospital with a significant drug overdose after an attempted suicide. This long-standing behavioral health (BH) patient has been managed "on and off" by a variety of BH professionals and has been receiving various psychotropic medications. In addition, the patient has a medical history that includes long-standing diabetes and CAD; other healthcare professionals have managed these aspects of the patient's healthcare. In fact, the medical professionals have not been in touch with the BH professionals, at the patient's request. In the ED, the BH professionals' role is preempted as the patient's overwhelming medical needs are the priority. When the patient is admitted to the intensive care unit (ICU), a host of consultants are brought to the case, and after being "cleared medically," the patient is transferred to the inpatient BH unit. Care is sometimes fragmented and the BH needs are addressed separately and apart from the medical needs of the patient. The PCP may not be involved until after discharge and may not have a clear sense of the many issues that play a role in the complete care of this patient. Although there is no question about the prioritization of care, there is also no integration of care. The patient's experience is divided into two distinctly different phases, in some ways compromising effective use of healthcare resources. Length of stay is clearly segmented into two sequential phases rather than managed in parallel.

Lack of care integration is a common problem on the outpatient side of the care continuum as well as on the inpatient side of care management. Processes of care that appropriately integrate care have been somewhat problematic in the U.S. healthcare system in the past. In recent years, it has become apparent that care integration needs to improve, which would improve the quality of care, resolve access issues, and reduce overutilization of healthcare resources (Deutschbein et al., 2020; Dillon et al., 2021).

Two recent initiatives bring these ideas into sharp perspective. The first is the concept of the patient-centered medical home (PCMH). Within this model, care integration services are well defined and the process of bringing care to the patients where, when, and how they need it becomes not only possible but also practical. The NCQA promulgates standards that describe this initiative (NCQA, 2023e). ACOs provide another model that incorporates these ideas into organized systems of care with healthcare providers, PCMHs, and hospitals partnering together. This is a program promulgated by the CMS (CMS, 2022).

NURSE-SENSITIVE PROCESS AND OUTCOME INDICATORS AT THE POPULATION LEVEL

Many authors have promulgated ways to organize measures, as taken together they represent a picture of quality. Kaplan and Norton (1992) suggest four generic categories that could work for any organization, including organizations that focus on healthcare. These perspectives include (a) internal business processes, (b) customer focus, (c) learning and growth, and (d) financing (Kaplan & Norton, 1992, 2005; Kober & Northcott, 2021; Shelton, 2021). The NCQA places the HEDIS measures into categories as well. The HEDIS categories include (a) effectiveness of care, (b) access/availability of care, (c) satisfaction with the experience of care, (d) use of services, and (e) cost of care (NCQA, 2023b).

Although the list of possible indicators used to measure population health and population health nursing may seem endless, four categories of measures, metrics, and indicators emerge. These broad categories are clinical quality, customer satisfaction, core business processes, and utilization of healthcare resources. Loosely based on the BSC model and the NCQA HEDIS frameworks, an organizing framework for evaluating population health nursing emerges (Kaplan & Norton, 1992, 2005; Kober & Northcott, 2021; NCQA, 2023c). As these categories are of use in organizing our thinking regarding quality in the inpatient setting, they also have merit in outpatient settings, and as we consider care of the entire population with a given disease condition, these categories continue to add value to this discussion as an organizing framework. For this discussion, the words *measures*, *metrics*, and *indicators* are used interchangeably. Healthcare organizational leaders may assemble a dashboard of these metrics. When a parsimonious set of measures are linked to the strategic plan, specific improvement techniques and goals and objectives metrics take on a deeper meaning for the organization.

Whenever possible, standardized data definitions are essential. This sets up a level playing field for comparisons. Since the late 1990s, data sets, external comparisons, and guidance for standardized numerator and denominator have emerged across the patient continuum of care. As our industry has become more accountable to the public for outcomes, this kind of standardization has been essential, facilitating external comparisons based on data. In addition, these numerators and denominators are described in detail, right down to the technical specifications. These technical specifications describe what types of codes are included in the numerator and which are included and excluded in the denominator. These codes have become widely accepted, the application of which results in fair and appropriate comparisons and rankings. Various groups (both governmental and private) have defined measures, specified the technical mechanics of counting and determining rates, and applied these measures across the industry to achieve standardization in data collection (NQF, 2023a). These include but are not limited to the following: (a) CMS (www.cms.gov/center/quality.asp), (b) TJC (www.jointcommission.org), (c) the AHRQ (www.ahrq.gov), (d) NCQA (www.ncqa.org), (e) the NQF (www.qualityforum.org), and (f) the National Database of Nursing Quality Indicators (NDNQI) (www.pressganey.com/platform/ndnqi).

Measures have emerged over time. As our foray into this area of accountability for outcomes has been heightened by legislators, policymakers, and the public at large, the connection between the cost of poor quality in healthcare and healthcare reform has become more explicit. Although it might require capital and operational outlay of funding to develop a specific product or service with the right features within the healthcare industry, the cost of poor quality adds a substantial burden to the cost of healthcare. For example, when a patient in a hospital setting experiences a delay in obtaining a diagnostic procedure that is essential to the appropriate management of their disease state, this core business process can delay decision-making, causing a longer length of stay (LOS) for the patient in the hospital. This delay may also lead to disease progression and result in complications that otherwise might have been prevented. Another question that should be addressed is whether these types of delays are due to the type of insurance, underinsurance, or lack of insurance. As discussed in Chapter 3, "Identifying Outcomes in Population-Based Nursing," an important component of APRN practice is the need to recognize and address issues related to healthcare disparities.

When patient safety is compromised in hospitals, the result can be substantial. The example of delayed diagnostic testing may not only hinder the determination of a patient's diagnosis but may also lead to patients receiving inaccurate medications or treatments or errors, such as a patient identification mix-up, that can result in loss of life. Over time, we are better able to identify the impact of the cost of poor quality by capturing and quantifying these indicators of quality in the aggregate. Sorting out "what counts and what doesn't" helps to provide clarity and a clearer view of quality across the board.

Clinical Quality

Nurse-sensitive indicators of population health that relate to clinical quality can be seen in several metrics recognized by external organizations with available external benchmarks. In the HEDIS data set created and maintained by the NCQA, there are several benchmarks that relate to chronic disease conditions (NCQA, 2023c). Nurses who are in the field or on the phone in telephone call centers reach out to patients with the intention of helping them wade through the various resources made available to them through private and public means to manage their overall health, given the presence of various disease states. The most common disease states managed by DM programs include the following: (a) diabetes mellitus, (b) persistent asthma, (c) COPD, (d) CAD, and (e) CHF. Other chronic disease conditions also may be of interest. In CM programs, the complexity of care is heightened by the number and acuity of the chronic conditions coexisting in a patient's profile. Social problems, housing, transportation, and pharmacy costs often emerge in CM programs. Similarly, the emphasis from a clinical quality perspective in H&W programs is on preventive care, early recognition of emerging disease, and use of appropriately placed screening tools.

With the agreement of the NCQA, the CMS has adopted the use of HEDIS in its STAR rating program for various types of MCOs. For example, each Medicare Advantage health plan licensed by the CMS is rated on a five-point star system. Clinical quality measures include process indicators collected through administrative means that contribute to a given health plan's STAR rating. For example, whether the patient with a diagnosis of diabetes mellitus has a glycosylated hemoglobin (HbA1C) test done at least annually tells us something about the care that a patient with diabetes receives. CMS weights each one of the STAR measures as to its importance. This process indicator of clinical quality that is determined by the presence or absence of an administrative claim or encounter for an outpatient laboratory test (in this case HbA1C) is weighted with one point toward the health plan's overall STAR rating. However, the actual value of HbA1C is a component of "comprehensive diabetes care," a HEDIS measure, which is included in HEDIS, and another STAR measure for Medicare Advantage health plans in Part C. We know from scientific research that patients who maintain lower HbA1C levels have fewer complications, a better quality of life, and longer life expectancy than do patients who are poorly controlled (NCQA, 2023a). This makes HbA1C levels a significant clinical outcome indicator. Health plans collect actual HbA1C levels through a rigorous process and through

> **BOX 9.3**
>
> **SAMPLE NURSE-SENSITIVE CLINICAL QUALITY MEASURES IN DM, CM, AND H&W PROGRAMS**
> 1. HEDIS Comprehensive Diabetes Mellitus Care: Did the patient have at least one HbA1C level drawn in a 12-month period?
> 2. CMS STARs HEDIS: Comprehensive Diabetes Care: Did the patient, aged 65 or older, show good control, through HbA1C levels of 8% or less?
> 3. HEDIS Asthma Care: Did the patient diagnosed with chronic persistent asthma have prescriptions for the appropriate medications to manage chronic persistent asthma?
> 4. AHRQ Prevention Quality Indicator of CHF: What is the annual inpatient admission rate per 100,000 (at the population level) for CHF?
> 5. AHRQ Prevention Quality Indicator of COPD: What is the annual inpatient admission rate per 100,000 (at the population level) for COPD?
> 6. HEDIS: Did the patient diagnosed with CAD and an LDL (low-density lipoprotein) level of greater than 100 mg/dL have a prescription for a statin or HMG-CoA (3-hydroxy-3-methylglutaryl-coenzyme A) reductase inhibitor?
> 7. HEDIS: Did the infant have appropriate well-child visits during their first year of life?
>
> *Source:* Adapted from Healthcare Effectiveness Data and Information Set. (2023). Narrative, technical specifications, and survey measurement (Vols. 1–3). Washington, DC: National Committee for Quality Assurance. Retrieved from www.ncqa.org/hedis/measures

a variety of means, including EHR data, providers' outpatient medical records, or actual laboratory data feeds. Most importantly, these data are weighted at three times the value of a process indicator in the overall STAR rating. To score at the highest, five-star rating, Medicare Advantage health plans strive to have a significant percentage of their patients score less than 8% on the HbA1C test.

Box 9.3 lists several examples of clinical quality measures that are sensitive to the APRN role at the population health level in DM, CM, and lifestyle management or H&W programs, whether their intervention is on the telephone, in person in any setting, or via a telehealth program. APRNs who have responsibilities regardless of the setting can strengthen a program design by ensuring that outcome measures are used in evaluating program effectiveness and incorporating a blend of process and outcome measures in quality program development.

Utilization of Healthcare Resources

One of the many important goals for nurses who work in DM, CM, and H&W programs is to direct patients to use healthcare resources in the most cost-effective way. In the context of population health, the most expensive healthcare resources include the use of the ED and inpatient stays. By ensuring that the patient's discharge plan coming out of the inpatient setting is fully executed, one can reduce the risk of rehospitalization. By ensuring that patients have transportation and other care coordination needs met, it is to be hoped that we can reduce or eliminate emergency medical service (EMS) use for a ride to the local ED for primary care issues. The two metrics that are the most useful and sensitive to the nursing role in DM and CM programs are inpatient admissions per 1,000 members and ED visits per 1,000 members. In some ways, this work is an extension of the work that nurses have participated in for years in UM programs based in hospitals, for health plans, and for other providers of healthcare benefits. However, DM, CM, and H&W nurses take UM to the next step and ensure that patients have the means, insight, and knowledge to carry out their healthcare needs with some degree of independence and autonomy. By reviewing care needs and targeting the right level of care and matching it to the appropriate venue, we reduce the inappropriate use of these very costly services.

An evaluation of healthcare resource use is often included in each DM or CM contract as a "return on investment" (ROI) analysis as evidence of financial performance. The bulk of the healthcare dollar primarily resides in the use of two resources: ED visits and inpatient stays. Both may be misused in the absence of an effective medical home or with poor access to primary care. At the population level, measuring the impact of population health models on the use of these two key healthcare resources is a very important component of any population health evaluation method. Three possibilities present themselves in a ROI evaluation; rigorous methodology is a component of well-designed DM and CM models. First, an estimation of cost avoidance involves using historical data to predict the number and percentage of ED users and inpatient admissions in a given patient population that are likely to occur after a year of DM intervention. For example, after 1 year of investment in a telephonic nursing DM program, it is reasonable to predict that patients will be linked into a medical home and lessen their risk of admissions for preventable primary care conditions such as uncontrolled diabetes, asthma, or even CHF. These strategies also have the potential to prevent the use of EDs for primary care. Another method to evaluate ROI is to predict a trend and trajectory based on the baseline history of a given set or population of patients. A typical data set for comparison is a 12-month period, used as the starting point or baseline for comparisons moving forward. A third option to calculate the ROI of a DM population health nursing program posits that because of DM intervention, certain specific events will not occur. These are examples of rate changes that could (potentially) be the subject of an ROI calculation: a reduction in the readmission rate, reduction of the rate of patients per 1,000 with multiple admissions, or reduction of patients with admissions for ambulatory-sensitive conditions (ASCs). ASCs are also described by AHRQ as preventive quality indicators. (Visit www.ahrq.gov/data/qualityindicators/index.html for more information on these important indicators.)

In recent years, two additional areas were identified for cost savings indicators: reducing the incidence of readmissions to the inpatient setting within 30 days of discharge and reducing the cost of pharmaceuticals by developing an appropriate formulary and applying rigorous criteria for pharmaceutical medical necessity determination. APRNs can take a key role in reducing inappropriate use of healthcare resources by ensuring that care coordination tasks are addressed across the continuum, particularly at the point of transition from one setting to another, and by building and tapping into community resources as well as medication management with pharmacy involvement (Harris et al., 2022).

All-cause readmissions within 30 days are a significant measure of healthcare resource usage and is another example of a CMS STARs outcome measure that is weighted more heavily in a given health plan's overall STAR rating (CMS, 2023a). Finally, although readmission after discharge from an acute care facility has long been an area of focus, in recent years, unplanned acute care readmissions within 30 days of discharge from a rehabilitation setting and from long-term care hospitals (LTCHs) have also received attention. In point of fact, LTCH has public reporting as most of the STAR ratings do (CMS, 2023e). Additionally, significant efforts have been made to reduce the utilization of expensive medications in pharmacy benefit programs and specialty pharmacy programs alike. Innovative programs, driven by pharmacists, which target long-term control of chronic conditions and the role of the clinical pharmacist, are emerging. Medication therapy management (MTM) programs for patients with chronic illness and complex medication profiles are becoming more of a mandate and less of a luxury (CMS, 2023f).

Measures that relate to medication usage such as medication reconciliation, particularly in the chronically ill and the elderly, are included in CMS STARs, as Plan D measures (part of the pharmacy benefit) and selected measures in Plan C, the medical benefit. There are also pharmacy measures that relate to special needs patient population plans for those patients who are dually eligible for both Medicare and Medicaid (CMS, 2023j).

It could be argued that many of these measures fall into both the clinical quality and the utilization of healthcare resource categories. They not only improve the clinical quality of care received and serve to prevent short- and long-term complications but also reduce inpatient hospitalizations for patients with chronic illness and an acute need, as well as reduce the cost of care. It is also interesting that many of these clinical and utilization of healthcare resource measures also emerge for Medicare patients who are members of ACOs. ACOs are formed to address the needs of direct, fee-for-service Part A and Part B Medicare patients. These ACOs mandate at least 5,000 Medicare patients for a 3-year term. To achieve the incentives, these ACOs must demonstrate the same type of improvement in similar measures as Medicare Advantage health plans (CMS, 2023h).

Customer Satisfaction

For many years, patients have been identified as important consumers of healthcare products and services and, accordingly, have been defined as "customers" and important stakeholders in DM and CM organizations (NCQA, 2023d; URAC, 2023). Accordingly, key metrics that are sensitive to the nursing role can tell us something about the degree to which our patients, as customers, have had a positive experience with our nurses, whether those nurses practice in hospitals, in DM organizations, or at MCOs. How frustrating is it when a customer makes a telephone call to any company and ends up in a hold queue for long periods of time? For many years, two call center metrics have been often cited as important: (a) average speed of answer (ASA) and (b) call abandonment rate (ABN) (Formichelli, 2007; Shadding, 2009). This literature is replete with guidance on how long it should take to answer inbound telephone calls to meet or exceed customers' expectations. The industry standard for ASA is fewer than 30 seconds and that for ABN is less than 5%, that is, less than 5% of calls should be lost when a customer abandons the call due to a prolonged waiting time (Formichelli, 2007). Akin to waiting for a response to a call light in an inpatient setting, prolonged wait times on the phone are a primary source of customer dissatisfaction. In recent years, the advent of multiple phone trees, predictive dialing, and interactive voice response (IVR) use in call centers has added technology and options aimed at improving the customer's experience. Call wait times and abandonment rates continue to be important drivers of customer satisfaction but in a more robust way, using statistical analyses and informatics (Jeunghyun et al., 2018; Selinka et al., 2022). Ensuring that staffing levels (for both licensed and nonlicensed staff members) are appropriate and that technology provides adequate tools for observing the call queue and using data down to the level of the staff member are important oversight supervisory functions for ensuring telephonic DM or CM care in a way that meets or exceeds customer satisfaction.

Monitoring, managing, and measuring complaints are additional ways to tap into the customer's experience. Customer complaints, whether from patient as customer or provider as customer, can be an insightful means to understanding patterns and trends of care delivery and can be the key to improvement. Customer complaints can be very serious and can lead to a written complaint or, if a patient is not satisfied with the resolution offered, the launching of a formal grievance process. Customer complaints that are resolved by the nurse on the call are important to document and are worth tracking. Sometimes, complaints come into a DM call center that might be serious, but the target of the complaint is not the DM organization. In this case, these complaints are also valuable indicators of quality and should be referred to an appropriate authority or organization. Again, tracking and trending the nature of the complaint and the agency or organization to which the complaint was referred (rather than resolution) may be all that is required.

Measuring customer satisfaction through a survey process has long been established as an important function, whether that measurement occurs in a hospital or in a population health setting, like a DM program. Many hospitals use a variety of prominent vendors for patient satisfaction monitoring such as Press Ganey™ Associates (www.pressganey.com/index.aspx) and many other research groups that specialize in healthcare survey processes. In recent years, the CMS has mandated the use of an agreed-upon set of questions administered in a consistent way regardless of the vendor. Vendors must be approved by CMS in order to serve a given organization and submit data to the CMS. In the inpatient venue, the CMS survey titled the Hospital Consumer Assessment of Healthcare Providers and Systems (HCAHPS) is required as part of the value-based purchasing program (CMS, 2023c). Although individual vendors, such as Press Ganey, offer comparisons based on various methods, the HCAHPS survey offers broad comparisons across the country on an agreed set of questions, worded the same and applied using the same mandated research methods.

Surveys targeted at PCPs, specialists, and other providers of healthcare services that evaluate the extent to which the DM organization provides services to them in the interests of their patients are another important tool to gauge overall effectiveness. Annual surveys of providers as customers can also be insightful to a DM organization, to large medical groups, and healthcare networks alike (American Medical Group Association [AMGA], 2023).

Phone automated surveys and IVR surveys are also available, and a variety of telephone services provide this capability. This type of data collection and these methods have been used extensively because they provide timely feedback that is relevant on an ongoing basis. They do present advantages over annual surveys in that a data stream is available with data summaries on six to eight items at weekly, monthly, or even daily frequency, with assignment right to the level of the nurse. Survey research is fraught with both opportunity and challenge. Careful attention must be paid to sample size, response rate, generalizability of the findings, frequency of assessment, reading level of written surveys, and so on. In short, survey research requires the same rigor as a well-designed research study if the results are expected to reflect services rendered accurately and point to quality improvement initiatives.

Another key component of the value-based purchasing program includes a customer satisfaction survey that taps into a given patient's level of satisfaction with their providers and healthcare systems. This tool, titled the Consumer Assessment of Healthcare Providers and Systems (CAHPS), has been developed in conjunction with the NCQA and launched using approved vendors across hospitals, health plans, home health organizations, CMS pharmacy programs, hemodialysis programs, hospice, outpatient and ambulatory surgery centers, and EDs. Surveys are customized to healthcare type (nursing home vs. hospital vs. healthcare system) and may vary by payer type (private, commercial insurance vs. Medicare or Medicaid). Items on the instruments may be nurse sensitive and may be of additional value because of available comparative data. Questions may ask about the extent to which advice has been offered by healthcare providers on such things as smoking cessation and hypertension or cholesterol management, all of which may relate to the nursing role in disease prevention/management or H&W programs that encourage self-care management, in addition to a consumer's primary experience with the service or system like ease of getting an appointment (CMS, 2023b).

Patient self-reported outcomes are captured in survey form by the CMS in the form of the Health Outcomes Survey (HOS), which is administered to a defined cohort of CMS members every 2 years. These self-reported outcomes include measures on the extent to which patients perceive their overall physical and emotional health status over the 2-year period. HOS measures also contribute to CMS STAR measures for managed Medicare health plans and for special needs plans for the dually eligible (CMS, 2023d).

Core Business Processes

Nurses are supported in many ways by the systems and processes through which they provide care. Although this is true in any direct care setting, it also has merit in telephone care and field-based DM and CM programs. While in hospitals, there might be some value to considering how acuity influences staffing levels; in the DM industry, acuity levels and ratios of staff to patients in DM programs are useful data. At the same time, because nurses are supported by job descriptions that are accurate and competency based, they are evaluated on their performance on a regular and ongoing basis. This is sound human resource practice, regardless of the setting or care type. Similarly, productivity levels are very important in all settings in which nurses practice. Can a given nurse manage a patient care assignment that is appropriate to the setting and meet all the patient care requirements? This important question in the DM and CM industry might be answered by examining not only how many patients can be cared for per nurse per day but also how many active minutes of the day the nurse is talking with patients on the telephone. Although in hospitals, outpatient settings, and rehabilitation facilities there is a *hands on* nature to the care, in telephonic DM programs, both *calls per nurse per day* and *talk time in minutes* are direct measures of nursing productivity. Clinical quality and utilization of healthcare resource outcomes may be the best overall indicators of the quality of care, but these indirect measures also have merit. In other words, for a nurse to be effective in managing the care of an entire population of patients across the continuum of care, volume, and focus matter. To measure overall effectiveness of a group of nurses in DM programs, these measures of core business processes, when taken with clinical quality, customer satisfaction, and utilization of healthcare resources, can add to the panel of metrics that bring depth and understanding to managing the care of hundreds of thousands of patients across an entire population.

Other measures that are reflective of core business processes have value in evaluating the role of the nurse. In population health, DM, and CM processes, APRNs are interested in finding those patients for whom they can have an impact on their healthcare behaviors and make a difference in the way in which they manage their day-to-day care. A patient with diabetes and advanced comorbidities, who has not been in an ED or admitted (even for short- or long-term complications) to an inpatient facility, may not have obvious gaps in treatment (i.e., this patient is well managed without any help from the DM nurse). Suppose that a given diabetic patient who is well managed (on their own) has an annual checkup with the PCP and their last HbA1C was less than 7%. This patient may have very little actionable need for a conversation with a nurse in a DM program other than an introduction, consent, a condition-specific assessment, written materials, and encouragement to stay the course. Contrast this to a newly diagnosed 55-year-old patient with an HbA1C of over 11%, with poor nutritional habits, who has just started on insulin and was just discharged from the hospital for "uncontrolled diabetes." Patients such as these have more actionable needs and are at risk for readmission if no DM assessments and interventions are put into place. Finding these patients, teeing them up for the nurse, and ensuring that we have accurate call information are all strategies that are collectively called "patient identification" and "acuity stratification" processes. Oftentimes, DM and CM companies and MCOs use sophisticated information technology processes to identify patients for the nurse to call. A resulting engagement rate that measures the percentage of patients who are identified with one or more of the disease conditions under study and the percentage of patients who complete an enrollment and condition-specific assessment process with a nurse is a useful indicator of the degree to which the DM and/or CM programs are reaching the intended population. This is a type of volume indicator that, when taken together with productivity metrics, can provide some evaluation of the impact of the role of the nurse on population health in DM and CM programs.

In summary, about 20 to 25 metrics in the four categories of (a) clinical quality, (b) customer satisfaction, (c) utilization of healthcare resources, and (d) core business processes taken together would provide an organization with a parsimonious panel of metrics. This panel of metrics described in detail earlier provides the reader with possibilities for evaluating the totality of any given population health nursing program, whether DM, CM, or all three program types. Kaplan and Norton (1992, 2005) describe this idea of a panel of metrics to guide the strategy of the organization as *the BSC*. The examples provided earlier and from these four categories fit the evaluation need in DM, CM, and H&W programs, but neither the categories nor the example metrics are the only possibilities. APRNs can apply these concepts to any venue and the type of measures developed could easily be adapted in a hospital or healthcare system, and outpatient clinic or a private practice and the population may vary in size. In general, metrics and measures should be easily found using existing measurement mechanisms and standardized data definitions, which can be compared against national standards and are representative of the nurse's role in improving the health of the population regardless of the care venue. A parsimonious set is useful; it is often the case that in healthcare we measure too many things. In tracking countless indicators without intention or purpose, we lose the ability to make the measures meaningful and may miss the overall strategic goals of the organization.

DATA SOURCES

In the past, administrative data sets had been criticized for not providing useful information and for not serving as accurate measures of quality. However, a broader understanding of the usefulness of administrative data has emerged in more recent times, particularly when evaluating quality at the level of the population (Jha et al., 2007; Schatz et al., 2005). Claims data has also been called "administrative data." Encounter data are another type of administrative data that are captured for patients in "at-risk" health plans, that is, plans that are capitated or partially capitated. Administrative data are rich in various coding types, including, but not limited to, the *International Classification of Diseases*, 10th Edition (ICD-10) codes (CDC, 2018c); Current Procedural Terminology or CPT codes; and the CMS's Healthcare Common Procedure Coding System (HCPCS) codes. Used as the basis for electronic billing, these codes are rich in information about the patient and have been refined through the years to provide even more information (American Academy of Professional Coders, 2018). In DM, the ICD-10 codes, demographics, and patient experiences, as captured through the administrative process, provide an outline of care that affords the opportunity not only to identify patients with the most actionable need but also to find patients with those gaps in treatment. In the past, the evaluation of quality required detailed and sometimes tedious chart reviews, with random samples of charts pulled from various patient types. The effective use of administrative data is providing a rich source of information on the effectiveness of DM programs in shaping patients' health behaviors and habits over time (NCQA, 2018a).

Organizations of all types have implemented EHR systems that have made documentation by clinicians both more available and more complex (Lorenzetti et al., 2018; Siegler et al., 2015). As reimbursement has become focused on both process and outcomes measures, reporting requirements for hospitals, health plans, and providers have escalated (AHRQ, 2023a; American Hospital Association, 2023). In addition, report writing has become not only useful but also essential. Hospital-based and health plans with DM, CM, and H&W programs alike are awash in reporting requirements to keep pace with financial rewards and regulatory mandates (NCQA, 2023c; NQF, 2023a).

In most DM programs, some type of documentation is required to track the patient's progress with an educational approach and the degree to which a behavior is shaped. So, although it is most important for the nurse to document an educational session on, for example, the importance of asthma controller medications, it may be just as important to hold a three-way call with the patient's PCP to identify the need to move from frequent use of a short-acting beta agonist to an inhaled corticosteroid and to document this action. The claim for the prescription may come through that administrative data set later, but the role of the nurse is and should be accurately captured in written or electronic documentation. The review of the nurse's documentation from a clinical perspective is no less important in call center and field-based DM programs than it is in the hospital, in an outpatient setting, or in a direct care home setting. This documentation needs to be audited on a regular and ongoing basis; this supervisory function can also provide rich evidence of the productivity and role of the nurse. It is an important precursor to those metrics that may be measured through claims or other sources.

Patient self-reported data may also be useful, but this source of information may be risky as it introduces bias (recall bias, information bias, etc.; see Chapter 5, "Epidemiological Methods and Measurements in Population-Based Nursing Practice: Part II"). Patients' recollection of a given result may be colored by their own resistance to a change in health behavior, by their lack of knowledge, or by very strong denial defense mechanisms that develop along with what may be a very difficult diagnosis to accept. Consequently, there are times when self-report data may not be useful. For the NCQA to award the status of Accredited with Performance Reporting, certain measures must be met that include actual laboratory results, and patient self-report is not permitted. Data collection methods using the HEDIS "hybrid" method require actual provider-held chart reviews (for a random sample) or data on laboratory results that come directly through a link to the laboratory that performed the test. Two examples that exemplify the use of laboratory data include the collection of HbA1C annual results in the patient with diabetes and the annual LDL levels in the CAD patient. The HEDIS technical specifications provide a depth of rigor on these data collection methods that is intense and appropriate. On the other hand, HEDIS recognizes that claims data on flu shots are very unreliable. Appropriately, patients are offered flu shots on a seasonal basis at health fairs, county-run clinics, during an inpatient stay, or at a local pharmacy (Pollert et al., 2008). It may be the case that, in these venues, there may be no claim submitted for the flu shot, considerably reducing the accuracy of the claims data on the incidence of obtaining flu shots in various patient populations. For most adults, the accuracy of the data on whether a patient has received a seasonal flu shot may be maximized by asking them. Self-report may be the best source of data available but is still not ideal (Government of Canada, 2023; Grosholz et al., 2015; King et al., 2018). Data sources abound for key metrics in a panel of indicators that are both nurse sensitive and descriptive of population-based nursing. The CMS recognizes the value of self-reported data and has incorporated a variety of measures in the Health Outcomes Survey (CMS, 2023d).

QUANTITATIVE STRATEGIES FOR THE EVALUATION OF OUTCOMES

One significant advantage of the study of health at the population level is the ample access to large populations of electronic data, allowing for a large sample size for analysis. Certainly, nursing's role in population health is enhanced by our ability to measure and track key characteristics of the patient population that are indicative of clinical quality and utilization of healthcare resources. Administrative data sets and access to an electronic medical record (EMR) in a given venue or an EHR that has the potential to "follow" the patient across various inpatient and outpatient settings have enhanced our collective ability as a profession to evaluate nursing's role in providing care and service by allowing us to use large data sets to analyze patterns of care and disease in the populations we serve.

Data Availability

The advent of the universal electronic billing process became a reality many years ago in the United States with the advancement of Medicare legislation. The CMS, known at the time as the Healthcare Financing Authority (HCFA), launched an electronic billing process for hospitals in the early 1990s. The electronic format emerged from a device called the "universal bill." This universal bill, issued in 1992 (UB92), was the first vehicle to provide a rich source of demographic, diagnostic, and procedural data. In more recent years, ways and means to measure quality through this data set and other claims from individual providers, from outpatient venues of all types, and from rehabilitation settings and other posthospital venues have been continually refined. Administrative data do provide some practical application, especially when linked to the EHR. Although the usefulness of these data has been qualified and challenged over time, there is a fair amount of consensus that the information included in claims and encounters can be useful in determining the overall health of a given population of patients with certain chronic conditions (e.g., CHF, CAD, asthma, COPD, and diabetes). These data also illustrate nursing's role regardless of venue in influencing outcomes for these patients.

Because of the very nature of lifestyle management (H&W), DM, and CM programs, data collection becomes possible using extraordinarily large data sets. Although there are methodological considerations for appropriate hypothesis testing of these data, developing processes for determining the impact of the nursing role on outcomes becomes possible without extensive and tedious chart review and manual data collection.

Electronic systems for facilitating EHR elevate the potential for outcomes research related to nursing's role in population health. In H&W, DM, and CM programs, the nursing role in providing guidance for patients' self-management of their disease conditions is documented in such a way that these *self-reported* data on milestones for patient care management are adequately captured for electronic reporting, theory testing, and hypothesis evaluation. For example, nurses who are involved in lifestyle management and H&W programs that include such things as smoking cessation programs can interact with patients telephonically to ascertain their progress with smoking cessation, and these interactions are captured in electronic reporting for later analysis. Our ability to evaluate whether the patient has filled a smoking cessation prescription or is using a smoking cessation treatment may be facilitated if pharmacy claims are available, but in general, we have no idea whether the patient filled the prescription and is taking it without a self-report. The patient's report on 7-day prevalence (e.g., *Have you smoked a tobacco product in the past 7 days?*) is the type of data available only through self-report or direct observation. These data can also be easily captured in EHR databases, and although it is still patient self-reported data, it is extremely useful and can be used in measurement submission, for example, in selected HEDIS measures (NCQA, 2023c).

In 2009, and through the Affordable Care Act (ACA), incentive monies became available to organizations to implement electronic means and to advance the use of the EMR and EHR systems as part of the HITECH (Health Information Technology for Economic and Clinical Health) Act. The program was initially called *Meaningful Use*, and organizations were required to use implemented information systems to submit data to the CMS on quality process and outcomes measures (American Medical Association [AMA], 2023; CMS, 2023i).

Hybrid data collection is a method proffered in the HEDIS data collection model. For some of the metrics, securing the data may require samples of outpatient charts with designated data collectors to provide specific data that are not available through electronic means. Here is an example: some programs may have the ability to secure electronic results of laboratory data. The HEDIS measure called *comprehensive diabetes care* includes several components. One measure includes the extent to which patients who have been diagnosed with diabetes were able to secure an HbA1C test within a 12-month period. This HEDIS metric can easily be compiled through quantitative methods if claims data are available. However, unless laboratory data are also available, the actual value of the HbA1C is not forthcoming. An alternative to this is found in the hybrid method of data collection. HEDIS provides for a method of random sample selection and sample size. Data collectors are deployed and collect the needed information by hand. For this measure and for several others in the HEDIS data set, patient self-reported data are not acceptable. To sort out the impact of a nursing DM strategy on patients' ongoing diabetes management, it is essential to be able to determine not only whether the patients have an annual HbA1C test performed but also the results of that test. More important, once you have those data, one can analyze which patients have good control (HbA1C less than 7% or 8%, depending on defined metrics for your population) and which patients have poor control (HbA1C >9%), and this can lead to identification of the strengths or weaknesses in a DM program. Without actual laboratory results in an electronic feed or hybrid data collection, claims data are limited in providing this insight. With good reason, and because of the significant dollars at risk, as incentives are provided for those organizations demonstrating improved outcomes in population health, audit validation procedures are rigorous (NCQA, 2023a, 2023c).

The CMS has, over time, refined billing practices and requirements for appropriate documentation in the electronic invoicing processes for inpatient facilities and independent providers of care. Accordingly, these changes have helped to capture useful information not only in claims and encounters but also in provider practices and to make connections for patients across the continuum of care. Incentives have been developed in recent years to reward positive practices and to better align payment with outcomes. For example, years ago, UM practices for Medicare required payment only when the appropriate patient placement and level of care in an acute care setting occurred, whereas individual provider reimbursement for an inpatient stay occurred regardless of denied payment to the facility. TJC and the CMS have now aligned their processes around the core measures project, holding hospitals accountable for process of care measures (e.g., getting the AMI patient with ST elevation to the catheter laboratory within 90 minutes of arrival to the hospital). In the past, no incentives were given to physicians who achieved the less-than-90-minute goal. Similarly, keeping a patient in the hospital longer for a hospital-acquired complication (e.g., removal of a retained instrument) had no consequences.

In 2009, the CMS began to limit reimbursement to hospitals that demonstrate these "never events." As a result, 14 conditions were identified in this category. Similarly, in 2006 a drive by the CMS to "pay for performance" was launched, encouraging individual providers to capture data in their billing practices that demonstrate patient outcomes and preventive measures in their outpatient practices, with a resultant financial reward. Despite these changes, after 10 years, only a 2% reduction in patient safety harm events was realized (U.S. Department of Health and Human Services Office of Inspector General, 2022). This notwithstanding, the OIG report suggests more aggressive reporting in its recommendations. Providers who can demonstrate (through their CMS billing) that a certain percentage of their diabetic patients have had an HbA1C test done annually and that a significant proportion of that patient population had results below 7% or 8%, depending on the nature of their patient population, receive additional reimbursement (CMS Quality Payment Program, 2023).

The ease of access to administrative data sets and claims data has appropriately led to legislation that is intended to protect the integrity of these electronic data. The Health Insurance Portability and Accountability Act (HIPAA) was passed in 1996 and has resulted in a number of requirements across the country and in any venue or service related to the patient's right to confidentiality and privacy protections. Highlights of these regulatory requirements include the following concepts: (a) annual training for all staff members (whether involved in patient care or not) regarding protected health information; (b) signed business associate agreements ensuring that these protections transverse various vendors and clients; and (c) adequate auditing, policies, and procedures to ensure that the extent and spirit of the regulations are met. Since its inception, HIPAA continues to influence data management processes and systems (CMS, 2023g)

National Trends and Healthcare Reform

Data availability, whether from electronic, self-report, or hybrid data, has changed the nature of the healthcare landscape, and the accessibility and reliability of these data have been influenced by powerful market pressures. Certainly, the CMS has had a significant impact on healthcare in the United States since Medicare legislation in the 1960s first guaranteed healthcare as a right to all Social Security recipients over the age of 65. In recent years, evolving legislation linked the issue of availability of healthcare to the quality of healthcare and recognized the inherent relationship between cost and quality. As quality improves, the cost of care is reduced. As measurement mechanisms and the availability of data have developed over the past 20 years, so has the collective wisdom. At the end of 2009, it was almost impossible to pick up a newspaper or read about the latest political debate without time and attention brought to "healthcare reform." Although pundits deconstruct the key elements of the current need for healthcare reform, all agree that the cost of providing healthcare in the United States has escalated. One can only hope that accessibility has improved for increasing segments of our society, but there are still significant disparities throughout regions of the country with a shortage of both primary care and subspecialty providers. There continues to be broad disagreement over the way in which healthcare reform was enacted despite the legislation passed in 2010. Regardless of the ongoing debate about this legislation, data availability because of claims, patient self-reporting, in hybrid data collection, and as a result of provider P4P (pay for performance) initiatives makes the measurement of quality considerably more elegant, more reliable, and clearer than it has ever been in the United States in estimating the impact of nursing's role in improving population health.

Since its enactment in 2010, the debate regarding healthcare reform has continued to mark the political landscape. By the end of 2014, a few states had chosen to refrain from opting into the program. The consequences of these states' decisions remain controversial 10 years after the ACA was signed into law. After the presidential election in 2016, the ACA continued to be the source of debate and efforts to legislate the reversal of the ACA were largely unsuccessful. As of this writing, the ACA remains in force and provides healthcare insurance coverage for a disenfranchised segment of the U.S. population (CMS, 2021). Regardless of the political debate, data on clinical outcomes are equally available for Medicare and Medicaid programs across the United States.

Standardized Data Definitions and Comparative Databases

A theme that is consistent in this chapter on evaluation methods is that measurement methods have evolved for the better over the course of the past 20 to 30 years. Clearly, the information technology age and the availability of administrative data sets are related to the present state of data availability. In addition, clinicians have provided adequate guidance through professional organizations on both process and outcome indicators of quality and have evolved data definitions that have methodological rigor and standardization (AHRQ, 2023a, 2023b; CMS, 2023b, 2023d; NCQA, 2023a, 2023c, 2023d). This agreement and standardization give rise to the potential for comparisons that are methodologically sound.

Standardized data definitions are made available by the NCQA (HEDIS volumes are available for purchase at www.NCQA.org) and include detailed technical specifications. The NCQA is a leader in the field and provides not only technical specifications and guidance on hybrid data collection and sample size but also certifications for HEDIS auditing capabilities. In addition to this functionality, the NCQA provides annual data comparisons with actual percentile rankings on the HEDIS measures for Medicare, Medicaid, and commercial lines of business. These are published on its website annually. Purchase of the Quality Compass makes regionalized comparisons possible and provides the percentile ranking comparisons a little sooner than they become public. Metrics with standardized data definitions are available from private and public groups, including, but not limited to, the NQF (www.qualityforum.org/Home.aspx), the CMS (www.cms.gov/center/quality.asp), TJC (www.jointcommission.org), and specialty groups such as the American College of Cardiology (see www.acc.org/Guidelines#/tab3), the Society of Thoracic Surgeons (see www.sts.org/quality-safety/performance-measures), and many others.

QUALITATIVE STRATEGIES FOR THE EVALUATION OF PROGRAM OUTCOMES

In the last 40 years, significant strides in nursing have been made to improve measurement methods and use quantitative means to evaluate population health. This notwithstanding, qualitative methods are also a source of rich and useful information in this evaluation process.

Accreditation and Certification

Accreditation and certification programs offer a systematic review of a given organization's ability to provide evidence of compliance with standards. Standards define the required elements to accreditation success, and these organizations provide both rigor and agreed-upon methodologies in pursuit of organizational distinction. Although many would argue that the process itself is more quantitative than qualitative, most would agree that the result is a credential that is desirable, often sought after, and sometimes a mandate. Most accreditation and certification programs provide various levels of review and accept both depth and breadth in terms of evidence permitted. (See Chapter 10, "The Role of Accreditation and Certification in Validating Population-Based Practice/Programs," for more information on accreditation and certification.)

Community Advisory Boards

As DM, CM, and UM programs have within their essential construct the total health of the population at large as a key benefit, oftentimes, representative members of that patient population are sought after to provide insight into the effectiveness and usefulness of these programs as benefits. These committees or boards meet on a regular basis (as frequently as quarterly to as seldom as annually or "ad hoc," depending on the need) and provide qualitative insight as to the impact of the program on patients' lives, as well as insight into enhancements. Telephonic services, written materials, field-based options, communication devices, and program changes are often reviewed with these boards to anticipate patient response. Certainly, members of the benefit program (patients and families) and local community groups representing the various segments of the community affected by the benefit might be included in the membership roster.

Provider Advisory Committees

Providers across specialties and venues, from nurses to physicians to hospitals, health systems, public health agencies, and managed care plans, are key components to the overall success in improving the health of the patient population in its entirety. Telephonic nursing provides options for care that did not exist in the past. However, face-to-face communications from nurse to PCP become more complex in this environment. In addition, quantitative methods have the potential to supply providers with data on their care practices that may or may not demonstrate the achievement of improvements in patient outcomes. Providing feedback to PCPs in a systematic and patient-centered way is a strategy that can be of tremendous benefit. Consequently, devising a vehicle to enhance communications with healthcare providers in a formal setting, such as through committees, can be of significant value.

Provider advisory committees come in all shapes and sizes and meet with varying frequency. Wakefield et al. (2021) advise that APRNs who are in private practice represent an important enhancement to our ability to extend primary care capacity across the country. Representative providers, including APRNs, can comment on data presentation; they can provide advice on ways and means to make sound use of these data in a global way, as well as help to anticipate reaction. These forums serve as educational opportunities for total population health and can enhance practice management as well as demonstrate how the EHR across the continuum of care can enhance communication processes among all members of the healthcare team and maximize patient outcomes. Provider advisory committees provide depth to population health, which may not be found through traditional quantitative methods.

SUMMARY

APRNs play an increasingly important role in evaluating the quality and effectiveness of healthcare delivery systems. As APRN roles have expanded into this area, it is paramount that APRNs understand the ways and means used to evaluate population health outcomes, as well as the systems of care that provide population health services. Various definitions of quality have been presented, and several theoretical frameworks are available for evaluating quality. Nurse-sensitive indicators of quality can be described using the following categories: (a) clinical quality, (b) utilization of healthcare resources, (c) core business processes, and (d) customer satisfaction. APRNs hold various roles, both clinical and administrative, in a variety of settings. Regardless of role or setting, measurement and improvement of quality with its broad definitions remain paramount. In the past, measurement systems were limited, and manual data collection was the primary method of gaining insight and information as to the outcomes of clinical care, management of chronic illness, and the patient's experience. As nurses strive to make an impact on the overall health of the population, reduce the cost of care, and improve the patient's experience of their healthcare, APRNs' roles expand.

END-OF-CHAPTER RESOURCES

EXERCISES AND DISCUSSION QUESTIONS

EXERCISE 9.1 You are a staff nurse working in a busy internist's medical practice. You have been a nurse for more than 30 years, and about 3 years ago, you decided to pursue an advanced degree in an RN to DNP program. You have about 2 years to go; you have just finished a course in Epidemiology, and you are intrigued by the total population health model. You believe it could serve as a good framework for your DNP project. The physician who you work for is excited about your educational advancement and is willing to support your idea of constructing your DNP project in this practice. You have noticed that you have quite a few patients with type 2 diabetes mellitus in the practice; many of these patients have Medicare, some have Medicaid, and most have been diagnosed for more than the 5 years that you have been with the practice.

The practice is not automated; though there is a beginning EMR, this practice has a 30-year track record, and most of the files are handwritten. This notwithstanding, you have a good relationship with the practice manager, who does the billing for the practice.

To further the possibility of framing your DNP project and to better grasp how to evaluate this practice at the population level, answer the following questions:

1. What measurements would be important to framing a DNP practice problem, and how would you go about doing this in your practice?
2. How could you determine, more specifically, the nature of the problem?
3. What is the gap in your practice and what qualitative and quantitative measures can shed insight?

EXERCISE 9.2 You are a staff nurse working in a large community hospital on a medical-surgical unit that has primarily elderly cardiac patients. You have worked part time at this hospital for more than 20 years, and now that your children have finished college, you have decided to pursue an advanced degree. You enrolled in an RN to DNP program as you have always wanted to remain clinically connected. You have no interest in pursuing an administrative role, but cardiac patients have always interested you. You note that many of your cardiac patients are familiar; there seems to be a bit of a revolving door, and many patients seem to be readmitted.

Your nurse manager knows that you are pursuing an advanced degree and has suggested that reducing readmissions within 30 days for CHF would make a good DNP project. Furthermore, she's mentioned that the quality improvement (QI) department is very interested in this and will be supportive of your efforts as this is an organizational priority.

To further the possibility of framing your DNP project and to better grasp how to evaluate this practice at the population level, answer the following questions:

1. What measurements would be important to framing a DNP practice problem, and how would you go about doing this for the patients in the hospital and on your unit?
2. How could you determine, more specifically, the nature of the problem?
3. What is the gap in practice at your organization (and on your unit), and what qualitative and quantitative measures can shed insight?

EXERCISE 9.3 You are a practicing nurse practitioner (NP) in a private practice with two other NPs and two internal medicine PCPs. You work in an affluent practice and most patients have insurance of some kind. For the past 10 years, you have used an EHR system that provides easy access to reports. You care for one patient at a time but cannot help but notice the large number of overweight and obese patients in your practice, some with diabetes and hypertension, some on the brink of developing. You think perhaps an evidence-based clinical practice guideline (CPG) that employs the use of SMART phone technology would help patients track their weight and increase exercise. Use of weight-reducing medications and bariatric surgery may be options for this patient population as well. You have not fleshed out your ideas, but in a recent staff meeting, your colleagues have expressed an interest. How would you go about developing and implementing a CPG for your practice?

A robust set of instructor resources designed to supplement this text is located at http://connect.springerpub.com/content/book/978-0-8261-4377-8. Qualifying instructors may request access by emailing textbook@springerpub.com.

REFERENCES

Affentranger, A., & Mulkey, D. (2023). Standardizing tobacco cessation counseling using the 5 A's intervention. *Journal of Nursing Care Quality, 38*(2), 146–151. https://doi.org/10.1097/NCQ.0000000000000671

Agency for Healthcare Research and Quality. (2023a). *Improving data collection across the health care system.* AHRQ. Retrieved 3/7/2023 from https://www.ahrq.gov/research/findings/final-reports/iomracereport/reldata5.html

Agency for Healthcare Research and Quality. (2023b). *Patient safety and quality improvement.* AHRQ. Retrieved 3/1/2023 from https://www.ahrq.gov/patient-safety/index.html

AHRQ. (2018, March 2018). *Toolkit for reducing central line-associated blood stream infections.* AHRQ. Retrieved 2/23/2023 from https://www.ahrq.gov/hai/clabsi-tools/index.html

American Association of Colleges of Nursing. (2023). *AACN essentials.* AACN. Retrieved 2/22/2023 from https://www.aacnnursing.org/DNP/DNP-Essentials

American Hospital Association. (2023). *Regulatory overload report.* Retrieved 3/7/2023 from https://www.aha.org/guidesreports/2017-11-03-regulatory-overload-report

American Medical Association. (2023). *Meaningful use: electronic health record (EHR) incentive programs.* AMA. Retrieved 3/7/2023 from https://www.ama-assn.org/practice-management/medicare-medicaid/meaningful-use-electronic-health-record-ehr-incentive#:~:text=Meaningful%20Use%3A%20Overview-,Meaningful%20Use%3A%20Overview,electronic%20capturing%20of%20clinical%20data

American Medical Group Association. (2023). *Provider satisfaction benchmarking survey.* AMGA. Retrieved 3/6/2023 from https://www.amga.org/performance-improvement/best-practices/benchmarking-surveys/provider-satisfaction-benchmarking-survey/

American Society for Quality. (2023). *What is six sigma?* ASQ. Retrieved 2/24/2023 from https://asq.org/quality-resources/six-sigma

Bagchi, S., Watkins, J., Pollock, D. A., Edwards, J. R., & Allen-Bridson, K. (2018). State health department validations of central line–associated bloodstream infection events reported via the National Healthcare Safety Network. *American Journal of Infection Control, 46*(11), 1290–1295. https://doi.org/10.1016/j.ajic.2018.04.233

Balanced Scorecard Institute. (2023). *Balanced scorecard basics.* Balanced Scorecard Institute. Retrieved 3/1/2023 from https://balancedscorecard.org/bsc-basics-overview/

Berwick, D. M., Godfrey, A. B., & Roessner, J. (1990). *Curing health care: New strategies for quality improvement.* Joasey-Bass.

Buetti, N., Marschall, J., Drees, M., Fakih, M. G., Hadaway, L., Maragakis, L. L., Monsees, E., Novosad, S., O'Grady, N. P., Rupp, M. E., Wolf, J., Yokoe, D., & Mermel, L. A. (2022). Strategies to prevent central line-associated bloodstream infections in acute-care hospitals: 2022 Update. *Infection Control and Hospital Epidemiology, 43*(5), 553–569. https://doi.org/10.1017/ice.2022.87

Carnut, L., & Narvai, P. C. (2020). A meta-summarization of qualitative findings about health systems performance evaluation models: Conceptual problems and comparability limitations. *Inquiry, 57*, 1–19. https://doi.org/10.1177/0046958020962650

Centers for Disease Control and Prevention. (2017). *Data summary of HAIs in the US: Assessing progress 2006–2016.* CDC. Retrieved 2/23/2023 from https://www.cdc.gov/hai/data/archive/data-summary-assessing-progress.html

Centers for Disease Control and Prevention. (2021). *2020 National and state healthcare-associated infecctions progress report.* CDC. Retrieved 2/22/2023 from https://www.cdc.gov/hai/data/archive/2020-HAI-progress-report.html

Centers for Medicare and Medicaid. (2021). *Affordable care act implementation FAQs set 5.* CMS. Retrieved 3/14/2023 from https://www.cms.gov/CCIIO/Resources/Fact-Sheets-and-FAQs/aca_implementation_faqs5

Centers for Medicare and Medicaid. (2022). *Accountable care organizations (ACOs).* CMS. Retrieved 3/1/2023 from https://www.cms.gov/priorities/innovation/innovation-models/aco

Centers for Medicare and Medicaid. (2023a). *2023 Medicare advantage and part D star ratings.* CMS. Retrieved 2/23/2023 from https://www.cms.gov/newsroom/fact-sheets/2023-medicare-advantage-and-part-d-star-ratings

Centers for Medicare and Medicaid. (2023b). *Consumer assessment of healthcare providers and systems (CAHPS).* CMS. Retrieved 3/6/2023 from https://www.cms.gov/Research-Statistics-Data-and-Systems/Research/CAHPS

Centers for Medicare and Medicaid. (2023c). *HCAHPS: Patient perspectives of care survey.* CMS. Retrieved 3/6/2023 from https://www.cms.gov/Medicare/Quality-Initiatives-Patient-Assessment-Instruments/HospitalQualityInits/HospitalHCAHPS

Centers for Medicare and Medicaid. (2023d). *Health outcomes survey (HOS).* CMS. Retrieved 3/6/2023 from https://www.cms.gov/Research-Statistics-Data-and-Systems/Research/HOS

Centers for Medicare and Medicaid (CMS). (2023e). *Long-term care hospital (LTCH) quality reporting program (QRP) public reporting.* CMS. Retrieved 3/1/2023 from https://www.cms.gov/medicare/quality-initiatives-patient-assessment-instruments/ltch-quality-reporting/ltch-quality-public-reporting

Centers for Medicare and Medicaid. (2023f). *Medication therapy management.* CMS. Retrieved 3/1/2023 from https://www.cms.gov/medicare/coverage/prescription-drug-coverage-contracting/medication-therapy-management

Centers for Medicare and Medicaid. (2023g). *Privacy and security information.* CMS. Retrieved 3/7/2023 from https://www.cms.gov/Regulations-and-Guidance/Administrative-Simplification/HIPAA-ACA/PrivacyandSecurityInformation

Centers for Medicare and Medicaid. (2023h). *Program guidance & specifications.* CMS. Retrieved 3/3/2023 from https://www.cms.gov/medicare/medicare-fee-for-service-payment/sharedsavingsprogram/program-guidance-and-specifications#quality-resources-and-information

Centers for Medicare and Medicaid. (2023i). *Promoting interoperability programs.* CMS. Retrieved 3/7/2023 from https://www.cms.gov/regulations-and-guidance/legislation/ehrincentiveprograms

Centers for Medicare and Medicaid. (2023j). *Special needs plans.* CMS. Retrieved 3/1/2023 from https://www.cms.gov/Medicare/Health-Plans/SpecialNeedsPlans#:~:text=A%20special%20needs%20plan%20(SNP,A%20dual%20eligible%2C%20or

Centers for Medicare and Medicaid Quality Payment Program. (2023). *Participation options overview.* CMS QPP. Retrieved 3/7/2023 from https://qpp.cms.gov/mips/overview

CMS. (2023). *Hospital acquired conditions.* Retrieved 2/22/2023 from https://www.cms.gov/Medicare/Medicare-Fee-for-Service-Payment/HospitalAcqCond/Hospital-Acquired_Conditions

Core Quality Measures Collaborative. (2023). *CQMC core sets.*

Crossing the Quality Chasm. (2003). National Academy Press.

DeFeo, J. A. (2019). *The Juran trilogy.* Juran. Retrieved 2/22/2023 from https://www.juran.com/blog/the-juran-trilogy-quality-planning/

Deming, W. E. (2000). *Out of the crisis.* MIT Press.

Deutschbein, J., Grittner, U., Schneider, A., & Schenk, L. (2020). Community care coordination for stroke survivors: Results of a complex intervention study. *BMC Health Services Research, 20*(1), 1–13. https://doi.org/10.1186/s12913-020-05993-x

Dillon, E. C., Kim, P., Li, M., Qiwen, H., Colocci, N., Cantril, C., & Hung, D. Y. (2021). Breast cancer navigation: Using physician and patient surveys to explore nurse navigator program experiences. *Clinical Journal of Oncology Nursing, 25*(5), 579–586. https://doi.org/10.1188/21.CJON.579-586

Donabedian, A. (1980). *The definition of quality and approaches to its assessment; exploration in quality assessment and monitoring* (Vol. 1). Health Administration Press.

Donabedian, A. (2005). Evaluating the quality of medical care. 1966. *Milbank Quarterly, 83*(4), 691–729. https://doi.org/10.1111/j.1468-0009.2005.00397.x

Drew, J. R., & Pandit, M. (2020). Why healthcare leadership should embrace quality improvement. *BMJ, 368,* m872. https://doi.org/10.1136/bmj.m872

Formichelli, L. (2007). By the numbers. *Multichannel Merchant, 3*(4), 44–45. https://login.proxy.libraries.rutgers.edu/login?url=https://search.ebscohost.com/login.aspx?direct=true&db=buh&AN=24795741&site=ehost-live

Goldberg, Z. N., & Nash, D. B. (2022). The emerging value-based care industry: Paving the road ahead. *American Journal of Medical Quality: The Official Journal of the American College of Medical Quality, 37*(5), 472–474. https://doi.org/10.1097/JMQ.0000000000000067

Government of Canada. (2023). *Highlights from the 2021–2022 seasonal influenza (flu) vaccination coverage survey.* Public Health Agency of Canda. Retrieved 3/7/2023 from https://www.canada.ca/en/public-health/services/immunization-vaccines/vaccination-coverage/seasonal-influenza-survey-results-2021-2022.html

Grosholz, J. M., Blake, S., Daugherty, J. D., Ayers, E., Omer, S. B., Polivka-West, L., & Howard, D. H. (2015, September). Accuracy of influenza vaccination rate estimates in United States nursing home residents. *Epidemiol Infect, 143*(12), 2588–2595. https://doi.org/10.1017/s0950268814003434

Guru Guide: Six thought leaders who changed the quality world forever. (2010). *Quality Progress, 43*(11), 14–21.

Hampe, H. M., Graper, L., Hayes-Leight, K., Olszewski, D., Moffa, M., & Bremmer, D. N. (2017). Accurate identification of infection source in burn trauma patients with central line infection to determine appropriate treatment option as well as proper public reporting. *Critical Care Nursing Quarterly, 40*(1), 16–23. https://doi.org/10.1097/CNQ.0000000000000136

Hansen, A. R., McLendon, S. F., & Rochani, H. (2022). Care coordination for rural residents with chronic disease: Predictors of improved outcomes. *Public Health Nursing, 39*(4), 760–769. https://doi.org/10.1111/phn.13038

Harris, M., Moore, V., Barnes, M., Persha, H., Reed, J., & Zillich, A. (2022). Effect of pharmacy-led interventions during care transitions on patient hospital readmission: A systematic review. *Journal of the American Pharmacists Association: JAPhA, 62*(5), 1477–1477. https://doi.org/10.1016/j.japh.2022.05.017

Heidary Dahooie, J., Mohammadi, N., Meidutė-Kavaliauskienė, I., & Binkytė-Velienė, A. (2021). A novel performance evaluation framework for new service development in the healthcare industry using hybrid ISM and ANP. *Technological and Economic Development of Economy, 27*(6), 1481–1508. https://doi.org/10.3846/tede.2021.15699

Hummer, R. A., & Hamilton, E. R. (2019). *Population health in America.* University of California Press. https://doi.org/10.1525/9780520965294

Institute for Healthcare Improvement. (2012). *How-to guide: Prevent central line-associated bloodstream infections (CLABSI).* https://www.ihi.org/resources/Pages/Tools/HowtoGuidePreventCentralLineAssociatedBloodstreamInfection.aspx

Institute for Healthcare Improvement. (2023a). *IHI scientific advisory group.* Retrieved 2/24/2023 from https://www.ihi.org/about/Pages/ScientificAdvisoryGroup.aspx

Institute for Healthcare Improvement. (2023b). *Population health.* IHI. Retrieved 2/22/2023 from https://www.ihi.org/Topics/Population-Health/Pages/default.aspx

Institute for Healthcare Improvement. (2023c). *QI essentials toolkilt: Plan-do-study-act (PDSA) worksheet*. IHI. Retrieved 2/28/2023 from https://www.ihi.org/resources/Pages/Tools/PlanDoStudyActWorksheet.aspx

Institute for Healthcare Improvement. (2023d). *Quality improvement essentials toolkit*. IHI. Retrieved 2/28/2023 from https://www.ihi.org/resources/Pages/Tools/Quality-Improvement-Essentials-Toolkit.aspx

Institute for Healthcare Improvement. (2023e). *Science of improvement*. Retrieved 2/24/2023 from https://www.ihi.org/about/Pages/ScienceofImprovement.aspx

Institute for Healthcare Improvement. (2023f). *Triple aim for populations*. IHI. Retrieved 2/22/2023 from https://www.ihi.org/Topics/TripleAim/Pages/default.aspx

Institute of Medicine. (2000). *To err is human: Building a safer health system* (1st ed.). National Academies Press.

Jeunghyun, K., Randhawa, R. S., & Ward, A. R. (2018, Spring). Dynamic scheduling in a many-server, multiclass system: The role of customer impatience in large systems. *Manufacturing & Service Operations Management, 20*(2), 285–301. https://doi.org/10.1287/msom.2017.0642

Joint Commission Resources. (2023). *Cardiac care measures*. Joint Commission Resources. Retrieved 2/22/2023 from https://www.jointcommission.org/measurement/measures/cardiac-care/

Juran. (2023). *Results in healthcare*. Retrieved 2/24/2023 from https://www.juran.com/results/case-studies/

Kalata, S., Howard, R., Diaz, A., Nuliyahu, U., Ibrahim, A. M., & Nathan, H. (2023). Association of skilled nursing facility ownership by health care networks with utilization and spending. *JAMA Network Open, 6*(2), e230140. https://doi.org/10.1001/jamanetworkopen.2023.0140

Kaplan, R. S., & Norton, D. P. (1992). The balanced scorecard: Neasures that drive performance. *Harvard Business Review, 70*(1), 71–79.

Kaplan, R. S., & Norton, D. R. (2005). The balanced scorecard: Measures that drive performance. *Harvard Business Review, 83*(7–8), 172–180. https://login.proxy.libraries.rutgers.edu/login?url=https://search.ebscohost.com/login.aspx?direct=true&db=buh&AN=17602418&site=ehost-live

King, J. P., McLean, H. Q., & Belongia, E. A. (2018). Validation of self-reported influenza vaccination in the current and prior season. *Influenza and Other Respiratory Viruses, 12*(6), 808–813. https://doi.org/10.1111/irv.12593

Kober, R., & Northcott, D. (2021). Testing cause-and-effect relationships within a balanced scorecard. *Accounting & Finance, 61*, 1815–1849. https://doi.org/10.1111/acfi.12645

Lorenzetti, D. L., Quan, H., Lucyk, K., Cunningham, C., Hennessy, D., Jiang, J., & Beck, C. A. (2018). Strategies for improving physician documentation in the emergency department: A systematic review. *BMC Emergency Medicine, 18*(1), 36. https://doi.org/10.1186/s12873-018-0188-z

Messinger, B. L., Rogers, D. N., & Hawker, C. D. (2019). Automation and process re-engineering work together to achieve six sigma quality: A 27-year history of continuous improvement. *Laboratory Medicine, 50*(2), e23–e35. https://doi.org/10.1093/labmed/lmy081

Mukherji, A. B., Lu, D., Qin, F., Hedlin, H., Johannsen, N. M., Chung, S., Kobayashi, Y., Haddad, F., Lamendola, C., Basina, M., Talamoa, R., Myers, J., & Palaniappan, L. (2022). Effectiveness of a community-based structured physical activity program for adults with type 2 diabetes: A randomized clinical trial. *JAMA Network Open, 5*(12), e2247858. https://doi.org/10.1001/jamanetworkopen.2022.47858

National Academies of Sciences, Engineering, and Medicine; Health and Medicine Division; Board on Population Health and Public Health Practice; Roundtable on Population Health Improvement, & Wizemann, T. M. (Eds.). (2021). *Population health science in the United States: Trends, evidence, and implications for policy: Proceedings of a joint symposium*. National Academies Press.

National Committee for Quality Assurance. (2023a). *Comprehensive diabetes care*. NCQA. Retrieved 3/1/2023 from https://www.ncqa.org/hedis/measures/comprehensive-diabetes-care/

National Committee for Quality Assurance. (2023b). *HEDIS measures*. NCQA. Retrieved 3/1/2023 from https://www.ncqa.org/hedis/

National Committee for Quality Assurance. (2023c). *HEDIS measures and technical resources*. NCQA. Retrieved 2/22/2023 from https://www.ncqa.org/hedis/measures/

National Committee for Quality Assurance. (2023d). *HEDIS medicare health outcomes survey*. NCQA. Retrieved 3/3/2023 from https://www.ncqa.org/hedis/measures/hos/

National Committee for Quality Assurance. (2023e). *Patient-centered medical home*. NCQA. Retrieved 3/1/2023 from https://www.ncqa.org/programs/health-care-providers-practices/patient-centered-medical-home-pcmh/

National Institutes of Standards and Technology. (2023). *Baldrige excellence framework health care 2023–2024 edition*. NIST. Retrieved 2/23/2023 from https://www.nist.gov/baldrige/publications/baldrige-excellence-framework/health-care

National Quality Forum (NQF). (2023a). *Core quality measures collaborative*. NQF. Retrieved 3/1/2023 from https://www.qualityforum.org/cqmc/

National Quality Forum. (2023b). *Serious reportable events*. NQF. Retrieved 2/22/2023 from https://www.qualityforum.org/topics/sres/serious_reportable_events.aspx

NIST. (2023). *Baldrige award recipients listing*. NIST. Retrieved 2/23/23 from https://www.nist.gov/baldrige/award-recipients?year=All&sector=1939011&title=&state=All

Pyzdek, T., & Keller, P. (2018). *The six sigma handbook* (5th ed.). McGraw Hill Education.

Sampath, B., Rakover, J., Baldoza, K., Mate, K., Lenoci-Edwards, J., & Barker, P. (2021). *Whole system quality*. IHI White Paper. https://www.ihi.org/resources/Pages/IHIWhitePapers/whole-system-quality.aspx

Selinka, G., Stolletz, R., & Maindl, T. I. (2022, Winter). Performance approximation for time-dependent queues with generally distributed abandonments. *INFORMS Journal on Computing, 34*(1), 20–38. https://doi.org/10.1287/ijoc.2021.1090

Sfantou, D. F., Laliotis, A., Patelarou, A. E., Sifaki-Pistolla, D., Matalliotakis, M., & Patelarou, E. (2017). Importance of leadership style towards quality of care measures in healthcare settings: A systematic review. *Healthcare (Basel), 5*(4), 73. https://doi.org/10.3390/healthcare5040073

Shadding, F. (2009). Are you watching the farm? *Response, 17*(6), 58–58. https://login.proxy.libraries.rutgers.edu/login?url=https://search.ebscohost.com/login.aspx?direct=true&db=buh&AN=36888386&site=ehost-live

Shelton, J. (2021). The balanced scorecard. *Facility Management Journal (FMJ), 31*(5), 113–117. https://login.proxy.libraries.rutgers.edu/login?url=https://search.ebscohost.com/login.aspx?direct=true&db=buh&AN=152663993&site=ehost-live

Siegler, J. E., Patel, N. N., & Dine, C. J. (2015, March). Prioritizing paperwork over patient care: Why can't we do both? *Journal Graduate Medical Education, 7*(1), 16–18. https://doi.org/10.4300/jgme-d-14-00494.1

The Deming Institute. (2023). *Enriching society through the Deming philosophy*. The W. Edwards Deming Institute. Retrieved 2/23/2023 from https://deming.org/

The Joint Commission. (2020). *Root cause analysis in health care: A joint commission guide to analysis and corrective action of sentinel and adverse events* (7th ed.). Joint Commission Resources.

Tossaint-Schoenmakers, R., Versluis, A., Chavannes, N., Talboom-Kamp, E., & Kasteleyn, M. (2021). The challenge of integrating eHealth into health care: Systematic literature review of the Donabedian model of structure, process, and outcome. *Journal of Medical Internet Research, 23*(5), e27180. https://doi.org/10.2196/27180

University of California San Francisco. (2023). *The kidney project statistics*. Retrieved 2/22/2023 from https://pharm.ucsf.edu/kidney/need/statistics

URAC. (2023). *Performance measurement results*. URAC. Retrieved 3/3/2023 from https://www.urac.org/outcomes-measures/research-and-measurement-reports/

U.S. Department of Health and Human Services Office of Inspector General. (2022). *Adverse events in hospitals: A quarter of medicare patients experienced harm in october 2018*. HHS OIG. Retrieved 3/7/2023 from https://oig.hhs.gov/oei/reports/OEI-06-18-00400.asp

Wakefield, M. K., Williams, D. R., LeMenestrel, S., & Flaubert, J. L. (2021). *The future of nursing 2020–2030*. National Academy of Medicine.

INTERNET RESOURCES

Accreditation Commission for Health Care, Inc. (ACHE): https://www.hfap.org/why-achc/. Formerly: Healthcare Facilities Accreditation Program (HFAP): https://www.hfap.org

Agency for Healthcare Research and Quality (AHRQ): www.ahrq.gov

ASQ: www.asq.org/learn-about-quality/iso-9000/overview/overview.html

Baldrige Performance Excellence Program: www.nist.gov/baldrige/publications/hc_criteria.cfm

CMS Accountable Care Organizations (ACOs): https://www.cms.gov/Medicare/Medicare-Fee-for-Service-Payment/ACO/index.html

CMS Hospital-Acquired Conditions (Present on Admission Indicator): www.cms.gov/HospitalAcqCond

CMS Quality Care Center: www.cms.gov/center/quality.asp

CMS, The Center for Consumer Information & Insurance Oversight: https://www.cms.gov/cciio/resources/regulations-and-guidance/index.html

HealthStream: https://www.healthstream.com/index.aspx

National Committee for Quality Assurance (NCQA): www.ncqa.org
National Database of Nursing Quality Indicators (NDNQI; https://www.pressganey.com/platform/ndnqi/
National Quality Forum (NQF): www.qualityforum.org
NCQA HEDIS and Performance Measurement: http://www.ncqa.org/hedis-quality-measurement/hedis-programs
Population Health Alliance: www.populationhealthalliance.org
Press Ganey™: www.pressganey.com/index.aspx
Rand Health Factors Affecting Physician Professional Satisfaction and Their Implications for Patient Care, Health Systems, and Health Policy: www.rand.org/content/dam/rand/pubs/research_reports/RR400/RR439/RAND_RR439.pdf
The Commission on Accreditation of Rehabilitation Facilities (CARF): www.carf.org/Accreditation
The Joint Commission (TJC): http://www.jointcommission.org
The Joint Commission Resources: https://www.jcrinc.com/
Triple Aim: www.ihi.org/Topics/TripleAim/Pages/default.aspx
URAC: www.urac.org

CHAPTER 10

THE ROLE OF ACCREDITATION AND CERTIFICATION IN VALIDATING POPULATION-BASED PRACTICE/PROGRAMS

GAIL M. JOHNSON

INTRODUCTION

This chapter addresses the role of specialty accreditation and certification in population-based healthcare. The scope of advanced practice nursing continues to evolve and expand throughout a variety of clinical practice sites such as acute care hospitals, long-term care facilities, subacute/rehab facilities, long-term acute care (LTAC), ambulatory health, public health, and behavioral health settings. Irrespective of the setting, the expectation for the advanced practice registered nurse (APRN) is a working knowledge of the required program accreditations for licensing and reimbursement. Also important is an understanding of the role of certification in validating patient care and quality outcomes.

The Institute of Medicine's (IOM) seminal work, *The Future of Nursing* (2010), defines the roles that APRNs should have in the design of future healthcare models. The IOM report identifies the need for healthcare organizations to support nurses as leaders in the development and adoption of innovative models of patient-centered care. The report further specifies all the responsibilities of agencies, including the federal government, to support these efforts. APRNs receive significant academic preparation focusing on advanced clinical practice. Such nurses also require knowledge of operationalizing and implementing clinical programs.

The American Association of Colleges of Nursing (AACN) (2021) identifies the 10 domains of educational content for nursing education. Developing programs and working toward program accreditation requires competence in each of these. Domain 5:

Quality and Safety at the advanced level notes three competencies and 15 sub-competencies that focus on using national safety references, benchmarks, data, evidence-based interventions, and business plan development aimed at improving the quality of care. This core competency for advanced nursing education best addresses the abilities that are required to lead organizations seeking external accreditations and certifications.

A set of standards is the primary hallmark of a credentialing program. Whether evaluation of a given program is housed in a facility (like an acute care hospital accredited through The Joint Commission [TJC] or Det Norske Veritas [DNV]), a public health agency, or a disease management (DM) program, both accreditation and certification are measures of quality. For example, TJC's certification program for congestive heart failure (CHF) is offered in conjunction with the American Heart Association (AHA) and is offered based on standards and outcomes (TJC, 2023a, 2023b). As nurses practice and provide nursing care within and throughout these facilities and programs, accreditation is an indirect measure of the quality of nursing practice. The processes used within an accrediting program are also variable, but characteristics include the following: (a) written documentation to support program infrastructure, including population served, volumes, leadership requirements, staffing, staff experience, and credentials; (b) standards of care or clinical practice guidelines in use and specific to the population served; (c) measures of success (often prescribed and reported regularly to the accrediting body); and (d) a site visit and follow-up with corrective action plans and measured improvements.

Accreditation and certification are mechanisms for evaluating the processes and outcomes of clinical programs. Accreditation is positively associated with the establishment of organizational structures and processes, the existence of quality and safety cultures, improved patient care and outcomes, and other benefits. During the process of accreditation/certification, organizations must produce metrics, many of which will be sensitive to the nursing role; demonstrate patient characteristics; and quantify patient outcomes. The accrediting process becomes qualitative as the evaluation of the quality of the program seeks to show improvement and sustain high quality of care in defined patient care indicators. Some accrediting bodies are less prescriptive in the exact application of their standards; this is in no way a detracting characteristic. In fact, the latitude in the application of the standards (the how) is often desirable as there are many ways to achieve the same outcome. Examples of accrediting bodies and the type of programs that they accredit or certify are provided in Exhibit 10.1. This list is not intended to be exhaustive but simply illustrative. Each includes standards that evaluate the outcome of nursing care in some way.

The effectiveness of patient care is evaluated by measuring patient outcomes; similarly, clinical programs are validated by measuring programmatic outcomes. Some accreditation and certification programs are essential requirements for clinical practice while others are voluntary additional credentials. The following information is a sampling of the various types of credentials that need to be considered when developing a new population-based clinical program or working within an established program that is seeking external validation.

EXHIBIT 10.1

EXAMPLES OF ACCREDITING BODIES AND THE TYPES OF PROGRAMS THEY ACCREDIT

The Joint Commission (TJC) accredits acute care hospitals and provides certification to several specialty hospitals and programs, many of which have a patient focus that goes well beyond the patient's inpatient experience. Accordingly, these accreditation programs have an influence on the health of the total patient population, as well as nursing's role in the experience. TJC is often designated by state licensure for hospital review. TJC holds deemed status for the Centers for Medicare and Medicaid Services (CMS). Having deemed status means that the healthcare facility has provided evidence to their accreditation body that they meet or exceed the CMS Conditions of Participation (CoPs; ecfr.gov/current/title42/chapterIV/subchapter-G/part-488/subpart-A). Hospitals seeking to achieve or maintain provider status with CMS must be both accredited and licensed. Find more information about TJC at www.jointcommission.org. TJC offers both accreditation of facilities for deemed status purposes and disease-specific care programs for a variety of disease entities.

The National Committee for Quality Assurance (NCQA) offers numerous recognition, accreditation, and certification programs, including, but are not limited to, health plans, utilization management (UM) programs, DM programs, Healthcare Effectiveness Data and Information Set (HEDIS) auditing, and many other types. Information regarding the programs offered by this organization can be found at www.ncqa.org.

The Utilization Review Accreditation Commission (URAC) formally adopted the acronym URAC in 1996. It is an organization with a long track record in offering accreditation for total population health. UM, DM, and case management (CM) programs and other types of accreditations that are related to the nursing role in total population health are among the many types offered. More information on this organization can be found at www.urac.org.

The Commission on Accreditation of Rehabilitation Facilities (CARF) is yet another organization with a focus on evaluating the quality of various programs, including behavioral health services across the rehabilitation continuum, durable medical equipment providers, aging programs, and other program types. The CARF website at www.carf.org/Accreditation provides a wealth of useful information.

Det Norske Veritas (DNV; formerly DNV-GL) provides healthcare facility accreditation based on National Integrated Accreditation for Healthcare Organizations (NIAHO) standards. Additionally, organizations choosing this route to CMS accreditation with deemed status must achieve certification by the International Organization for Standardization (ISO) at the first reaccreditation visit (year 4). Like TJC, DNV offers both accreditation of facilities for deemed status purposes (compliance with the CMS CoPs) and disease-specific care programs for a variety of disease entities. Although this organization specializes in managing risk for many types of industries, their recent focus on the healthcare industry (achieving the ability to grant deemed status to facilities by CMS CoPs in 2008) has opened a new option for accreditation for hospitals. Like TJC, DNV has CMS approval to accredit healthcare facilities. DNV focuses on accrediting hospitals, critical access hospitals, and facilities offering other specialty services; and they offer a variety of disease-specific certifications for stroke, diabetes management, and a variety of cardiac and other programs. More information can be sought at www.dnv.us/supplychain/healthcare/index.html.

(continued)

> **EXHIBIT 10.1**
>
> **The Healthcare Facilities Accreditation Program (HFAP)** was originally created in 1945 to conduct an objective review of services provided by osteopathic hospitals; HFAP has maintained its deeming authority through CMS and meets or exceeds the standards required by the CMS CoPs to provide accreditation to hospitals, ambulatory care/surgical facilities, mental health facilities, physical rehabilitation facilities, clinical laboratories, and critical access hospitals. HFAP also provides certification reviews for Primary Stroke Centers. Find more information about HFAP at www.hfap.org/about/overview.aspx.
>
> **The Public Health Accreditation Board (PHAB)** accredits tribal, state, local, and territorial public health departments. PHAB is a nonprofit entity created in 2007 to accredit public health departments following a Robert Wood Johnson Foundation initiative, *Exploring Accreditation*. PHAB has created standards and measures as a framework for evaluating the performance of public health departments. More information on PHAB can be found at www.phaboard.org/accreditation-overview/what-is-accreditation.
>
> **Community Health Accreditation Partner (CHAP)** has the CMS deeming authority by CMS for home health, hospice, and home care medical equipment. CHAP standards are designed for home and community-based care and are helpful for new and developing programs. Information about CHAP can be found at chapinc.org.

GOVERNMENTAL PROGRAMS

CENTERS FOR MEDICARE AND MEDICAID SERVICES

Reimbursement is a critical element for any program. CMS is the largest payer for most adult populations, and its role will continue to grow as the population in the United States ages. To receive payment from Medicare and Medicaid, healthcare programs/organizations must meet the CoPs and Conditions for Coverage (CfCs) identified by CMS. The intent of these regulations is to protect patient health and safety and to promote quality of care. Organizations that can provide CMS accreditation are noted in Box 10.1 (notably, DNV, [Healthcare Facilities Accreditation Program (HFAP)], and TJC). Certifying that the CoPs and CfCs are met is achieved via a survey conducted by one of these organizations on behalf of the federal government. These CMS-approved accrediting organizations are identified as having *deeming authority*. In effect, when a healthcare entity is successfully accredited by a deeming body, it is granted deemed status, which certifies that the organization has met the Conditions of Participation (CoPs).

Organizations seeking CMS approval may choose to be surveyed either by an approved accrediting organization, such as TJC, DNV, or HFAP, or by state surveyors on behalf of CMS. A TJC, DNV, or HFAP survey may be followed by a random state validation survey conducted by the state's Department of Health entity on behalf of CMS. These validation surveys are used to evaluate the effectiveness of the accrediting organization's review process.

> **BOX 10.1**
>
> **CONDITIONS FOR COVERAGE (CFCS) AND CONDITIONS OF PARTICIPATION (CoPs)**
>
> Ambulatory surgery centers (ASCs)
>
> Community mental health centers (CMHCs)
>
> Comprehensive outpatient rehabilitation facilities (CORFs)
>
> Critical access hospitals (CAHs)
>
> End-stage renal disease facilities
>
> Federally qualified health centers
>
> Home health agencies
>
> Hospices
>
> Hospitals
>
> Hospital swing beds
>
> Intermediate Care Facilities for Individuals with Intellectual Disabilities (ICF/IID)
>
> Organ procurement organizations (OPOs)
>
> Portable X-ray suppliers
>
> Programs of All-Inclusive Care for the Elderly (PACE) organizations
>
> Clinics, rehabilitation agencies, and public health agencies as providers of outpatient physical therapy and speech-language pathology services
>
> Psychiatric hospitals
>
> Religious nonmedical healthcare institutions
>
> - Rural health clinics
> - Long-term care facilities
> - Transplant centers
>
> Specific information about each of these categories can be found on the CMS website using the following address/link: www.cms.gov/medicare/health-safety-standards/conditions-coverage-participation.
>
> *Source:* From Centers for Medicare and Medicaid Services (CMS). (2018a). *Conditions for coverage (CfCs) & conditions of participations (CoPs)*. Retrieved from www.cms.gov/Regulations-and-Guidance/Legislation/CFCsAndCoPs/index.html?redirect=/CFCsAndCoPs

In addition to facility accreditation, CMS requires organizations to be certified as Medicare approved to perform certain procedures such as carotid artery stenting, ventricular assist device (VAD) destination therapy, certain oncologic PET scans in Medicare-specified studies, and lung volume reduction surgery. Information on Medicare-approved facilities/trials/registries can be found at www.cms.gov/medicare/coverage/approved-facilities-trials-registries. Early clinical program planning should include a review of the national coverage determination to identify the criteria for certification by CMS.

Controlling the growth of healthcare spending is a major focus of the federal government. Pay for performance (P4P) or value-based purchasing (VBP) is an evolving innovation initiative instituted by CMS whereby reimbursement is based on performance that results in quality patient outcomes. Hospital-acquired conditions (HACs) provide an example of a P4P focus. Postoperative surgical site infections (SSIs), central line-associated bloodstream infections (CLABSIs), catheter-associated urinary tract infections (CAUTIs), methicillin-resistant *Staphylococcus aureus* (MRSA), and *Clostridium difficile* (*C. diff*) are several examples of HACs. To fund the program, each year CMS withholds a percentage of inpatient payments from hospitals. While this program was suspended briefly during the coronavirus disease 2019 (COVID-19) pandemic, for 2022, the withholding percentage was 2%. A hospital can earn back more than the withheld amount (effectively earning a bonus) if it performs well with VBP metrics (www.advisory.com/Resources/value-based-care-should-be-more-than-a-buzzword). Accordingly, VBP continues to expand to include more indicators annually across the continuum of care. Private payers frequently use CMS guidelines as a basis for their protocols, and as a result, value-based care and reimbursement has expanded outside of CMS. Following the lead set by CMS, private insurance companies, such as Aetna, Blue Cross, and United, to name just a few, have implemented VBP contracts with providers. The Triple Aim model developed by the Institute for Healthcare Improvement (IHI) is consistent with trends in VBP. For more on Triple Aim, see Chapter 3, "Identifying Outcomes in Population-Based Nursing," and Chapter 9, "Evaluation of Practice at the Population Level."

The focus of VBP is not just on acute care hospitals. The Medicare Access and CHIP Reauthorization Act (MACRA) is a piece of legislation that created merit-based incentive payment system (MIPS) and advanced alternative payment models for other clinical settings. One such alternative payment model is the oncology care model (OCM). It serves as a good example for APRNs who practice outside of acute care hospitals. Practices that participate in the OCM have agreed to a payment model that includes financial and performance accountability related to chemotherapy administration for cancer patients (CMS, 2018a). The model essentially rewards high-quality evidence-based coordinated care. Performance accountability includes data from quality measures, claims data, and patient satisfaction surveys. The Oncology Nursing Society (ONS) has identified the need for oncology APRNs to be familiar with MIPS and OCM and to take leadership roles in participating in these programs (Galioto, 2017). More information on these CMS programs can be found at www.cms.gov/priorities/innovation/innovation-models/enhancing-oncology-model.

Home health agencies provide skilled care to homebound patients. TJC and Community Health Accreditation Partner (CHAP) have CMS deeming authority for accrediting home health, hospice, and home care medical equipment. CHAP *Standards of Excellence* (education.chaplinq.org) are designed for home and community-based care and provide a useful guide for developing and implementing new programs. Likewise, TJC has the *Comprehensive Accreditation Manual for Home Care* (www.

jcrinc.com/health-care-settings/home-care), which provides standards and measures for home care programs.

STATE DESIGNATIONS

It is important for APRNs who are developing clinical programs to review state (as well as federal) requirements for licensure of organizations, which may include requirements for accreditation and/or certification. APRNs should be knowledgeable about the state regulations for their clinical practice location (e.g., acute care, ambulatory care, long-term care, etc.), as well as the specialty in which they are practicing. Like federal designations, state designations are also premised on the concepts of patient safety and quality. Many states, for example, have formal requirements for licensing and certification of trauma, cardiac, stroke, and perinatal care, to name just a few. An example of a clinical area that has been in the spotlight and that has evolved in many states into one of the most formalized processes for approval is stroke care. This focus is likely due to the large amount of healthcare dollars spent on stroke, cardiovascular, and heart disease care in the United States. The Centers for Disease Control and Prevention (CDC) estimates that about $1 of every $7 spent on healthcare is related to these diseases (www.cdc.gov/dhdsp/docs/DHDSP_Investment_Factsheet-508.pdf). In 2004, New Jersey and Florida became the first states to legislate stroke care. Massachusetts and New York subsequently also developed regulations for care (Centers for Disease Control and Prevention [CDC], 2023). Other states quickly followed suit and there is much discussion on the national level for universal standards adoption. The focus has not been limited to the hospital care of stroke patients. Stroke prevention programs, as well as follow-up care, are also addressed in many of the more formalized stroke continuum of care regulations.

The process for providing stroke care varies from state to state. In some states, there are no requirements for providing stroke care, and in others, the requirements are prescriptive and require state licensing. In some states, the requirements for licensing include achieving some level of external stroke program certification or accreditations (e.g., through DNV or TJC). States, such as Massachusetts, have developed and implemented a state-designed and state-administered Stroke Designation Program. Many states have enacted stroke center legislation, require external accreditation of stroke programs, or have criteria for designation as a primary stroke center or as a comprehensive stroke center. In most cases, legislation or administrative policy gives a state agency, typically the state's Department of Health or Emergency Management Services (EMS), the authority to develop designation criteria. Many stroke programs voluntarily choose program certification for stroke to validate the quality of their program even without a state requirement. Hospitals can achieve stroke certification from several national organizations, including TJC, DNV, HFAP, and the AHA.

One of the major features of any disease-specific certification is data collection and analysis. Measures are typically both process and outcome based and are designed to drive compliance with evidence-based practice (EBP) standards. While the results are mixed, much focus in the literature has been placed on the value of certifications and accreditations to improve patient care. In one study, using systematic literature review methodology, Hussein et al. (2021) found that the accreditation process itself was stressful, but it had a positive effect on the organizations' culture of safety, improved data related to process measures, enhanced efficiency, and shortened patient length of stay. Employee as well as patient satisfaction and readmissions were found to be unrelated to accreditation status.

ACCOUNTABLE CARE ORGANIZATIONS

Credentialing as an Accountable Care Organization (ACO) is not a traditional accreditation or certification program, but there are similarities that make a review of the program noteworthy to include here. Although ACOs started as a mechanism for reducing the cost of healthcare, the basis for achieving reduced costs is a focus on quality patient care that results in optimal outcomes. According to CMS, ACOs were designed under the Affordable Care Act (ACA) as a strategy to reduce overall Medicare costs (innovation.cms.gov). Under the fee-for-service Medicare payment system, providers are rewarded based on the tests that are ordered. This is an area with a high potential for waste and abuse. Patients often seek care from multiple providers which can result in repeated testing due to a lack of coordinated care. Under the traditional fee-for-service payment system, providers are compensated based on the care and services provided, which can result in billing for duplicate services. It is easy to find examples of fee-for-service abuse. Newspapers often publish articles that report on providers or facilities being investigated for Medicare/Medicaid fraud for over testing or for providing and billing for unnecessary care. A 2018 article published online reported on a national healthcare fraud takedown carried out by the Department of Justice (DOJ). This investigation resulted in charges against more than 600 defendants, including 165 doctors, nurses, and other licensed medical professionals in districts across the United States (Stewart, 2018). Charges included fraud related to unnecessary testing, billing, and medication prescribing. The goals of the ACO model are to monitor and coordinate care to prevent such abuse while maintaining quality of care. A 2022 *The New York Times* article reported insurers "exploited Medicare for billions" (Abelson & Sanger-Katz, 2022) by incentivizing doctors to inflate diagnoses to make their patients appear sicker, therefore enabling them to bill Medicare at a higher rate. A 2022 *The Washington Post* article reported that a COVID-19 testing center located at an international airport overbilled Medicare more than $1.5 million by inflating the time spent with each patient being tested, claiming that the 5-minute clinic visit was 30 minutes or longer and involved higher levels of medical care and decisions (Thompson, 2022).

The ACO model is of particular interest to APRNs as it is largely focused on wellness and preventive care. The goal of an ACO is to coordinate care to ensure that patients get the right care at the right time, prevent medical errors, and, at the same time, avoid duplication of services (CMS, 2018b).

Technology is a key feature of ACOs because coordination and tracking of care is critical to success. The primary care provider is the one essential member of an ACO. Other members of the ACO can include specialists, hospitals, post-acute care providers, federally qualified health centers (FQHCs), joint venture partners, insurers, and drug stores, to name a few. To become an ACO, the applicant must meet the following requirements (CMS, 2023):

- Be a legal entity formed under state, federal, or tribal law.
- Handle a minimum of 5,000 Medicare lives annually.
- Have an organizational structure with clinical and administrative effectiveness.
- Demonstrate evidence-based medicine and coordination of care, with data reporting tied to performance and cost.
- Have a legal structure to receive and distribute payments.
- Make a 3-year commitment to the program.

There are also several shared saving tracks for which the ACO applicant can apply. Details on such tracks can be found at www.cms.gov/Medicare/Medicare-Fee-for-Service-Payment/sharedsavingsprogram/for-acos. Shared savings payments are based on financial performance and quality outcomes separately. The ACO model is complex with a detailed application process and significant reporting requirements that require a knowledgeable coordinator. APRNs working with populations covered by Medicare and Medicaid should become familiar with ACOs in their geographical area, as well as opportunities for participating in ACOs. The advantage of an ACO for patients is improved outcomes as the result of coordinated evidence-based care. This model of care delivery continues to evolve as the CMS Innovation Center adjusts the ACO option to enhance safety and quality in patient care, improve access to care, and enhance benefits for covered lives, all while providing payment incentives to providers and demonstrating overall reduction in healthcare costs (innovation.cms.gov/innovation-models/next-generation-aco-model).

NONGOVERNMENTAL PROGRAMS

There are a host of nongovernmental population-based programmatic certifications. It is generally accepted that program certification by professional organizations and accrediting organizations improves the functioning and outcomes of clinical programs. Numerous studies have been conducted over the years to qualify and quantify the value of accreditation (Melo, 2017; Procaccini et al., 2018). Even the process of preparing for and achieving accreditation is believed to improve performance. This is likely because accrediting organizations generally focus on organizational structure and processes, the environment in which care is provided, the qualifications of staff, evidence-based best practice, policies for care, and high-quality patient outcomes (Lin et al., 2017). Patient outcomes are typically evaluated in the context of benchmarking, which includes analyzing performance against peer organizations. The following is a sampling of the types of clinical programmatic accreditations/certifications in existence.

THE JOINT COMMISSION AND DNV DISEASE-SPECIFIC CARE CERTIFICATIONS

While many organizations offer certifications, TJC has perhaps the most diverse opportunities for programmatic and disease-specific certifications. In 2002, TJC started the Disease-Specific Care (DSC) Certification Program, which is designed to evaluate and certify the care of patients with any chronic disease or condition across the continuum (TJC, 2023). Although TJC can certify any clinical program based on a condition-based model, there are multiple procedures or diseases and areas for which TJC offers certification (Box 10.2). TJC cites many benefits to DSC, with the most important being the improvement of quality patient care by reducing clinical variation through a standardized approach. Best-practice protocols and data-driven performance are the foundation of DSC.

BOX 10.2

TJC DISEASE-SPECIFIC CARE CERTIFICATIONS

Ambulatory care certifications
- Advanced orthopedic
- Primary medical home

Behavioral healthcare

Healthcare staffing

Home care
- Community-based palliative care

Hospital
- Cardiac
- Orthopedic
- Stroke
- Medication compounding
- Perinatal care
- Palliative care
- Patient blood management
- Primary medical home

Nursing care center
- Memory care
- Post-acute care

Source: www.jointcommission.org/what-we-offer/certification/certifications-by-setting

COMMUNITY HEALTH

Community healthcare is an important component of population health, with a long history of providing crucial services (primary, secondary, and tertiary care) to vulnerable groups. Public health is an essential element of the healthcare system. The focus of public health is in the community where people work, live, and play. Public health agencies can be state, local, territorial, or tribal and are accredited by the PHAB. PHAB is a nonprofit organization that was created specifically to accredit public health departments. The goal of PHAB is to "advance and transform public health practice by championing performance improvement, strong infrastructure, and innovation" (PHAB, 2023).

PROFESSIONAL ORGANIZATIONS

American College of Surgeons

The American College of Surgeons (ACS) has a long history of validating the quality of clinical programs. The ACS first issued minimum standards for hospitals in 1917. The creation of these standards led to the program now known as TJC. Additional achievements include the creation of the Commission on Cancer (CoC) in 1922 and the Committee on Trauma (COT) in 1950. More recently in 2005 the ACS initiated programs for breast care (National Accreditation Program for Breast Centers [NAPBC]) and bariatric surgery. The bariatric surgery certification known as Metabolic and Bariatric Surgery Accreditation is run jointly by the ACS and the American Society for Metabolic and Bariatric Surgery (ASMBS) (ACS, 2018). Although these programs appear to be focused exclusively on hospitals, they are all concerned with the continuum of care including pre- and post-hospital care. These programs also have comprehensive data registries that focus on the continuum of care. Patient outcomes are evaluated against benchmark data. APRNs need to be knowledgeable about these programs and specifically about how their patient populations can benefit by following best-practice recommendations. According to the ACS (2018), facilities that have implemented these programs have improved surgical quality, prevented complications, reduced costs, and saved lives. The ACS principles for quality are found on their website (www.facs.org/quality-programs/about). These principles are like the foundations of many accreditation and certification processes.

American Nurses Credentialing Center

Magnet® designation by the American Nurses Credentialing Center (ANCC) is considered by many to be the highest recognition for nursing excellence. The term *Magnet hospital* dates to 1983 when the American Academy of Nursing (AACN) Task Force on Nursing Practice in Hospitals conducted a study of 163 hospitals to identify work environments that attract and retain (therefore, the term *Magnet*) well-qualified nurses. These organizations were also evaluated on their quality of care. Of the 163 hospitals in the initial study, 41 were identified as having qualities that attracted and retained nurses and were therefore described as Magnet Hospitals (Nursing World, 2018).

In 1990, the American Nurses Association (ANA) incorporated the ANCC as a subsidiary nonprofit organization. The ANCC was created to provide a body responsible for credentialing clinical nursing programs and services. Later that same year, the ANA Board of Directors approved a proposal to recognize excellence in hospital-based nursing services known as the Magnet Hospital Recognition Program. This program built upon the earlier work of the 1983 ANA Task Force. In 1994, the University of Washington Medical Center in Seattle, Washington, became the first ANCC Magnet-designated organization and was recognized in redesignation in 2022 for their seventh consecutive award (Nursing World, 2018; www.nursingworld.org/organizational-programs/magnet/find-a-magnet-organization).

Over the years, the Magnet Recognition Program® has continued to evolve and expand to include long-term care facilities, home health agencies, and healthcare organizations outside of the United States. While the number of hospitals currently designated is constantly changing, as of October 2022, there were 601 Magnet hospitals (less than 10% of all hospitals in the United States), including 13 outside the United States and four that provide ambulatory care services only (www.nursingworld.org/organizational-programs/magnet/find-a-magnet-organization). The Magnet Model depicts components that include transformational leadership, structural empowerment, exemplary professional practice, and new knowledge and is linked by the common thread of empirical outcomes (ANCC, 2021).

Shared decision-making is a critical feature of Magnet organizations. Shared decision-making may take many forms, but its hallmark is "a dynamic partnership between leadership, nurses, and other healthcare professionals that promotes collaborations, facilitates deliberation and decision making, and fosters accountability for improving patient outcomes, quality, and enhancing work life" (ANCC, 2021, p. 203). In addition to unit-based councils (UBCs), typically there are a few other councils in which clinical nurses and nurse leaders partner in shared decision-making. These might include professional practice, nursing research, quality and safety, education, peer review, and collaborative practice (among others). As clinical practice leaders, APRNs can play a significant role in the Magnet process as active members of these various councils. The academic preparation of the APRN and other nursing professionals with advanced nursing degrees, which includes skills in EBP, biostatistics, translational science, systems management, technology, and healthcare economics, makes these nurses uniquely qualified to support the important activities of shared decision-making councils.

The 2023 *Magnet Application Manual* (ANCC, 2021) includes some changes in standards which further support the need for APRN leadership in organizations seeking Magnet recognition. There is an emphasis on "diversity, equity, inclusion, and well-being of healthcare workers, patient and communities" (ANCC, 2021, p. 3). Additionally, the current revisions to standards have a focus on ambulatory care nursing and the use of new knowledge and EBP (ANCC, 2021).

Nursing research is another area of focus where the APRN's skills are necessary. When applying for Magnet designation/resignation, a table is submitted that lists all nursing research activities. These must be Institutional Review Board (IRB)-approved studies in which the principal investigator or coinvestigator is a nurse. Clinical nurses must be involved in nursing research and provided opportunities to present their research both internal and external to the organization. APRNs are considered clinical nurses by definition and are academically prepared for these activities, including acting as mentors or preceptors to stimulate interest in research by clinical bedside nurses (AACN, 2021).

For many years, research and evidence to support the impact of nursing care on patient outcomes has been a focus in the healthcare professional literature. A study by Bilgin and Ozmen (2022) used a systematic review methodology to examine the impact of Magnet designation on patient mortality. They concluded that Magnet designated hospitals overall have lower mortality rates and concluded that this outcome provides evidence of the value of Magnet designation for its impact on quality of patient care and cost savings. A study conducted by Bekelis et al. (2017) evaluated patients admitted for ischemic stroke and concluded that patients admitted to Magnet facilities were associated with decreases in fatality, shorter length of stay, and need for discharge to a long-term care facility, thereby demonstrating the value of Magnet designation.

Specialty Organizations

Many professional organizations offer certification for clinical programs. The following is a brief sampling of specialty organizations and the programs that they certify:

- American Heart Association (AHA): Cardiovascular care and stroke
- American College of Cardiology/Society of Cardiovascular Patient Care: Cardiovascular care and chest pain
- National Committee of Quality Assurance (NCQA): Many certifications, including Patient-Centered Specialty Practice (PCSP) recognition, diabetes care, oncology care, and behavioral healthcare
- National Hospice and Palliative Care Organization: Community palliative care
- The American Society for Gastrointestinal Endoscopy (ASGE): Gastrointestinal and endoscopy care
- American Academy of Pediatrics (AAP): Pediatric medical home
- American Congress of Obstetricians and Gynecologists (ACOG): Safety Certification in Outpatient Practice Excellence (SCOPE)
- Alzheimer's Association: Dementia care

The World Health Organization Baby-Friendly Hospital Initiative

In addition to professional organizations, national and international organizations offer certifications/designations for specific health initiatives. One such designation is the World Health Organization (WHO) Baby Friendly Hospital Initiative (BFHI), which was created in 1991 to protect, promote, and support breastfeeding and to reduce worldwide malnutrition. BFHI designation is based on the *Ten Steps to Successful Breastfeeding* and the International Code of Marketing of Breast-Milk Substitutes. By 2021, there were 160 countries and more than 20,000 facilities that have earned Baby-Friendly designation (www.babyfriendlyusa.org/about), including all 50 states and more than 600 facilities in the United States. For more information on BFHI, go to www.babyfriendlyusa.org.

THE ROLE OF ADVANCED PRACTICE REGISTERED NURSES IN PROGRAM ACCREDITATION

APRNs need to be aware of the opportunities to obtain program credentialing for their population-based area of practice. They should identify such opportunities by reviewing programs offered by governmental and nongovernmental agencies. An essential first step is knowledge about the state of your clinical program. Does your organization measure critical programmatic outcomes? Does it enter data into a national database to track performance? Many organizations, such as the AHA and the ACS, have databases that allow organizations and programs to participate and benchmark performance against other programs. The vast majority of Magnet recognized facilities (95%) use the National Database of Nursing Quality Indicators® (NDNQI®) to assess performance on nurse-sensitive indicators (NSIs; Press Ganey, 2018). Information on NSI can be found in Chapter 2, "Identifying Outcomes in Population-Based Nursing." It is critically important to know how well your organization performs in comparison to others on a broader (particularly national) level and not just within your local area.

Clinical program accreditation/certification frequently rests on the documentation of the prioritization of EBP within an organization. APRNs are academically prepared to serve as champions for the use of EBP. Best practices in nursing are evidenced by measurable outcomes. An important element of implementing EBP is to measure outcomes before and after any changes in practice in order to evaluate the impact of the change.

Doctor of Nursing Practice (DNP)-educated nurses and APRNs performing in a variety of roles and settings may become the standard for leading organizational efforts toward accreditation. Using Magnet designation as an example, agencies applying for designation are required to have a Magnet program director (MPD). Although qualifications for the MPD are not specified, nor is there a specified educational requirement, the academic preparation of the DNP-educated APRN includes the competencies necessary for leading efforts to achieve Magnet designation. DNP programs that are designed using AACN's 10 domains of educational content for nursing education that provides the APRN with the academic preparation and skills that are critical for the MPD role. Specific essentials that prepare the APRN for the MPD role include knowledge; person-centered care; population health; scholarship; quality and safety; interprofessional partnerships; systems-based practice; informatics and technologies; professionalism; and personal, professional, and leadership development (AACN, 2021). Finally, APRNs are well-recognized by members of the healthcare team as internal consultants and a resource for nursing staff and other members of the care team as clinical experts.

CREATING THE PLAN

A major part of program development in preparation for accreditation is planning and creating an action plan. Program design and the development process is discussed in detail in Chapter 8, "Concepts in Program Design and Development." The goal of every clinical program should be to benefit the population being served. If the program under development requires accreditation, then the requirements or standards of such a designation are essential in early consideration within the planning process. Ideally, the planning team should include at least one member who has expertise in the requirements for accreditation, members who demonstrate strong writing skills, and, in some cases, an outside expert/consultant who may be of value if there is no internal team member with significant experience and knowledge of the accreditation program. There are often resources at the accreditation organization that can be of assistance. For example, both TJC and Magnet assign liaisons to participating organizations. Many healthcare entities have contracts with best-practice consulting firms, which often have clinical content experts that are available to member organizations. These companies typically have teams for the prominent clinical foci of the current marketplace, such as cardiovascular, oncology, post-acute, orthopedics, neuroscience, and new and emerging areas of focus.

During the earliest stages of planning for accreditation, accreditation standards and clinical practice guidelines must be identified and understood. Performance of a gap analysis is another critical first step and should be performed using an interdisciplinary team approach. An action plan with goals, timelines, and accountabilities should be created. This action plan is then integrated into the overall program design and development plan to ensure success. An executive sponsor who is a senior member of administration should serve as a champion for the initiative. This role can be extremely useful in maintaining focus and eliminating barriers. When preparing to apply, applicants should be sure to provide only the information that is specifically required; more is not always better. Once the document has been accepted and a site visit is imminent, it is essential to prepare for the visit. Who will escort the surveyors? Who should surveyors meet with? What should surveyors see? What space will be dedicated for use by the surveyors? Remember that the site visit is used to validate the information presented in the application. Plan every aspect of the site visit carefully. A detailed agenda is essential, including the details of each session, attendees, and location. Participants should have ample advance notice of the site visit day(s) so that their calendars can be cleared. Some sessions may require a dress rehearsal so that all participants can engage, know what is expected of them, and prepare for the type of questions that the surveyors/appraisers are likely to ask. Such use of mock site visits can be a useful tool and help make the site survey go more smoothly. Once accreditation is achieved, organizations should formally celebrate the accomplishment. This provides the perfect opportunity for recognition of the participants at every level of the organization that helped to make the accreditation/certification process a success.

SUMMARY

The healthcare marketplace is extremely competitive. Achieving good rankings from external agencies such as Leapfrog, CMS Star Ratings, and *U.S. News and World Report*, to name a few, has become a desired and necessary goal for healthcare organizations. Administrators are constantly on the lookout to identify opportunities to differentiate and validate their organization. Achieving accreditation helps to validate programs and organizations in the context of national and professional standards. Consumers are increasingly savvy in assessing programs and often look to external rankings for help in deciding where to seek care. Payers, both private and governmental, are looking for value-based care in their efforts to reduce healthcare costs. Accreditation offers healthcare providers an opportunity to qualify and quantify the quality of clinical programs.

Accreditation is recognized to assess, build, and validate clinical programs and it requires extensive preparation and dedication. The process itself provides an opportunity to develop a framework for quality improvement and to create a culture which focuses on outstanding care that requires staff engagement.

In the past, accreditation was viewed as a process separate from the everyday functioning of an organization, but organizations cannot be successful with standards compliance when such compliance is only reviewed in cycles prior to the application for accreditation. The current paradigm requires a continuous, ongoing focus on meeting standards of excellent clinical practice, analyzing performance, achieving optimal outcomes, and producing sustainable change. Accreditation provides APRNs with the opportunity to be leaders in clinical care and champions for validation of clinical practice.

END-OF-CHAPTER RESOURCES

EXERCISES

EXERCISE 10.1 Identify an accreditation and/or certification designation applicable to your area of practice/population-based program. Conduct a gap analysis to identify areas requiring additional focus/changes to achieve the accreditation. Create an action plan for each matter that is identified as an impediment to accreditation/certification.

EXERCISE 10.2 Imagine you are going to lead a team to obtain accreditation and/or certification for your population-based program. Identify the interdisciplinary team members you would select and provide an explanation for each selection. Identify where you may need external resources to supplement the team. Why do you need these external resources? What are your goals for these consultants?

EXERCISE 10.3 Identify two evidence-based nursing protocols that you want to implement at your organization. What are the performance metrics you will measure? What is your current performance? What national benchmarks can you use to measure your performance?

A robust set of instructor resources designed to supplement this text is located at http://connect.springerpub.com/content/book/978-0-8261-4377-8. Qualifying instructors may request access by emailing textbook@springerpub.com.

REFERENCES

Abelson, R., & Sanger-Katz, M. (2022). The cash monster was insatiable: How insurers exploited Medicare for billions. *The New York Times*, October 8, 2022. Retrieved from https://www.nytimes.com/2022/10/08/upshot/medicare-advantage-fraud-allegations.html

American Nurses Credentialing Center. (2021). *2023 Magnet application manual*. American Nurses Credentialing Center.

American Association of Colleges of Nursing. (2021). *The essentials: Core competencies for professional nursing education*. Retrieved from http://www.aacnnursing.org/Portals/42/AcademicNursing/pdf/Essentials-2021.pdf

American College of Surgeons. (2018). *American College of Surgeons: 100-year history of leading quality improvement*. Retrieved from https://www.facs.org/quality-programs/about

Bekelis, N., Missios, S., & MacKenzie, T. (2017). Association of Magnet status with hospitalization outcomes for ischemic stroke patients. *Journal of the American Heart Association, 6*. E005880. https://doi.org/10.1161/JAHA.117.005880

Bilgin, N., & Ozmen, D. (2022). Mortality in Magnet hospitals: A systematic review. *Nigerian Journal of Clinical Practice, 25*, 1203–1210. https://doi.org/10.4103/njcp.njcp_183_22

Centers for Disease Control and Prevention. (2023). *Stroke systems of care: State policy interventions by evidence level*. Retrieved from: https://www.cdc.gov/dhdsp/policy_resources/stroke_systems_of_care/evidence_interventions.htm

Centers for Medicare and Medicaid Services. (2018a). *Oncology care model*. Retrieved from https://www.cms.gov/priorities/innovation/innovation-models/enhancing-oncology-model

Centers for Medicare and Medicaid Services. (2018b). *Accountable care organizations (ACOs)*. Retrieved from https://www.cms.gov/priorities/innovation/innovation-models/aco

Centers for Medicare and Medicaid Services. (2023). *For ACOs*. Retrieved from https://www.cms.gov/medicare/payment/fee-for-service-providers/shared-savings-program-ssp-acos

Galioto, M. (2017). APRNs have a role in leading value based care. *Oncology Nursing Society – ONS Voice*. Retrieved from https://voice.ons.org/news-and-views/apns-have-a-role-in-leading-value-based-care

Hussein, M., Pavolova, M., Ghalwash, M., & Grooy, W. (2021). The impact of hospital accreditation on the quality of healthcare: A systematic literature review. *BMC Health Research, 21*, 1057. https://doi.org/10.1186/s12913-021-07097-6

Institute of Medicine. (2010). *Future of nursing leading change, advancing health: Report recommendations*. Retrieved from https://nap.nationalacademies.org/catalog/12956/the-future-of-nursing-leading-change-advancing-health

Lin, P., Chandra, F., Shapiro, F., Osman, B. M., Urman, R. D., & Ahn, S. S. (2017). The need for accreditation of office-based interventional vascular centers. *Annals of Vascular Surgery, 38*, 332–338. https://doi.org/10.1016/j.avsg.2016.06.010

Melo, S. (2017). The impact of accreditation on healthcare quality improvement: A qualitative case study. *Journal of Health Organization and Management, 30*(8), 1242–1258. https:/doi.org/10.1108/JHOM-01-2016-0021

Nursing World. (2018). *Magnet Recognition Program®*. Retrieved from https://www.nursingworld.org/organizational-programs/magnet/about-magnet/

Press Ganey. (2018). *Nursing quality – NDNQI*. Retrieved from http://www.pressganey.com/solutions/clinical-quality/nursing-quality

Procaccini, D., Curley, A. L. C., & Goldman, M. (2018). Baby-Friendly practices minimize newborn infants weight loss. *Breastfeeding Medicine: The Official Journal of the Academy of Breastfeeding Medicine, 13*(3), 189–194. https://doi.org/10.1089/bfm.2017.0182

Public Health Accreditation Board. (2023). *What is public health accreditation*? Retrieved from http://www.phaboard.org/accreditation-overview/what-is-accreditation

Stewart, A. (2018). *Providers from 35 states charged in healthcare fraud crackdown: Here's the breakdown*. Retrieved from https://www.beckersasc.com/asc-coding-billing-and-collections/providers-from-35-states-charged-in-healthcare-fraud-crackdown-here-s-the-breakdown.html

The Joint Commission. (2023a). *Facts about Joint commission*. Retrieved from https://www.jointcommission.org/what-we-offer/certification/what-is-certification

The Joint Commission. (2023b). *Certifications by healthcare setting*. Retrieved from https://www.jointcommission.org/what-we-offer/certifications-by-setting

Thompson, S. (2022, April 22). Doctor overseeing coronavirus testing at BWI accused of health-care fraud. *The Washington Post*. https://www.washingtonpost.com/dc-md-va/2022/04/23/maryland-covid-fraud/

INTERNET RESOURCES

Advisory Board: https://www.advisory.com/
Alzheimer's Association: https://www.alz.org/
American Academy of Pediatrics (AAP): https://www.aap.org/
American Association Colleges of Nursing (AACN): https://www.aacnnursing.org/
American College of Cardiology (ACC)/Society of Cardiovascular Patient Care: https://www.acc.org/
American College of Surgeons (ACS): https://www.facs.org/
American Congress of Obstetricians and Gynecologists (ACOG): https://www.acog.org/
American Heart Association (AHA): https://www.heart.org/
American Nurses Credentialing Center (ANCC): https://www.nursingworld.org/ancc/
American Society for Gastrointestinal Endoscopy (ASGE): https://www.asge.org/
American Stroke Association (ASA): https://www.stroke.org/
Baby-Friendly Hospital Initiative (BFHI): https://www.babyfriendlyusa.org/
Centers for Disease Control and Prevention (CDC): https://www.cdc.gov/
Centers for Medicare and Medicaid Services (CMS): https://www.cms.gov/
Centers for Medicare and Medicaid Services (CMS)/CMS Star Ratings: https://www.cms.gov/medicare/provider-enrollment-and-certification/certificationandcomplianc/fsqrs

Community Health Accreditation Partner (CHAP): https://www.chapinc.org/
Coode of Federal Regulations. Title 52, Chapter IV, Subchapter G, Subpart-A. Definitions: https://ecfr.gov/current/title42/chapterIV/subchapter-G/part-488/subpart-A
Das Norske Veritas (DNV): https://www.dnv.com/services/hospital-accreditation-7516/
Institute of Medicine (IOM)/National Academy of Medicine (NAM): https://nam.edu/
International Organization for Standardization (ISO): https://www.iso.org/home.html/
Leapfrog: https://www.leapfroggroup.org/
National Database of Nursing Quality Indicators (NDNQI): https://ojin.nursingworld.org/table-of-contents/volume-12-2007/number-3-september-2007/nursing-quality-indicators/
National Hospice and Palliative Care Organization (NHPCO): https://www.nhpco.org/
The Commission on Accreditation of Rehabilitation Facilities (CARF): www.carf.org/
The Healthcare Facilities Accreditation Program (HFAP): https://www.hfap.org/
The Joint Commission (TJC): www.jointcommission.org/
The National Committee for Quality Assurance (NCQA): www.ncqa.org/
The Public Health Accreditation Board (PHAB): http://www.phaboard.org/
The Utilization Review Accreditations Commission (URAC): https://www.urac.org/
U.S. News and World Report Best Hospitals: https://health.usnews.com/best-hospitals
World Health Organization (WHO): http://www.who.int/

CHAPTER 11

BUILDING RELATIONSHIPS AND ENGAGING COMMUNITIES THROUGH COLLABORATION

SONDA M. OPPEWAL

One silver bracelet does not make much jingle.

—African proverb

INTRODUCTION

Let us consider this adage when we think of community health assessment (CHA). The primary purpose of building relationships and engaging communities through collaboration, essential for CHAs, is to facilitate ongoing dialogue with diverse community partners to help assess, plan, implement, and evaluate priority community issues from assessment through program design and development. By working *with* the community, healthcare professionals have the opportunity to collaborate on issues relevant to community members to ensure the sustainability and long-term success of community-based programs. This type of collaboration fosters bidirectional communication, deep understanding, and knowledge in the quest to ensure compassionate, relevant, high-quality, and culturally sensitive interventions. For collaboration to be successful, advanced practice registered nurses (APRNs) need specialized knowledge and skills to build rapport, foster trust, respect differences, and involve diverse community partners on an ongoing basis through all phases of the CHA. Returning to the adage, many bracelets are needed to make a melodic jingle that is rich and beautiful to hear.

FOUNDATION FOR COLLABORATION AND COMMUNITY ENGAGEMENT

All APRNs are charged with improving the health of communities, improving population health, decreasing health disparities, and improving health equity. Working actively with community members and organizations is part of nursing's rich history. Consider the work of Lillian Wald, founder of public health nursing in the United States. She collaborated with community members, agencies, and philanthropists from industry, housing, recreation, and education to improve health outcomes (Buhler-Wilkerson, 1993). In more recent times, Dr. Ernest Grant, president of the American Nurses Association (ANA), is known internationally for his nursing work in burn care and prevention which has required collaboration with numerous community members and agencies (Nelson, 2019). Collaboration and community engagement are critical strategies for all nurses involved with population-based nursing regardless of one's work setting. The foundation for these skills is grounded in the work of numerous professional nursing organizations and legislation; three are highlighted in this chapter. They include the American Association of Colleges of Nursing's (AACN) *The Essentials: Core Competencies for Professional Nursing Education* (2021), competencies from APRN organizations, and the Patient Protection and Affordable Care Act (ACA).

AMERICAN ASSOCIATION OF COLLEGES OF NURSING

The AACN published *The Essentials of Doctoral Education for Advanced Practice Nurses* in 2006. This seminal curricular framework provided guidance to the faculty of baccalaureate, master's, and doctoral education. A major update occurred in 2021 when AACN revised *The Essentials* by articulating ten professional nursing practice domains and competencies for all levels of education, including sub-competencies that build upon and move from entry to advanced practice.

Building relationships and engaging communities through collaborations are skills that are clearly outlined in two of the domains. Domain 3 of *The Essentials* is specific to population health; the importance of collaborative activities from numerous partners is described. The competency related to managing population health includes sub-competencies that are relevant to this chapter including data analysis from primary and secondary sources, stakeholder collaboration, and implementing interventions that are culturally and linguistically appropriate. Engaging in effective partnerships is a second competency associated with the population health domain. One of the advanced nursing sub-competencies articulates the role of leadership when partnering with others to improve health outcomes (AACN, 2021).

Domain 6 of *The Essentials* is specific to interprofessional partnerships. It specifies collaboration with diverse partners and stakeholders. Specific competencies focus on communicating to facilitate partnerships, performing in various team roles effectively, using knowledge of other professions to help deal with healthcare needs, working with others respectfully, sharing values, and demonstrating a culture of mutual learning (AACN, 2021).

PROFESSIONAL APRN COMPETENCIES

After the AACN (2006) published *The Essentials of Doctoral Education for Advanced Nursing Practice* with the recommendation to establish the Doctor of Nursing Practice (DNP) as the highest practice degree in nursing, advanced practice nursing organizations started developing practice doctorate competencies. The National Organization of Nurse Practitioner Faculties (NONPF) was the first to publish competencies for doctorate nursing practice in 2006 (Pohl et al., 2009). The most recent competencies were published in 2022, titled "Nurse Practitioner Role Core Competencies," to align with the 2021 AACN *Essentials*. The new competencies are considered essential for all nurse practitioners (NONPF, 2022).

The National Association of Clinical Nurse Specialists (NACNS) is the only national nursing organization dedicated to nurses who are clinical nurse specialists (CNSs). NACNS endorsed the DNP as entry into CNS practice in 2015 (Saunders, 2022). Hence, faculty who teach CNS students are expected to use *the Essentials* curriculum fully. Furthermore, *the Essentials* align well with the CNS role competencies set forth in the 2019 statement on CNS practice and education (Saunders, 2022). Like NONPF and NACNS, professional organizations for nurse midwives, the American College of Nurse-Midwives (ACNM), and nurse anesthetists, the American Association of Nurse Anesthesiology (AANA), recognize collaboration as an important professional attribute for its members (AANA, 2016; ACNM, 2020). More specifically, one of the doctoral-level competencies in midwifery is to "Collaborate with other health care leaders in the development of systems that improve the standard of care for persons seeking midwifery care" (ACNM, 2021, p.3).

THE PATIENT PROTECTION AND AFFORDABLE CARE ACT

The foundation for collaboration and community engagement is grounded in legislation in addition to professional nursing organizations. The ACA was the first comprehensive health reform legislation passed by Congress in more than 50 years before President Barack Obama signed it into law on March 23, 2010. The purpose of this Act was to expand access to health insurance coverage, improve systems delivering healthcare, and keep healthcare costs controlled (Kaiser Family Foundation, 2013). One requirement of the ACA specifically applies to nonprofit hospitals with a federal tax exemption. These hospitals must conduct a community health needs assessment (CHNA) every 3 years and plan and implement strategies to meet the community health needs identified from the assessment. The CHNA must include input from persons who represent the broad interests of the community, including those with special knowledge of, or expertise in, public health, such as local health departments (LHDs) (Carlton & Singh, 2018; Rozier, 2020). Collaboration among healthcare agencies and public health agencies is vital. The Internal Revenue Service (IRS) specifies that a hospital must solicit input from entities that represent the broad interests of the community including three required sources: a governmental public health department, medically underserved members or individuals of organizations serving these populations, and written comments on the hospital's most recently conducted CHNA and adopted implementation strategy. Other sources of input to assure broad community input include local government officials and school districts, private businesses, healthcare consumers, nonprofit community-based agencies, academic experts, healthcare providers from various settings including community health centers, health insurance and managed care organizations, and labor and workforce representatives (IRS, 2022).

The terms CHA and CHNA may be used interchangeably. However, a CHNA must meet certain requirements specific for tax-exempt hospitals as outlined by the ACA and IRS regulations. The purpose of a CHA or CHNA is to identify health problems, needs, gaps, strengths, and assets and to be used as a stimulus for action to improve health by addressing priority needs based on community input and with community partners.

Community Health Assessment Compliance

In many states, nonprofit hospitals have joined with LHDs to fulfill the requirement to conduct a CHNA. Health departments are also required to conduct community assessments on a regular basis and have the expertise to do so. For example, in urban Wake County, North Carolina (where the capital of the state, Raleigh, is located), more than 80 agencies and community partners collaborated to complete the 2022 CHNA (Live Well Wake, 2022). One intent of this large collaborative effort was to avoid duplication of efforts among the LHDs, different hospitals, and community health centers that received federal money under Section 330 of the Public Health Service (PHS) Act. The CHNA was led by Live Well Wake, which is a collaborative that formed from the 2018 CHNA and Population Health Task Force Initiatives with the goal of building strong cross-sector partnerships among the county's major healthcare systems, county agencies, and community-based organizations (Live Well Wake, 2022). Key players in this collaborative CHNA included Wake County Health and Human Services (local public health department); three hospitals, WakeMed Health and Hospitals, Duke Raleigh Hospital, and UNC Health; Advance Community Health, a federally qualified health center (FQHC); Alliance Health, a managed care organization for public behavioral healthcare (members are insured by Medicaid or are uninsured); the North Carolina Institute for Public Health which is part of the UNC Gillings School of Global Public Health; United Way; the Wake County Board of Commissioners; Citrix, a large business; and the Wake County Medical Society. Also participating were other nonprofit, faith-based, educational, government, and business organizations, as well as Wake County residents (Live Well Wake, 2022).

Researchers recently examined the involvement of LHDs with hospitals' CHNAs to better understand collaboration and hospital investment in community health. They found that LHDs that collaborated with hospital CHNAs were more likely to be involved in jointly planning implementation strategies to tackle the identified problems than LHDs that were not. Furthermore, they found that hospitals were more likely to invest in community health improvement initiatives when LHDs were involved with hospital implementation strategies (Carlton & Singh, 2018).

Advance Community Health is a (FQHC that, like other FQHCs, receives grants under Section 330 of the PHS Act. These safety net providers provide comprehensive outpatient care in medically underserved areas or populations and must meet specific requirements for enhanced reimbursement from Medicare and Medicaid, as well as other benefits. FQHCs must serve an underserved area or population, offer a sliding fee scale, provide comprehensive services, have an ongoing quality assurance program, and have a governing board of directors with the majority of members receiving client care at the FQHC (Centers for Medicare and Medicaid Services [CMS], 2018). In addition, health centers must conduct a needs assessment every three years of available health resources, health status indicators, and economic and demographic factors that impact health in order to assess the unmet need for health services among the population served by the center (Health Resources and Services Administration [HRSA], 2018).

Collaborative efforts for conducting CHNAs in rural areas may occur on a regional level across several counties. For example, in Western North Carolina, the Western North Carolina (WNC) Health Network is an alliance of 33 hospitals, health departments, and health centers. The mission of WNC Health Network is to improve health and healthcare across their region of 16 counties (WNC Health Network, 2023a). One of its components, the WNC Healthy Impact, is a partnership of coordinated efforts between hospitals, public health agencies, and key community partners in the western part of the state. The WNC Healthy Impact collaborative works on a CHNA to assess community needs, develop plans collaboratively, coordinate action, and evaluate the impact and progress of the action plans (WNC Health Network, 2023b).

As these examples demonstrate, in many places, health departments, hospitals, and healthcare agency professionals in outpatient clinics can collaborate to assess and address health issues relevant to their community. Such efforts help to ensure sustainability and the long-term success of both hospital and community-based programs. Not only is collaboration needed for IRS compliance for 501(c)(3) hospitals under the ACA, but it also makes sense to work together to avoid duplicate efforts. Successful collaborative efforts between community partners, agencies, stakeholders, and residents reflect the active involvement of diverse partners. Such CHNAs are more likely to be relevant, culturally responsive, and successful in achieving high-quality healthcare and reducing health disparities and inequities than those developed by less diverse working groups.

In summary, the essential or core competency work of the AACN, NONPF, NACNS, AANA, and ACNM represents a comprehensive foundation for APRN practice in population-based nursing and expertise in collaboration and community engagement. Federal legislation enacted by the ACA supports CHNAs carried out by hospitals and public health departments with the engagement or active involvement of diverse community partners. To build relationships with communities and to be successful in population health endeavors, APRNs require skills in leadership, collaboration, research, and policymaking. APRNs can take lead roles in engaging communities in activities to assess and improve health. These efforts require time; trust; teamwork; and active collaboration with community leaders, members, and stakeholders.

COMMUNITY HEALTH ASSESSMENT
WHY ASSESS THE COMMUNITY?

CHA and analysis are a cornerstone of effective population-based nursing care and are the first step in improving community health. For many healthcare organizations, it is also a legislative requirement, as discussed for nonprofit hospitals. FQHC ambulatory care centers are also required to perform a community needs assessment every 3 years (Burns et al., 2020), and state health departments conduct state CHAs for their state health improvement plans as a requirement of Public Health Foundation Board accreditation (Fromknecht et al., 2021). The end product of a CHA is the identification of community assets and needs that are congruent with the cultural diversity of the community, which will then be used to drive needed changes to improve health and health equity (Ryan-Ibarra et al., 2018). It involves community member participation and collaboration throughout the process, during planning, data collection, analysis, priority setting with community validation, and evaluation. CHAs can reveal critical information about what works and what does not work for a community.

While conducting a CHA, APRNs may work with various community partners in hospitals, health departments, faith-based organizations, local housing authorities, social services, and first responders, as well as stakeholders from various community groups and members of different disciplines. Leadership requires the ability to collaborate with individuals and leaders from different groups and agencies who may have different perspectives about health and healthcare needs. Centering dialogue on common overarching goals is one of the first steps to achieving them. CHAs may be considered a type of community-based participatory research (CBPR) because it is a systematic process and it requires trusting relationships among researchers (or healthcare professionals) and community members. Mutually identified goals must be identified and agreed upon. It may take years for researchers and community members to build the trusting relationships needed to identify mutually identified goals and to conduct community-based participatory research, especially in communities that have been marginalized (Fitzpatrick, 2016).

Any plan to meet the needs of a community that is derived from data synthesized into a CHA may truly be considered an evidence-based practice plan. According to the Centers for Disease Control and Prevention (CDC), addressing health improvement has a greater impact when it is a shared responsibility of federal, state, and local governments and with diverse community agencies, faith-based organizations, philanthropists and investors, healthcare and public health professionals, health insurers, nonprofits, and community members (CDC Community Health Improvement Navigator, 2022). If health improvement is the goal, many sectors of the community must be involved in a CHA.

A CHA may focus on a community as defined by its geopolitical boundaries (e.g., towns, cities, counties) or on an aggregate of a community (Gibson & Thatcher, 2020, pp. 370–394). CHAs are most often conducted for communities with specific geographical boundaries. These assessments can be used to identify populations that need more intensive study of specific problems or of subpopulations that require an aggregate assessment.

For example, a health needs assessment was conducted for five different Plain Communities in Pennsylvania and compared with the general PA population because these Old Order Amish and Old Order Mennonite groups were more isolated and often not assessed as part of larger geographical assessments (Miller et al., 2019).

While some CHAs have a narrow focus based on specific questions, other CHAs are more comprehensive. A comprehensive CHA addresses the characteristics of the community's physical environment, infrastructure, and population characteristics. Regardless of the scope and breadth of a CHA, APRNs need to work with community members to identify community strengths, weaknesses, and priorities. Such collaboration and community engagement leads to mutually agreed-upon goals for improvement, targeted outcomes, and "buy in" by communities to act together to improve health.

CONDUCTING THE ASSESSMENT

CHAs are not done in isolation; no one should attempt a CHA alone. The APRN may lead a CHA, serve as a member of the CHA team by representing their practice organization, or provide expert information or other assistance. A key function of the planning committee of the CHA is to work collaboratively with a diverse group of community partners, solicit input from multiple sources, agree on the purpose of the assessment, identify partnership responsibilities, and agree on the choice of assessment methods best suited for the specific community. For a CHA to be successful, it is essential to work collaboratively with community partners and stakeholders from the very beginning of the planning process through the CHA's completion (Money et al., 2020).

APRNs can mobilize diverse community partners and stakeholders within the community to assist with the CHA by "thinking out of the box." The CHA team should consider soliciting input from representatives of businesses; schools; agencies who work with youth; faith-based organizations; health and social service agencies; emergency services; environmental agencies; and other cross-sector partners in transportation, economic development, and legal systems. Ultimately, CHA team members should represent diverse ages, populations, interests, and points of view so that different perspectives about health and community issues will be obtained and considered. Community members have valuable contributions to make to the CHA and are concerned and interested in the community where they live and/or work, and they are familiar with the needs and resources of the community (Institute for Healthcare Improvement [IHI], 2019). Furthermore, in order to achieve health equity, it is imperative to engage diverse cross-sector partners and stakeholders, so their various needs are considered, as well as the social determinants of health that impact the community (Fromknecht et al., 2021).

Assessment methods include the analysis of primary data, data directly collected, and secondary data that was collected by someone else and may be obtained from online databases and websites. A literature review can be done to help identify current information on health topics. CHA team members can obtain primary data from participant observation, windshield and walking surveys (WWS), key informant interviews, surveys, and focus groups. Each method has advantages and disadvantages that must be considered along with available resources such as personnel, budget, time, and expertise.

Fortunately, there is a plethora of information available at one's fingertips on the Internet. Tools exist that quickly provide data for communities, counties, states, and nations. Information that is available from online databases and various websites, such as county and municipal home pages, provides important data elements for consideration. APRNs are well-positioned to help find data from a variety of sources given their experience and education.

Data collected from CHAs may be organized in different ways to facilitate analysis and synthesis. One comprehensive framework is the community assessment wheel. CHA data can be organized into nine components represented by a wheel with an inner circle and eight hubs (Anderson & McFarlane, 2019). The community core is the inner circle that is surrounded by eight hubs or components that together form a larger circle. The community core includes data that describes the people in the community in terms of their history, demographics, ethnicity, vital statistics, values, beliefs, and religion. The hubs of the community assessment wheel include the categories of physical environment, health and social services, safety and transportation, communication, politics and government, education, recreation, and economics (Anderson & McFarlane, 2019). CHA team members can use the nine components of the wheel to identify questions that need to be answered about the community and to organize data in a systematic and comprehensive manner. This type of CHA can provide insight into the root causes of community health problems, as well as community resources and strengths (Anderson & McFarlane, 2019).

Anderson and McFarlane (2019) recommend that assessments be conducted in incremental fashion to better manage the enormity of the task. For example, CHA team members can stop at predetermined intervals to analyze and synthesize the data as they are collected. While the process of conducting a CHA is ongoing, concurrent generation and analysis of data will identify recurrent themes that may signal that sufficient data are collected. Alternatively, the APRN may discover that further information is needed because of the appearance of inconsistencies within the data and gaps needing additional clarification. Qualitative or contextual information derived from participant observation, focus groups, key informant interviews, and windshield surveys provides rich and valuable information that can bring clarity to the information gleaned from surveys, literature reviews, and secondary data analyses. For example, parents and caregivers who are interviewed about childhood obesity may offer insight into family and community values and beliefs about eating and physical activity. This is important contextual information. In addition, parents may be able to describe why some strategies are not helpful and identify alternate strategies that align better with the characteristics of the family, neighborhood, or community.

ASSESSMENT TOOLS AND METHODS

ASSESSMENT TOOLS

Numerous CHA resources exist to help guide CHAs and to make the process efficient. They provide useful information on how to build relationships and trust with communities, work through the CHA process, gather data, and design evidence-based interventions.

This chapter highlights five such CHA resources: (a) the *Healthy People 2030* website, (b) the Community Tool Box, (c) the American Hospital Association Community Health Improvement (ACHI) Community Health Assessment Toolkit, (d) the County Health Rankings and Roadmaps, and (e) the CDC Community Health Improvement Navigator.

Healthy People 2030

Developed by the Office of Disease Prevention and Health Promotion (ODPHP), the *Healthy People* website outlines America's roadmap for achieving good health and well-being. Its vision is to achieve health equity, create healthy environments, and engage cross-sector stakeholders in designing strategies to improve health (Hasbrouck, 2021; Ochiai et al., 2021). It includes a treasure trove of data and resources for APRNs who are charged with working on a CHA. The *Healthy People 2030* Tools for Action section (ODPHP, n.d.a) includes examples of partnership and community stories that highlight how they are working to improve health and help achieve *Healthy People* objectives. A pathway for using *Healthy People 2030* in one's own community is outlined with four steps (ODPHP, n.d.b). The first step is to identify needs and priority populations by reviewing the objectives and considering how national goals compare with one's priorities and using this information to help build partnerships. The second step is to set one's own targets by finding local data to compare with the national data available on *Healthy People 2030*. The third step is to find inspiration and practical tools by exploring the evidence-based interventions and resources. The fourth step is to monitor national progress and use the *Healthy People 2030* data as a benchmark, to compare progress and use data to inform healthy programs and policies (ODHP, n.d.b).

The *Healthy People 2030* website provides data from a variety of reliable data sources for each of 355 core objectives. Each objective includes specific data sources that meet data requirements to ensure accuracy and reliability and a baseline value at the national level (Giroir, 2021). The objectives are easily found as they are organized by topics under the headings of health conditions, health behaviors, populations, settings and systems, and social determinants of health. Refer to health.gov/healthypeople/objectives-and-data/browse-objectives. APRNs can easily locate and interact with detailed data for the objectives by reviewing data that may be available by age group, country of birth, disability status, educational attainment, family income, geographical location, health insurance status, marital status, race/ethnicity, sex, sexual orientation, and veteran status. Trend data may also be available for specific objectives. The *Healthy People 2030* website can be accessed at health.gov/healthypeople.

Community Tool Box

Initiated in 1994, the Community Tool Box is an online resource for people working to improve community health. This free public service was developed by the Center for Community Health and Development at the University of Kansas along with both national and international partners. It includes more than 300 educational modules and numerous free tools to provide guidance for community assessment and other components of community practice, such as planning, intervention, evaluation, and advocacy.

Its resources have been widely used not only in the United States but also in more than 230 countries throughout the world (Center for Community Health and Development, 2022a). The Community Tool Box allows for quick location of specific skills needed by using the table of contents which is organized into 13 focus areas with 46 chapters or by locating one of the 16 toolkits (Center for Community Health and Development, 2022b). One of the focus areas is community assessment. Some examples from chapters in this section include *Assessing Community Needs and Resources* and *Getting Issues on the Public Agenda*. A related toolkit for the community assessment focus is titled *Assessing Community Needs and Resources* (Center for Community Health and Development, 2022c). The Community Tool Box can be accessed at ctb.ku.edu/en.

The American Hospital Association Community Health Improvement Community Health Assessment Toolkit

The ACHI is a national association for healthcare professionals interested in community health, community benefit, and population health. It is affiliated with the American Hospital Association (AHA). ACHI's mission is to advance community health by providing education, resources, professional development, and other opportunities for engagement and growth (AHA Community Health Improvement, 2023). The *Community Health Assessment Toolkit* outlines nine steps (and includes resources) for conducting CHNAs. The primary purpose of the toolkit is to help nonprofit hospitals meet the ACA requirement to conduct a CHNA every 3 years. The nine steps in the framework are meant to be cyclical and include the following: (a) reflect and strategize, (b) identify and engage stakeholders, (c) define the community, (d) collect and analyze data, (e) prioritize community health issues, (f) document and communicate results, (g) plan implementation strategies, (h) implement strategies, and (i) evaluate progress. Each step has a brief purpose and key components that are succinctly outlined and includes resources to help conduct the CHNA (AHA Community Health Improvement, 2017). The Community Health Assessment Toolkit can be accessed at www.healthycommunities.org/resources/community-health-assessment-toolkit.

County Health Rankings and Roadmaps

This online tool is a free resource that provides a large amount of county-level data on important health factors, allowing for easy comparisons with other counties and states. APRNs can quickly find population-based data on education, income, the quality of air and water, smoking, obesity, healthy food access, teen births, and much more. Over 30 data measures organized by length of life, quality of life, health behaviors, clinical care, social and economic factors, and physical environment are presented in a similar format for each county in each state from various national sources (University of Wisconsin Population Health Institute, 2023a).

The County Health Rankings started in 2010 when the University of Wisconsin Population Health Institute collaborated with the Robert Wood Johnson Foundation to release county-level data about health outcomes and associated health indices, such as environmental, economic, and social risk factors. It also provides information on clinical care factors. Each year, these data are updated and released to the public. APRNs can use these data to quickly identify the community needs, problems, strengths, and assets of a county. In addition to locating comprehensive data easily, the roadmaps component of the website provides resources to help understand the county data and suggests evidence-based strategies and resources for action that will lead to healthier change (Remington et al., 2015; University of Wisconsin Population Health Institute, 2023b). County Health Rankings and Roadmaps can be accessed at www.countyhealthrankings.org.

Centers for Disease Control and Prevention Community Health Improvement Navigator

The CDC Community Health Improvement Navigator, known as the CHI Navigator, is a particularly good resource for CHA teams that are comprised of numerous agencies and stakeholders. The underlying assumptions of the CHI Navigator are that it is important to work together with diverse and numerous partners, engage communities in the CHA process, keep lines of communication open, and sustain results. Tools and resources are organized into four key areas: (a) the who, what, and where of improving community health; (b) collaborative approaches to CHI; (c) establishing and maintaining effective collaborations; and (d) finding interventions that are effective (CDC, 2022a). Numerous tools and resources are available that explain the steps for successful CHA efforts. These include assessing needs and resources, focusing on what is important, choosing effective policies and programs;,acting on what is important, and evaluating action (CDC, 2022b). APRNs will discover that this resource provides a "one-stop shop," with expert tools and resources to refer to when leading or participating in CHA and improvement efforts. The CHI Navigator can be accessed at www.cdc.gov/chinav/index.html.

ASSESSMENT METHODS
Focus Groups

CHA teams can use focus groups to obtain valuable contextual data about communities. Through the focus group format, community members can provide input about what they think their community needs. Sometimes specific stakeholders in a community form the focus group, such as members of government agencies, first responders, clergy, or representatives from senior or youth groups. More often, the focus groups are open meetings to which all members of a community are invited. Several community destinations such as faith-based organizations or public libraries provide appropriate settings, and a variety of meeting times optimize the opportunities for community members to participate.

A well-trained and prepared moderator leads the focus group. The moderator should guide the group so that it does not stray from the issues or topics being addressed, and the moderator should ask explicit questions that are specifically worded to elicit public input. Without an experienced moderator, group member focus can vacillate or become lost, and the discussion may become tangential and too diffuse to extract useful information.

An experienced moderator will prompt or cue the members in a way that elicits descriptions of the problem and its root causes, as well as innovative and constructive ideas and creative solutions. Many focus groups are recorded for transcription or later review to avoid missing any thoughts and ideas or nuances from the discussion.

During focus group discussions, it may become apparent that projects under consideration are not important or viewed as a high priority by the community members in the meeting. Subsequently, the focus of the assessment may shift. This should be considered a successful outcome of the focus group and not a negative outcome. It is critically important for community members to prioritize their own assets and needs so they will be more likely to "buy into" agreed-upon projects and assist with long-term sustainability efforts (Center for Community Health and Development, 2022d).

A team working with the Center for Healthy African American Men through Partnerships used focus groups to generate information to guide the development of prevention programs to reduce disparities in education, violence, and premature mortality experienced by African American males (Phillips et al., 2018). Parents of African American male children enrolled in a middle school received a letter of invitation to participate in discussion groups about risk-taking behaviors. Experienced African American moderators facilitated the groups. The following is an example of one script topic: "What are the most important issues affecting the well-being and future success of young people in the African American community?" A total of nine related topics were discussed (Phillips et al., 2018, p. S84).

Those who participated in the focus groups revealed that a lack of social support and male parental presence in homes, anger among their sons, and insufficient licensed counselors to assist their sons in school were major factors impacting the health and success of their children. The parents cited a need for young males to assume more leadership roles. Information elicited from the parents provided insight into the needs of this aggregate group. The study team planned to combine focus group data with key informant interviews of community stakeholders and data from a school-wide youth survey to select and "refine" an evidence-based intervention to support the future academic success and healthy development of young African American males in the community (Phillips et al., 2018). Another study that used focus groups explored what Black and Hispanic inner-city boys thought were the most important community needs because this group's input is often overlooked (Rigg et al., 2019).

Key Informant Interviews

Key informant interviews are useful for obtaining information from people who are well-acquainted with a topic or subject that is being explored by the CHA team. Key informant interviews can provide useful contextual data and insight about community issues, problems, and assets. Key informants are most often selected from people representing different sectors of the community and who have the knowledge and experience to fill in gaps from data collected using other methods. Depending on time and resources, interviews may be conducted face-to-face, via telephone, through email, or in a focus group format. CHA team members are tasked with identifying what information is needed for the CHA and compiling the questions to ask informants. Key informant interviews can be highly to loosely structured depending on the type of information that is being sought. The most common interview format type for eliciting information from key informants is semi-structured where the interviewer does not follow a formalized list of questions but asks open-ended questions to allow more flexibility with the discussion. This is a more common method than a straightforward question-and-answer format because informants can digress and elaborate on answers. An additional bonus of a more loosely structured format is that informants have the freedom to raise issues of concern that CHA team members may not yet have become aware of (Center for Community Health and Development, 2022e).

In 1992, this author participated in a CHA of a rural county in Tennessee. CHA data were derived using several methods, including 48 key informant interviews with people who were well-acquainted with the county. These key informants were recommended by community members. They included beauticians, country store owners, teachers, pastors, and law enforcement personnel. These initial informants led the CHA team members to other people who had additional information and knowledge of the community. A semi-structured interview format was used (Oppewal & Shuman, 1992). Although the CHA was completed many years ago, the action that resulted from that CHA exists today in the form of two school-based health centers that are FQHCs. The Hancock County Elementary School-Based Health Center and the Hancock County Middle/High School Health Center are outpatient clinics that are part of a faculty practice network of nurse-managed health centers operated by East Tennessee State University's College of Nursing (refer to www.etsu.edu/nursing/clinics). APRNs and other professionals provide primary care, mental health services, health education, and urgent care to school students and community members. The need for the school-based health centers was identified through the key informant interviews (Oppewal & Shuman, 1992).

Surveys

Surveys offer another assessment method for generating data for a CHA. Surveys are not always used by CHA teams because they are expensive to carry out, and it can be difficult to find a reliable and valid survey tool related to the topic of interest. When surveys are used in a CHA, they are most often employed to survey either a subgroup of a population or the entire community to reach people who might not otherwise have the opportunity to provide input. For example, part of the Hancock County CHA included the administration of the CDC Youth Risk Behavior Survey (YRBS) to students who attended the one high school in the county. It allowed high school students to have a voice in the CHA. Data from the YRBS provided compelling rationale to develop a school-based health center (Oppewal & Shuman, 2022).

CHA surveys can be conducted using different sampling approaches, from a convenience sample carried out in various locations of the community to one that is randomized and clustered. They can be used to elicit both quantitative and qualitative data related to community concerns, resources, and strengths. Often, numerous methods for distributing surveys are used depending on the resources available to the CHA team and the characteristics of the community. Surveys can be conducted at different community locations like faith-based organizations, grocery stores, or other places where people gather. They may be distributed via email, postal mail, newspaper, QR codes, or social media. They can also be carried out through telephone interviews or by offering assistance to people who may, for one reason or the other, not be able to complete surveys independently. Often, the aim of a survey is to include information from as many community members as possible in the CHA if the group is small to moderate in size. Please refer to more specific information about how to conduct surveys in the Community Tool Box (Center for Community Health and Development, 2022f, 2022g).

Windshield and Walking Surveys and Participant Observation

A *windshield survey* refers to information gleaned from purposeful observations made from a moving vehicle; a *walking survey* has the same purpose, but data are obtained by walking. These collection methods can help CHA teams to obtain an overall feel or impression of a community, and they also aid in the identification of community challenges, problems, assets, and strengths. The APRN can use WWSs to make observations about the physical environment; the amount of green space; the type and condition of available housing, public spaces, and businesses (including both retail stores and commercial developments); and other details that can reveal information about a community (Gibson & Thatcher, 2020). Before implementing a WWS, CHA team members should first identify the purpose of the WWS and then decide on questions that will guide the scope and structure of the WWS. For example, the survey may be guided by a broad question about the nature of a community or by narrower questions such as types and conditions of physical activity options, including sidewalks, parks, and recreational centers (Center for Community Health and Development, 2018h).

One CHA windshield survey that undergraduate students conducted in a small industrial town revealed a large number of taverns. The students discovered that many of the men who patronized them smoked cigarettes. Students learned that it was the usual custom for the men in this community to stop on their way home after work to enjoy some socialization. A review of LHD data also revealed a high incidence of oral cancer in this town. This is an example of how a windshield survey, combined with health-related data, can be used to identify potential areas for intervention in a community. The interventions that ensued included an oral screening clinic and a smoking cessation program that targeted the tavern patrons.

Participant observation is a research method used to obtain purposeful observations indirectly (or passively) or more directly by participating in community activities. CHAs may include participant observation as a data collection method when there is a need for direct observation or participation in community activities. A CHA team might decide to use participant observation to better understand information gleaned from surveys, key informant interviews, or focus groups. For example, the APRN may use participant observation to purposely observe a town hall meeting after key informants describe the meetings as tense and contentious. Observations can help CHA team members better understand community conflict or to follow up on information obtained from focus group discussions or key informant interviews.

Secondary Data Analysis and Literature Reviews

Secondary data sources and literature reviews are often used for CHAs because they are relatively inexpensive, efficient, and easy to use. *Secondary data* are data that are collected by someone other than the user. Common sources of secondary data used for CHAs include censuses, information collected by government departments (such as the CDC), and organizational records (e.g., from churches, schools, or local government records). Such data can be used to describe demographic and socioeconomic characteristics of communities, as well as the health of a community. A general recommendation is for CHA teams to determine local assets and needs by using data and indicators at the smallest geographical level for counties such as census blocks or zip codes (CDC, 2022c). Analyses of existing data from various sources or from literature located for the purpose of better understanding a community or its problems should be done systematically. The five assessment tools highlighted in this chapter have many online resources to help CHA team members find relevant and meaningful community health data and indicators. Other sources of community-level indicators and benchmarking information are briefly highlighted in Table 11.1.

U.S. Census Data

The U.S. Census Bureau's mission is to provide Americans with quality data about its people, places, and economy. The decennial census is probably most familiar to Americans, but other censuses and surveys are completed to compile vast datasets. As required by the U.S. Constitution, the U.S. Census Bureau conducts a census of the entire population every 10 years. While basic data are collected on everyone, a selected sample of the population is surveyed in greater detail using the "long form." Those data provide a plethora of community characteristics (e.g., age, sex, race, education, employment, income, housing) to better describe the makeup of communities. The information gathered is compiled and analyzed and reported to the nation. It is used by the government to make planning decisions, including the allocation of funds to government agencies (U.S. Census Bureau, 2017). It should be noted that despite the efforts of census workers to be as inclusive as possible, low-income and migratory populations are often underrepresented in the data. Census data as a source of information are invaluable as a rich source of information with numerous details that will help identify important community characteristics related to social, economic, educational, housing, and demographic characteristics, among many other measures. Census information is available at www.census.gov and the website data.census.gov allows one to easily locate a wealth of community information.

Health Department Vital Statistics and Disease and Health Reports

Vital statistics are an excellent source of information about a community and are easily obtainable. Although considered "dry" by many community assessors, data on births, deaths, marriages, and divorces are vital statistics within a community and are collected

TABLE 11.1 Sources of Community-Level Indicators

SOURCE OF COMMUNITY-LEVEL INDICATORS	BRIEF DESCRIPTION	WEBSITE
BRFSS	Telephone survey to collect state data about U.S. community member health conditions, risk factors, and preventive serves	www.cdc.gov/brfss
CDC Wonder	Online databases to analyze public health data	wonder.cdc.gov
CMS Data Clearinghouse	Search tool of data and information resources of CMS programs health topics, settings of care	www.cms.gov/Research-Statistics-Data-and-Systems/Research-Statistics-Data-and-Systems
Community Commons	Data, tools, and stories for promoting community change	www.communitycommons.org
County Health Rankings and Roadmaps	County-level data related to health; evidence, guidance, and examples to improve health equity	www.countyhealthrankings.org
Dartmouth Atlas of Health Care	Data on distribution of medical resources using Medicare and Medicaid data	www.dartmouthatlas.org
DHDS	State-level adult disability-specific data	www.cdc.gov/ncbddd/disabilityandhealth/dhds/index.html
HealthData.gov	Searchable datasets of government data on a wide range of topics	healthdata.gov
HRSA Warehouse	Data and maps on HRSA's Health Care Programs	data.hrsa.gov
KIDS COUNT (Annie E. Casey Foundation)	Data, policies, and tools to help children	www.aecf.org/work/kids-count
National Center for Health Statistics	Statistical information to guide actions and policies to improve health	www.cdc.gov/nchs/index.htm
National Environmental Public Health Tracking Network	Environmental and health data from city, state, and national sources	ephtracking.cdc.gov
PLACES: Local Data for Better Health (CDC)	Health data on small areas across the country	www.cdc.gov/places/index.html
PRAMS	State-specific, population-based data on maternal attitudes and experiences before, during, and shortly after pregnancy	www.cdc.gov/prams/index.htm
U.S. Census Bureau	Population, housing, economic, and geographical information	www.census.gov
U.S. Food Environment Atlas	Food environment indicators that influence food choices and diet quality	ers.usda.gov/foodatlas

BRFSS, Behavioral Risk Factor Surveillance System; CDC, Centers for Disease Control and Prevention; CMS, Centers for Medicare and Medicaid Services; DHDS, Disability and Health Data System; HRSA, Health Resources and Services Administration; PRAMS, Pregnancy Risk Assessment and Monitoring System.

Source: From Centers for Disease Control and Prevention. (2022). *Public health professionals gateway. Data and benchmarks.* www.cdc.gov/stltpublichealth/cha/data.html

on an ongoing basis. There is also a wide spectrum of quantitative information on populations available on the Internet. Information from health departments, in combination with information gleaned from other sources such as surveys or focus groups, can help provide valuable data to consider for improving the health of communities.

The CDC publishes data in the *Morbidity and Mortality Weekly Report* (see www.cdc.gov/mmwr/index.html) that are not often available elsewhere; these reports are valuable sources of health information for APRNs. Morbidity and mortality data are also available from other U.S. Department of Health and Human Services (DHHS) and CDC websites. Information on notifiable diseases, adverse drug reactions, injuries, occupational health, and birth defects are some examples of the wide range of information that is available from these two government agencies.

Another useful resource is the public-use data files available through the CDC's National Center for Health Statistics (NCHS). Public-use data files include downloadable datasets and questionnaires that are organized as population surveys (the National Health and Nutrition Examination Survey, National Health Interview Survey, National Survey of Family Growth); vital records (National Vital Statistics System, National Death Index, Vital Statistics Rapid Release); provider surveys related to healthcare, ambulatory medical care, electronic health records, hospital care, and post-acute and long-term care studies; and historical surveys or surveys that have been completed (NCHS, 2023). The NCHS website can be accessed at www.cdc.gov/nchs/index.htm.

BUILDING RELATIONSHIPS

COLLABORATION/COMMUNITY PARTNERSHIP

A community is comprised of many people, and the APRN needs to have a comprehensive understanding of those people in order to build a trusting relationship. Understanding a community's culture is essential to program success. The APRN should expect this process to take time, patience, commitment, and persistence. Moreover, understanding the makeup of a community and its cultural norms, as well as being sensitive and respectful of differences, is essential for successful collaboration and community partnership.

Community involvement is the foundation of a successful CHA. The members of the community, including the people, the government, the health department, the churches, nonprofits and helping agencies, and the local businesses, to name a few, all need to be involved. Who are the leaders in the community? APRNs can identify the people who are respected and trusted and who encourage other community members to participate in activities. This is not always a political leader but can be a church member, a parent, a community advocate, or someone else. Many communities do not have an inherent trust in "outsiders" who come into their community. There may be a history in the county of well-intentioned CHA teams providing assessments and starting needed programs only to leave without providing community members with the tools (financial or otherwise) to sustain programs after they are gone. The APRN will have the most success with planning, conducting, and evaluating a CHA by working with and being guided by trusted members of the community rather than doing these activities without active community partnership.

It is also imperative that communities are not viewed as having a "problem" that needs to be fixed. Communities want to feel they are productive and cohesive and do not want someone to tell them how to fix their problems. They want partnership and understanding of who they are and what they stand for. When working on a CHA, it is essential to identify both the community's assets and weaknesses. By identifying the assets (or strengths), the APRN can elicit more trust from community members because they do not want to be defined only by their problems. This mutual understanding can build trust and cooperation. It requires listening by both parties involved; education and learning should be bidirectional. Program leaders such as the APRN should provide the community and its members with the tools to sustain programs on their own. A sense of independence and self-sufficiency is important for long-term success. This is the ultimate form of partnership—one that is built upon mutual trust, cooperation, effective communication, and authentic relationships.

CASE STUDY

The concept of community collaboration can be illustrated by discussing a CHA in Lee County, North Carolina. Lee County is a rural county located in the center of the state. It is one of the smallest counties in North Carolina, encompassing just over 255 square miles. It is comprised of eight townships and its population increased steadily to 64,138 as of July 1, 2021 (U.S. Census Bureau, 2022). The population is approximately 57% White, 20% African American, and 21% Hispanic or Latinx; 8.6% of the population was born outside of the United States. The percent of people living in poverty is 15.1% and the median household income is $57,674. About 86% of the county residents have a high school diploma and 21% have earned a bachelor's degree or higher (U.S. Census Bureau, 2022).

Lee County Public Health Department (LCPH) leads the county in a state-required CHA every 4 years using a variety of data collection methods. One of its first tasks was to form a CHA team charged with evaluating the health status of the county, identify and prioritize health concerns that could pose threats to community members, and develop strategies for the priority community health issues (LCPH & Lee County Community Action Network [LeeCAN], 2019). CHA team members were Health Department employees and members of the Healthy Carolinians Partnership in Lee County, known as the Community Action Network (LeeCAN). LeeCAN is a partnership with representation from government agencies, the local hospital, health and social service agencies, schools and Lee County Partnership for Children, senior services, the cooperative extension agency, the sheriff's office and police department, United Way, the YMCA, Parks and Recreation, and members from the faith-based communities. The mission of the LeeCAN is to use collaborative community effort to improve awareness of and resources to effectively deal with health and safety issues in the county (Lee County, North Carolina Government, 2022). One of the many strengths of Lee County is due to its rural nature. People know each other and work well with each other. The CHA process was led by the Lee County Health Department in partnership with LeeCAN

(continued)

partners, Central Carolina Hospital, Sanford Housing Authority, El Refugio, Cooperative Extension, and the Lee County Enrichment Center (LCPH & LeeCAN, 2019).

Mary Hawley Oates, the school nurse supervisor of Lee County Schools and a Lee County Board of Health member, provided insight into the collaborative efforts of the CHA (M. Oates, personal communication, January 27, 2023). The CHA team decided to use a survey to optimize community member participation. Members of the CHA team looked for an appropriate instrument for collecting information that would measure variables of interest consistently, dependably, and accurately. They selected a survey that had been originally used in three other rural North Carolina counties and that was previously validated for use as a health-focused data collection tool. The survey was made available in both paper copy, distributed in public locations like the library, clinics, churches, and the local food bank, and electronically, via social media sites and on a publicized website. It was distributed and made available in the local newspaper, through "open house" and "community forum" events, local churches, volunteer fire departments, and local businesses. A total of 225 surveys were collected and analyzed (LCPH & LeeCAN, 2019).

After analyzing the initial Community Health Opinion survey data, the CHA team noted that two areas in Lee County had a poor rate of survey returns. One location was in the incorporated town of Broadway, which has just over 1,000 residents. The second location, Lemon Springs, is a small community outside of these two areas; however, it is not incorporated into a town. Very few surveys (fewer than 10) were received from Broadway and Lemon Springs. The team thought that literacy or language barriers, distrust of government agencies, and general complacency were potential factors associated with the poor survey response rate.

Given the concern with the low input from community members in Broadway and Lemon Springs, the assessment team decided to conduct focus groups in each of the areas. Topics were preselected from the previous surveys, and a moderator familiar with the CHA process but not actively involved in the earlier data collection efforts was chosen. The meetings were held on a weekday in a central location during midday. Food and door prizes were incentives to attend; a record of attendees was not kept so that anonymity could be maintained.

The focus groups unearthed valuable information. Common themes were affordability of health insurance, lack of specialty care in Lee County, and the need to educate residents about public health services. Specific concerns included drugs and the subsequent negative impact on their communities. In addition, more activities or community facilities were requested to cater to older adults and children. In general, the focus group participants felt that their community was a good place to live and to raise a family. Participants stated that they wanted to know how to teach children about avoiding drug use and to provide parents who have problems in this area with help. They also commented about the need for the unemployed to have access to training that matched available employment in the area. Additionally, transportation was noted as "always an issue." More public transportation to access healthcare services in the community was identified as one of their priority needs.

(continued)

In addition to holding focus groups that targeted the community at large, focus groups were held to target low-income residents, older adults, Hispanic community members, and health professionals (LCPH & LeeCAN, 2019). The qualitative data collected from the focus groups provided rich information that confirmed and built on results from the previously completed surveys. Data obtained from surveys and focus groups were used to develop action plans to target the issues identified by community members. The CHA survey and the focus groups were helpful in revealing residents' perceptions about health and quality-of-life issues in Lee County.

The CHA team used secondary data analysis to validate findings from the surveys and to fill in gaps in information. According to the CHA report, the key sources of secondary data were the following (LCPH & LeeCAN, 2019, p. 11):

- North Carolina State Center for Health Statistics, including:
  - Health Stats for North Carolina
  - County Health Data Books
  - Behavioral Risk Factor Surveillance System (BRFSS)
  - Vital statistics
  - Cancer register
- U.S. Census
- NC Department of Medical Assistance
- UNC Cecil G. Sheps Center for Health Services

After analyzing the primary data collected from community members and secondary data, data were synthesized by key areas related to tobacco use, substance abuse, obesity, and teen pregnancy/STDs. CHA team members met with LeeCAN and Lee County Health Department members in August 2019 to review the assessment's results. They agreed that the health priorities for the next four years were tobacco use/substance abuse, obesity/overweight, and teen pregnancy (LCPH & LeeCAN, 2019). The 2022 CHA's data collection started in the spring of 2022 with a community opinion survey, and results from the CHA will be available in 2023 (Lee County, North Carolina Government, 2022).

The CHA team included numerous community partners and leaders. It engaged community members by providing a wide range of opportunities for community participation. The information garnered from the CHA helped community agencies in formulating program goals and objectives. Data obtained during the CHA process also supplied necessary information for grant proposals and documentation for the need for resources and funding for priority county issues. An additional benefit was the dissemination of a supportive services inventory that was created as Appendix B in the CHA report (LCPH & LeeCAN, 2019).

SUMMARY

The CHA process extends beyond collecting community data; it includes establishing trust and rapport with community partners and involving community members actively throughout the entire assessment process. Community programs are most successful when diverse community members from different sectors of the community participate in the planning, implementation, and evaluation of programs that address local health concerns. Building meaningful, trusting relationships, and engaging communities through collaboration is a rewarding experience for the APRN. The CHA must be totally inclusive and reflect the collaboration necessary to create an accurate and comprehensive depiction of the community. It is also a dynamic process and should incorporate multiple methods to assess and address a community's needs.

The CHA should be readdressed at regular intervals to identify changing needs. With the information obtained through a well-designed CHA, the APRN has the data needed to develop evidence-based projects that meet the needs of the community. Working with community leaders is critical for success, especially in engaging community members in the process. Only then can community programs be developed and integrated into a successful healthcare plan that will be acceptable and sustainable within the community. These strategies are not always easy, but they allow community members to become empowered and creative in their own approach to improving their community.

Building relationships and engaging communities through collaboration requires time, persistence, and patience. It does not happen quickly but is a process that builds over time and may involve years. The information collected in a CHA is used to spark action that will result in healthy policies, innovative and sustainable programs, and health promotion initiatives with active community involvement.

END-OF-CHAPTER RESOURCES

EXERCISES AND DISCUSSION QUESTIONS

EXERCISE 11.1 APRNs should recognize the value of collaboration and make it a regular part of their practice regardless of whether they will lead a CHA process or participate as a team member in a CHA.

   a. Describe ways that you anticipate using collaboration as an APRN or ways that you currently engage in collaboration in your practice.
   b. Consider how diverse your stakeholders and collaborators are. What additional partners might you collaborate with? How well do your partners reflect insight on the social determinants of health that impact your community members?
   c. What are potential barriers to collaboration?
   d. What are potential facilitators of collaboration?

EXERCISE 11.2 The APRN who practices in a primary care center is asked to participate on the CHA team. Choose a county for your practice and find the U.S. Census Data for it and then the County Health Rankings for that county to quickly obtain general information about the county. When reviewing this information, compare the county level data with state and national data. Next, find the most recent county CHA to learn more about how the CHA was previously conducted. Search the Internet using the title of your county and *Community Health Assessment*. Answer the following questions:

   a. What information can be found from the U.S. Census Bureau to help the team understand the demographic makeup of the county?
   b. What information does County Health Rankings provide related to health outcomes and the social determinants of health for your county? Refer to www.countyhealthrankings.org.
   c. What county assets or strengths were identified from the last CHA report?
   d. What were the significant priority areas identified by the analysis of findings in the Tyrrell County CHA report?

EXERCISE 11.3 A CHA team sets the goal of increasing a community survey response rate by 15% in an upcoming CHA.

   a. What strategies might be considered for reaching more respondents and achieving the survey response rate goal?

b. CHA team members used educational data as a proxy for literacy when reviewing the survey for appropriate reading level. According to the 2019 census data, 55% of county residents have a high school education, 42% have a bachelor's degree, and 8% have a graduate degree. How can health literacy be considered when selecting or adapting the survey?

c. How might CHA planning members identify additional distribution sites for the community survey?

> A robust set of instructor resources designed to supplement this text is located at http://connect.springerpub.com/content/book/978-0-8261-4377-8. Qualifying instructors may request access by emailing textbook@springerpub.com.

REFERENCES

AHA Community Health Improvement. (2017). *Community health assessment toolkit*. https://www.healthycommunities.org/resources/community-health-assessment-toolkit

AHA Community Health Improvement. (2023). *About ACHI*. https://www.healthycommunities.org/about-ACHI

American Association of Colleges of Nursing. (2006). *The essentials of doctoral education for advanced nursing practice*. Author. http://www.aacnnursing.org/Portals/42/Publications/DNPEssentials.pdf

American Association of Colleges of Nursing. (2021). *The Essentials: Core competencies for professional nursing education*. https://www.aacnnursing.org/Essentials

American Association of Nurse Anesthesiology. (2016). *Professional attributes of the nurse anesthetist: Practice considerations*. https://www.aana.com

American College of Nurse-Midwives. (2020). *Core competencies for basic midwifery practice*. https://www.midwife.org/ACNM-Documents

American College of Nurse-Midwives. (2021). *Competencies for doctoral education in midwifery*. http://www.midwife.org/default.aspx?bid=59&cat=2&button=Search&rec=49

Anderson, E. T., & McFarlane, J. (2019). *Community as partner: Theory and practice in nursing* (8th ed.). Wolters Kluwer Health.

Buhler-Wilkerson, K. (1993). Bringing care to the people: Lillian Wald's legacy to public health nursing. *American Journal of Nursing, 83*(12), 1778–1776. https://doi.org/10.2105/ajph.83.12.1778

Burns, J. C., Teadt, S., Bradley, W. W., & Shade, G. H. (2020). Enhancing adolescent and young adult health services! A review of the community needs assessment process in an urban federally qualified health center. *Health Equity, 4*(1), 218–224. https://doi.org/10.1089/heq.2019.0108

Carlton, E. L., & Singh, S. R. (2018). Joint community health needs assessments as a path for coordinating community-wide health improvement efforts between hospitals and local health departments. *American Journal of Public Health, 108*(5), 676–682. https://doi.org/10.2105/AJPH.2018.304339

CDC Community Health Improvement Navigator. (2022, October 18). *Making the case for collaborative CHI*. Centers for Disease Control and Prevention. https://www.cdc.gov/chinav/case/index.html

Center for Community Health and Development. (2018h). *Chapter 3, Section 21: Windshield and walking surveys*. Community Tool Box. https://ctb.ku.edu/en/table-of-contents/assessment/assessing-community-needs-and-resources/windshield-walking-surveys/main

Center for Community Health and Development. (2022a). *About the Tool Box*. Community Tool Box. https://ctb.ku.edu/en/about-the-tool-box

Center for Community Health and Development. (2022b). *Table of Contents*. Community Tool Box. https://ctb.ku.edu/en/table-of-contents

Center for Community Health and Development. (2022c). *[Toolkit 2] Assessing community needs and resources*. Community Tool Box. https://ctb.ku.edu/en/assessing-community-needs-and-resources

Center for Community Health and Development. (2022d). *Chapter 3, Section 6: Conducting focus groups*. Community Tool Box. https://ctb.ku.edu/en/table-of-contents/assessment/assessing-community-needs-and-resources/conduct-focus-groups/main

Center for Community Health and Development. (2022e). *Chapter 3, Section 12: Conducting interviews.* Community Tool Box. https://ctb.ku.edu/en/table-of-contents/assessment/assessing-community-needs-and-resources/conduct-interviews/main

Center for Community Health and Development. (2022f). *Chapter 3, Section 7: Conducting needs assessment surveys.* Community Tool Box. https://ctb.ku.edu/en/table-of-contents/assessment/assessing-community-needs-and-resources/conducting-needs-assessment-surveys/main

Center for Community Health and Development. (2022g). *Chapter 3, Section 13: Conducting surveys.* Community ToolBox. https://ctb.ku.edu/en/table-of-contents/assessment/assessing-community-needs-and-resources/conduct-surveys/main

Centers for Disease Control and Prevention. (2022a). *CDC community health improvement navigator.* Retrieved from https://www.cdc.gov/chinav/index.html

Centers for Disease Control and Prevention (2022b). *Tools for successful CHI efforts.* CDC Community Health Improvement Navigator. https://www.cdc.gov/chinav/tools/index.html

Centers for Disease Control and Prevention. (2022c). *Public health professionals gateway. Data and benchmarks.* https://www.cdc.gov/publichealthgateway/cha/data.html

Centers for Medicare & Medicaid Services. (2018). *Federally qualified health center. Medicare Learning Network (MLN) booklet.* Centers for Medicare & Medicaid Services. https://www.cms.gov/Outreach-and-Education/Medicare-Learning-Network-MLN/MLNProducts/Downloads/fqhcfactsheet.pdf

Fitzpatrick, J. (2016). Community-based participatory research: Challenges and opportunities. *Applied Nursing Research, 31*, 187. https://doi.org/doi:10.1016/j.apnr.2016.06.005

Fromknecht, C. Q., Hallman, V. A., & Heffernan, M. (2021). Developing state health improvement plans: Exploring states' use of Healthy People. *Journal of Public Health Management and Practice, 27* (Suppl. 6), S274–S279. https://doi.org/10.1097/PHH.0000000000001421

Gibson, M. E., & Thatcher, E. J. (2020). Community as client: Assessment and analysis. In M. Stanhope & J. Lancaster (Eds.), *Public health nursing: Population-centered health care in the community* (10th ed.). Elsevier.

Giroir, B. P. (2021). Healthy People 2030: A call to action to lead America to healthier lives. *Journal of Public Health Management and Practice, 27*(Suppl. 6), S222–S224. https://doi.org/10.1097/PHH.0000000000001266

Hasbrouck, L. (2021). Healthy People 2030: An improved framework. *Health Education & Behavior, 48*(2), 113–114. https://doi.org/10.1177/1090198121997812

Health Resources Services Administration. (2018, August). *Health center program compliance manual.* Bureau of Primary Health Care. https://bphc.hrsa.gov/compliance/compliance-manual

Institute for Healthcare Improvement. (2019). *Improving health equity: Partner with the community. Guidance for health care organizations.* Institute for Healthcare Improvement. Available at www.IHI.org

Internal Revenue Service. (2022, July 15.). *Community health needs assessment for charitable hospital organizations – Section 501(r)(3).* https://www.irs.gov/charities-non-profits/community-health-needs-assessment-for-charitable-hospital-organizations-section-501r3

Kaiser Family Foundation. (2013, April 25). *Summary of the Affordable Care Act.* Heath Reform. https://www.kff.org/health-reform/fact-sheet/summary-of-the-affordable-care-act

Lee County, North Carolina Government. (2022). *Community Action Network (LeeCAN).* https://www.leecountync.gov/departments/public_health/community_action_network_leecan.php

Lee County Public Health & Lee Community Action Network. (2019). *Lee County Community Health Assessment 2018.* https://leecountync.gov/departments/public_health/community_action_network_leecan.php

Live Well Wake. (2022). *Wake County community health needs assessment: April 2022.* https://livewellwake.org/wp-content/uploads/2022/09/LWW_CHNA-2022-FINAL.pdf

Miller, K., Berwood, Y., Abbott, C., Buckland, S. T., Dlugi, E., Adams, Z., Rajagopalan, V., Schulman, M., Hilfrank, K., & Cohen, M. A. (2019). Health needs assessment of five Pennsylvania Plain populations. *International Journal of Environmental Research and Public Health, 16*(13), 2378. https://doi.org/10.3390/ijerph16132378

Money, E. B., Williams, J., Zelek, M., & Amobi, A. (2020). Engaging the power of communities for better health. *North Carolina Medical Journal, 81*(3), 195–197. https://doi.org/10.18043/ncm.81.3.195

National Center for Health Statistics. (2023, January 31). Centers for Disease Control and Prevention. https://www.cdc.gov/nchs/index.htm

National Organization of Nurse Practitioner Faculties (NONPF). (2022). *National Organization of Nurse Practitioner Faculties' nurse practitioner role core competencies*. www.nonpf.org/page/NP_Role_Core_Competencies

Nelson, R. (2019). Ernest Grant breaks barriers. *American Journal of Nursing, 119*(1), 65–66. https://doi.org/10.1097/01.NAJ.0000552617.90814.d5

Ochiai, E., Kigenyi, T., Sondik, E., Pronk, N., Kleinman, D. V., Blakey, C., Fromknecht, C. Q., Heffernan, M., & Brewer, K. H. (2021). Healthy People 2030 leading health indicators and overall health and well-being measures: Opportunities to assess and improve the health and well-being of the nation. *Journal of Public Health Management and Practice, 27*(Suppl. 6), S235–S241. https://doi.org/10.1097/PHH.0000000000001424

Office of Disease Prevention and Health Promotion. (n.d.a). Tools for action. In *Healthy People 2030*. U.S. Department of Health and Human Services. https://health.gov/healthypeople/tools-action

Office of Disease Prevention and Health Promotion. (n.d.b). Use Healthy People 2030 in your work. In *Healthy People 2030*. U.S. Department of Health and Human Services. https://health.gov/healthypeople/tools-action/use-healthy-people-2030-your-work

Oppewal, S., & Shuman, P. (1992). *Community needs assessment of Hancock County*. Report prepared for the First Tennessee Community Health Agency, East Tennessee State University, School of Nursing, Department of Family/Community Nursing, Tennessee.

Phillips, J. M., Branch, C. J., Brady, S. S., & Simpson, T. (2018). Parents speak: A needs assessment for community programming for Black male youth. *American Journal of Preventive Medicine, 55*(5), S82–S87. https://doi.org/10.1016/j.amepre.2018.05.014

Pohl, J. M., Savrin, C., Fiandt, K., Beauchesne, M., Drayton-Brooks, S., Scheibmeir, M., Brackley, M., & Werner, K. E. (2009). Quality and safety in graduate nursing education: Cross-mapping QSEN graduate competencies with NONPF's NP core and practice doctorate competencies. *Nursing Outlook, 57*(6), 349–354. https://doi.org/10.1016/j.outlook.2009.08.002

Remington, P. L., Catlin, B. B., & Gennuso, K. P. (2015). The county health rankings: Rationale and methods. *Population Health Metrics, 13*, 11. https://doi.org/10.1186/s12963-015-0044-2

Rigg, K. K., McNeish, R., Schadrac, D., Gonzalez, A., & Tran, Q. (2019). Community needs of minority male youth living in inner-city Chicago. *Children and Youth Services Review, 98*, 284–289. https://doi.org/10.1016/j.childyouth.2019.01.011

Rozier, M. D. (2020). Nonprofit hospital community benefit in the U.S.: A scoping review from 2010 to 2019. *Frontiers of Public Health, 8*(Article 72). https://doi.org/10.3389/fpubh.2020.00072

Ryan-Ibarra, S., Pearlman, D., Grinnell, S., Hanni, K., Islas, G., & Teutsch, S. (2018). Core metrics pilot study: A case study. *Journal of Public Health Management and Practice, 24*(6), 578–585. https://doi.org/10.1097/PHH.0000000000000715

Saunders, M. M. (2022). The implications of the new *Essentials* on the CNS profession—Let's respond! *Clinical Nurse Specialist, The Journal for Advanced Nursing Practice, 36*(3), 129–130. https://doi.org/10.1097/NUR.0000000000000668

University of Wisconsin Population Health Institute. (2023a). *About us*. County Health Rankings & Roadmaps. https://www.countyhealthrankings.org/about-us

University of Wisconsin Population Health Institute. (2023b). *2022 measures*. County Health Rankings & Roadmaps. https://www.countyhealthrankings.org/explore-health-rankings/county-health-rankings-measures

U.S. Census Bureau. (2017). *U.S. Census Bureau at a glance*. https://www.census.gov/about/what/census-at-a-glance.html#censuses

U.S. Census Bureau. (2022). *QuickFacts: Lee County, NC*. Retrieved from https://www.census.gov/quickfacts/fact/table/leecountynorthcarolina,US/PST045221

WNC Health Network. (2023a). *Who we are*. https://www.wnchn.org/who-we-are/#mission

WNC Health Network. (2023b). *WNC Healthy Impact*. https://www.wnchn.org/wnc-healthy-impact/

CHAPTER 12

CHALLENGES IN PROGRAM IMPLEMENTATION

BARBARA A. NIEDZ

INTRODUCTION

The role of the nurse includes compassionate and quality care not only for the individual but also for the family and the community. Advanced practice registered nurses (APRNs) seek to improve the circumstances that contribute to poor population health. APRNs work in various roles and venues to improve population health, whether as a primary care provider, in a hospital, a community setting, health plan, or healthcare system. Improving population health requires change, evidence-based interventions, innovation, and astute implementation. In Chapter 9, "Evaluation of Practice at the Population Level," we discuss the role that planning, improvement, and control play in enhancing patients' experiences and outcomes. Those successes in segmented areas are well-documented. This chapter builds on Chapter 9, "Evaluation of Practice at the Population Level," and explores the potential for expanding those improvements as innovations and disseminating them broadly across many more patients, in communities, healthcare systems, and health plans; in short, larger and larger populations. The overall goal is to improve public health.

People want a better life. They want to be healthier, and they want to live longer, happier, and more productive lives. One challenge lies in changing the behaviors and attitudes of individuals. More importantly, changing healthcare systems in communities to improve the public health from a population health perspective is of primary concern and not easily accomplished by individual practitioners. Making healthcare more accessible, cost-effective, and safe for patients requires a specific skill set and tools and above all else, a multidisciplinary approach. For many, change is uncomfortable or difficult, but it is a necessary process to implement innovation broadly to create and spread improvement. The focus of this chapter falls in three of the domain essentials that frame nursing professional education: *population health, interprofessional partnerships, and a systems-based practice* (American Association of Colleges of Nursing [AACN], 2021).

IMPLEMENTATION SCIENCE

Healthcare organizations (whether large or small) and APRNs struggle with making a good idea real and spreading it throughout so that it effectively and measurably results in improvement across an entire practice, organization, or system. Oftentimes, the best ideas, even when supported by sound research, lay fallow and do not have the desired effects or outcomes for the practice, organization, healthcare system, or community. Though techniques may work effectively for one patient, spreading those interventions more globally can be challenging. An evidence-based approach is only as good as the outcomes it produces. This struggle is apparent in failed implementations of countless innovations that may have worked elsewhere but not in *this* organization. Maybe it worked on one nursing unit but just did not catch on in others. Is the fault in the innovation itself or in the implementation of it on a greater scale?

Implementation science provides a scientific approach using methods that enhance the uptake of research evidence in practice, closing the research to practice gap in healthcare, and ultimately improving health in communities (Bauer et al., 2015). Bauer and Kirchner (2020) explain that evidence-based clinical practice guidelines exist in abundance with sound high-quality research supporting them. However, many remain unimplemented (NIH National Cancer Institute, 2022).

In nursing, research abounds. However, expanding the practice implications may be stymied at the organizational level. A staff member in a major medical center successfully implements an evidence-based practice change, an innovation, on one nursing unit, but the change fails when an implementation attempt is made to expand the innovation to other units. Why? What accounts for this deficit? Similarly, two like-minded APRNs working in a primary care practice with a large type 2 Medicaid and Medicare diabetic patient population have great success over 1 year in improving Healthcare Effectiveness Data and Information Set (HEDIS) comprehensive diabetes care (CDC) rates for over 100 patients using an evidence-based practice guideline promulgated by the ADA (American Diabetes Association [ADA] Professionals, 2023). A year after this success, the two APRNs have achieved even greater success with their cadre of patients. However, none of the other six APRNs in the practice was able to make the same improvements in CDC, though the practice is similar in the number of diabetic patients and the need for improvement. Thus, the HEDIS scores for the practice remain low. What accounts for this failure? In both of these scenarios, tools to achieve practice change were not used and dissemination of the innovation was not replicated.

The purpose of this chapter is to present theoretical frameworks that can drive change and result in a more global expansion of evidence-based interventions that are known to improve outcomes. Accompanying these models, examples of success, as well as barriers, are included. Most importantly, the chapter includes tools which have been shown to be successful in achieving the kind of change that is needed for population health today.

LEWIN'S STAGES OF CHANGE

Lewin's Change Model is derived from the social sciences and provides a brief but profound approach to understanding how change occurs (Lewin, 1951). Change at the aggregate level whether it is needed on a small scale, for example, in a private practice, or on a larger scale, like an entire community, requires a planned and deliberate approach. Lewin (1951) explains that there are driving forces that move toward the desired state and, in counterpoint, restraining forces that push back against the change in favor of the status quo. In nursing, the model has often provided a framework for change (Hussain et al., 2018). Furthermore, Lewin's model is characterized by three distinct phases: *unfreezing, changing,* and *refreezing.* The model is linear and may not address all the complexities inherent in achieving a particular desired state as change scenarios, especially in nursing and healthcare, are often complex (Box 12.1).

In the role of a change agent, the APRN begins by destabilizing the group or community by asking questions to generate hope and visions of something different, something possibly better. Perhaps the group or community is already experiencing a desire for something different. In private practice, this can be a practicing APRN who sees scores

BOX 12.1

LEWIN'S CHANGE MODEL EXAMPLE

Driving Forces

- APRNs in private practice with six other providers identify low HEDIS CDC scores as an opportunity for improvement.
- These two APRNs drive a pilot within the practice and improve HEDIS CDC for a cadre of 100 patients over a 6-month period initially, which was sustained over a year.
- They shared the "toolkit", clinical practice guideline, and revised workflow process with the remaining providers to encourage participation in the new model.
- Improved scores can result in financial rewards through the MIPS program.
- Despite the pilot, overall practice HEDIS CDC is still below the 30th percentile and not eligible for financial rewards.

Desired State

- Achieve the 80% percentile for HEDIS CDC for the entire practice within the next calendar year in order to achieve financial gain and improve patient care

Restraining Forces

- The toolkit and clinical practice guideline require some IT savvy while the office depends on manual documentation.
- Two out of the four remaining providers are set to retire in 6 months and are not invested.
- Four out of the four remaining providers are intrigued by the pilot results but are wary of change.

on key metrics for the practice (through HEDIS or Merit-Based Incentive Payment System (MIPS); see Chapter 8, "Concepts in Program Design and Development") below par and not competitive. In a medical center, this could be observed at the practice council. For example, only two medical-surgical nursing units are hitting the benchmark comparisons for Hospital Consumer Assessment of Healthcare Providers and Systems (HCAHPS), while six other similar medical-surgical nursing units are not. On an even greater scale, one hospital in a healthcare system hits all the competitive outcomes for a primary stroke center, while three other similar hospitals in the same system do not. Disequilibrium in the current moment underscores the relevance and potential of change and of moving out of the current comfort zone.

UNFREEZING

The first stage of change is *unfreezing* and may arise from an assessment or it may be activated by the APRN through motivation, health education, advocacy, or other strategies (Hilton & Anderson, 2018; Institute for Healthcare Improvement, 2023). In the unfreezing phase, gathering information from stakeholder groups is vital to better understand how the change initiative will be perceived and the extent to which unfreezing attitudes, behaviors, and habits from key participants is needed to achieve the desired state. The current state of the culture is preeminent, and various tools are available to gain insight. A strengths, weaknesses, opportunities, and threats (SWOT) review can be insightful (MindTools, 2022). A stakeholder analysis is also useful in the unfreezing phase and tools are readily available (White et al., 2021). Resistance to change may be preeminent in this phase, particularly if attitudes are strong. For example, when electronic health records (EHRs) were first introduced in hospitals, resistance was modest; but when providers' practice was affected with mandated physician order entry, the IT change strategy needed to address providers' objections in a comprehensive and thorough way in order to achieve success. Focus groups or a qualitative approach (see Chapter 11, "Building Relationships and Engaging Communities Through Collaboration") can also further this goal and provide insight to potential barriers (Williamson et al., 2021).

CHANGING, MOVING, OR TRANSITION

The second stage in Lewin's model reflects an understanding that change is not a timed event but an ongoing process that can be facilitated by APRN actions. This stage is known variously as *changing, moving,* or *transition* (Hussain et al., 2018; Lewin, 1951). Change begins with individuals and builds to groups transitioning to new attitudes and behaviors as they acquire new skills and perspectives.

The combination of destabilizing the present state and the challenge of questioning the status quo can make the second stage the most difficult of Lewin's three phases. The support role of the APRN is very important, as the nurse must accept attempts at change against the risk of early failures. One approach is to design a pilot, start small, and achieve success. For example, when the practice reviews outcomes data at a staff meeting and realizes the very poor results for HEDIS (and for MIPS) on CDC, two nurse practitioners agree to try a series of smartphone applications for tracking nutrition, exercise, foot care, and eye care routinely with patients and, after 6 months' time, provide preliminary feedback to the rest of the practice. Other providers in the practice are encouraged to adopt the use of the tools but are close to retirement, do not have/use smartphones, and are significantly resistant to the change, demonstrating significant resistance to the status quo and an unwillingness to adopt the innovation. The practice presents the potential impact of improved HEDIS scores on financial rewards for the practice through MIPS (a driving force), but these retiring practitioners will not benefit from financial changes that will occur in the future (a restraining force). Even though the pilot appears to be successful, it will take significant effort to address the concerns of the resistant providers to expand the intervention across the entire practice and achieve the HEDIS and MIPS desired state for the entire practice and not just for the two successful APRNs who initiated the change process. This phase is dominated by complexity in terms of both driving and restraining forces and may not necessarily be linear or quick to resolve, even when a pilot is successfully used.

REFREEZING

The third stage of change is *refreezing* (or *freezing*), which reflects restabilization that follows making a change. This stage can also require an extended period of time, as the change or transition that team members experience can lead to a change in their daily work as they internalize what is now different. There is a myriad of tools that can assist the process, and many of them have been used in nursing processes. For example, Rew et al. (2020) uses project management tools in the nursing research process. White et al. (2021) advocate for the use of project management tools in the translation of nursing research evidence into practice. Shirey (2008) advises the use of project management tools to drive organizational change for leaders, entrepreneurs, and APRNs alike.

The change process is complex, and Lewin's model, though simple and straightforward, has been used successfully in nursing. Tools that can facilitate understanding the present state in terms of need for change (to unfreeze) can be unearthed using SWOT analysis or stakeholder analysis, focus group discussions, surveys, and other means. To try an innovation out on a small scale using the pilot approach can be a very compelling driving force in the changing phase, especially if it is successful. Expanding the change more globally can be addressed in the refreezing phase using project management tools.

ROGERS' DIFFUSION OF INNOVATIONS THEORY

An evidence-based change in practice can easily be considered an intervention or an innovation. Though definitions may vary slightly, they both can provide new guidance that can assist with improving outcomes in a particular site or setting and are certainly for patients regardless of venue. Even when evidence is available and might work effectively in one place, it is often not fully disseminated throughout the entire healthcare system (Berwick, 2003). This notwithstanding, there are many factors that influence the achievement of successful change. Rogers' Diffusion of Innovations Theory has been used extensively in healthcare, in nursing, and globally (Balas & Chapman, 2018; Dingfelder & Mandell, 2011; Mohammadi et al., 2018; Rogers, 2003). Although not a change theory per se, it has been widely used to achieve change by adopting research evidence (i.e., innovation) to achieve a change in practice and improved outcomes. In addition, evaluating and implementing research evidence to achieve improved outcomes is not always a straight path, as implementation may be constrained by various obstacles and barriers. Rogers' Diffusion of Innovations Theory provides a framework that can be applied to various scenarios, from private practice to public health (Rogers, 2003; Setswe & Zungu, 2022; White et al., 2021).

Rogers' social science theory is based on research from more than 60 years ago with the first edition published in 1962. The theory explains that one can make general observations about an individual's willingness to accept an innovation and categorized individuals into five categories: innovators (2.5%), early adopters (13.5%), early majority (34%), late majority (34%), and laggards (16%) (Rogers, 2003). This framework is helpful in implementing a change across a given venue or social system as each of the five types have characteristics which can be insightful for disseminating innovation. For example, the two APRNs who launched an evidence-based pilot project in a modestly sized private practice to achieve compliance in HEDIS CDC could be considered innovators in this specific primary care practice. However, their use of a toolkit to improve HEDIS CDC met resistance from other practitioners in the practice when they tried to disseminate the same techniques more broadly. There were two providers who were very conservative, a bit older, and considering retirement. They could be considered laggards. If this evidence-based change has any hope of succeeding across the entire practice, attention to the needs of the laggards who make up 33% of the entire practice is essential. The laggard group may be resistant to change anything in their practice and the motivating factor of an increased MIPS financial reward may occur after their retirement. However, the remaining four practitioners are willing to try the techniques, and although they may be slow to use them, they eventually come on board (late majority). The APRN change agents need to better understand how each staff member in the practice (including the medical assistants, receptionists, and staff RNs) might react and what will convince them to adopt the evidence-based change and incorporate this into their management of patients with diabetes.

The theory is characterized by five key elements that are used in describing the innovation itself: *relative advantage, compatibility, complexity, trialability,* and *observability* (Lien & Jiang, 2017). If the innovation is perceived by the individuals who might adopt it as having an advantage over present practice, that could be an enticement. Compatibility of an innovation is another important concern. This is the degree to which the innovation fits with an individual's values, experiences, and needs. Complexity is directly related to the speed needed to bring an innovation to fruition; breaking an innovation into component parts may be the key to implementing a complex innovation. Trialability is the ability of an intervention to be tried out with a portion of the population, like the APRNs did with the HEDIS CDC pilot. Some interventions or innovations might be trickier to pilot or to break down into its component parts for a trial. For example, if the private practice relies on all manual documentation and wants to move forward with an EHR, it may be very difficult to pilot in a small practice. The last characteristic of an innovation has to do with the observability of results. Changing a diabetic's A1C levels may take many weeks with constant support and intervention on the part of the primary care staff. Results in MIPS will be lagged even further, so both outcomes (better glucose control and financial rewards for same) may influence full staff participation in the innovation because results may not be immediately observable.

Scott et al. (2008) conducted a research study on the uptake of a cardiac patient education toolkit in Canada. The research endeavor was framed using Rogers' Diffusion of Innovations Theory and there were 153 interested physicians recruited to participate. Of the 115 physicians who completed the survey, relative advantage and observability of healthcare benefits were significantly associated with intention to use the toolkit. Practicing physicians who were in solo private practices reported more environmental barriers to using the toolkit than practitioners in larger practices.

Accelerating diffusion in any implementation endeavor can be challenging. However, there are tools that can guide the effort (Figure 12.1) (Tidd & Bessant, 2023). Scarbrough and Kyratsis (2022) explain that diffusing innovation is the task of implementation, and getting from a trial to scale especially in a large organization can be challenging. Some of these tools have been mentioned in Chapter 9, "Evaluation of Practice at the Population Level," and are useful whether implementing Lewin's Change Model or Rogers' Diffusion of Innovations Theory. For example, SWOT analysis and stakeholder analysis can help to identify readiness to change. Additional tools like a failure mode and effects analysis (FMEA) and project management tools like a Gantt chart are also tools that can guide an implementation effort and help to estimate time frame, examine obstacles, open communication channels, and prevent implementation challenges (ASQ, 2023a, 2023b).

THE REACH, ADOPTION, IMPLEMENTATION, AND MAINTENANCE MODEL AND THE PRACTICAL ROBUST IMPLEMENTATION AND SUSTAINABILITY MODEL

The reach, adoption, implementation, and maintenance model (RE-AIM) and the practical robust implementation and maintenance model (PRISM) have been identified as strategies to disseminate public health initiatives in order to positively influence population health with evidence-based innovation (Glasgow et al., 1999; RE-AIM, 2023a, 2023b). The RE-AIM model and tools are an integrated framework "developed to improve the adoption and sustainable implementation of evidence-based interventions in a wide range of health, public health, educational, community and other settings" (RE-AIM, 2023a, 2023b). These models are particularly useful when expanding an intervention or innovation that involves dissemination at a greater scale, perhaps even approaching the entirety of a population. These models are focused on health promotion behaviors and, most particularly, creating widespread application of evidence-based interventions that produce positive health outcomes in the population. When instituting change in a small venue, like a nursing care unit in a hospital or in a private practice, all of the tools presented in this chapter have usefulness and applicability. However, changing practice at the organizational or system level requires a broader focus.

The complexity of the problem cannot be understated, especially when change is needed globally. There could be national policy changes needed, a long-term legislative

FIGURE 12.1

Tools for diffusing innovation.

PRACTICAL TIPS FOR SUCCESSFUL SHARING

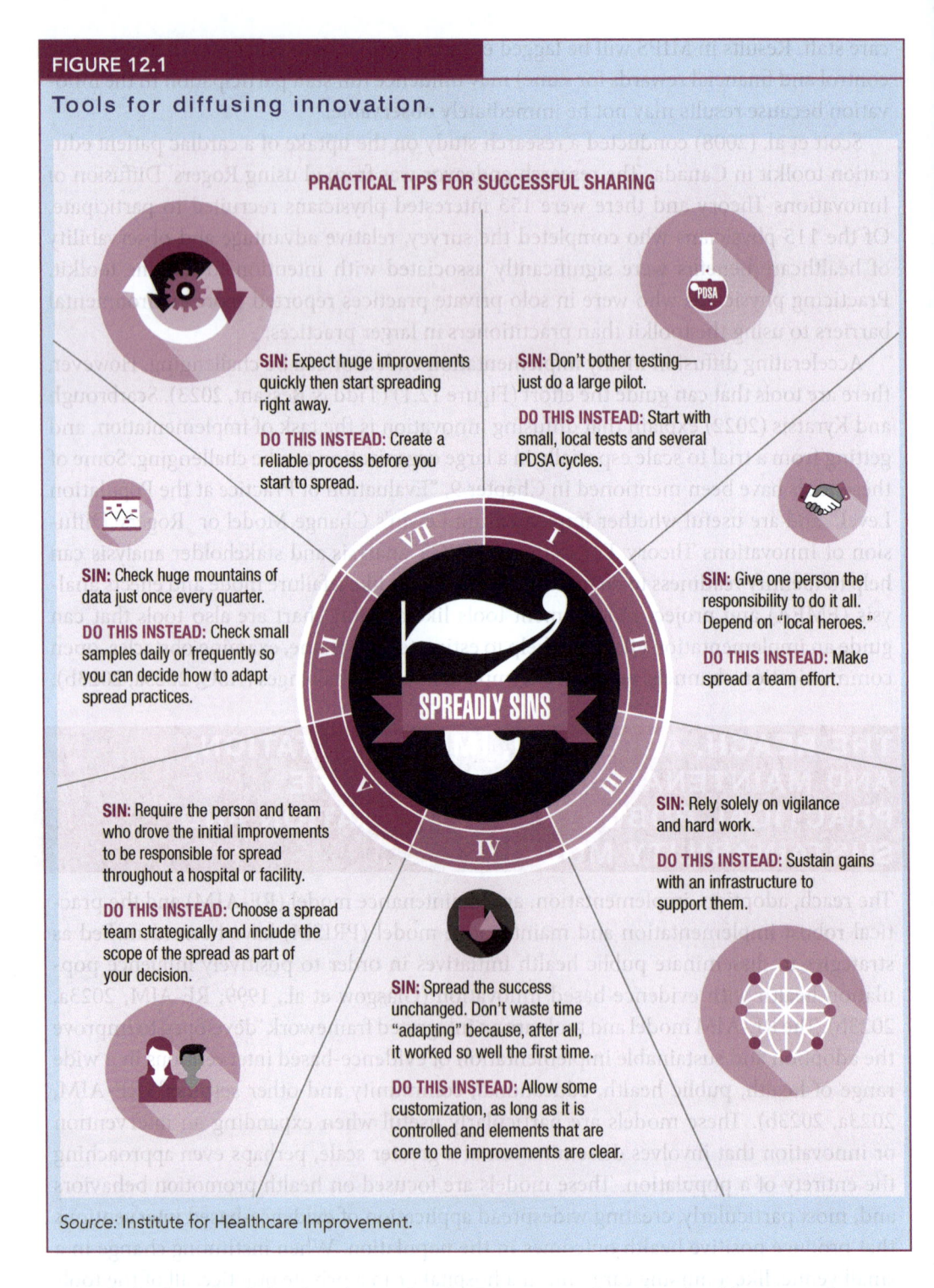

7 SPREADLY SINS

I. SIN: Don't bother testing—just do a large pilot.
DO THIS INSTEAD: Start with small, local tests and several PDSA cycles.

II. SIN: Give one person the responsibility to do it all. Depend on "local heroes."
DO THIS INSTEAD: Make spread a team effort.

III. SIN: Rely solely on vigilance and hard work.
DO THIS INSTEAD: Sustain gains with an infrastructure to support them.

IV. SIN: Spread the success unchanged. Don't waste time "adapting" because, after all, it worked so well the first time.
DO THIS INSTEAD: Allow some customization, as long as it is controlled and elements that are core to the improvements are clear.

V. SIN: Require the person and team who drove the initial improvements to be responsible for spread throughout a hospital or facility.
DO THIS INSTEAD: Choose a spread team strategically and include the scope of the spread as part of your decision.

VI. SIN: Check huge mountains of data just once every quarter.
DO THIS INSTEAD: Check small samples daily or frequently so you can decide how to adapt spread practices.

VII. SIN: Expect huge improvements quickly then start spreading right away.
DO THIS INSTEAD: Create a reliable process before you start to spread.

Source: Institute for Healthcare Improvement.

agenda both at the federal and state levels. Education of existing healthcare professionals may be required as well as change in academic curricula for nurses, providers, and assistive staff. The role of corporations may also come into play, helping or hindering the public health agenda. Change of this magnitude could be a significant undertaking far

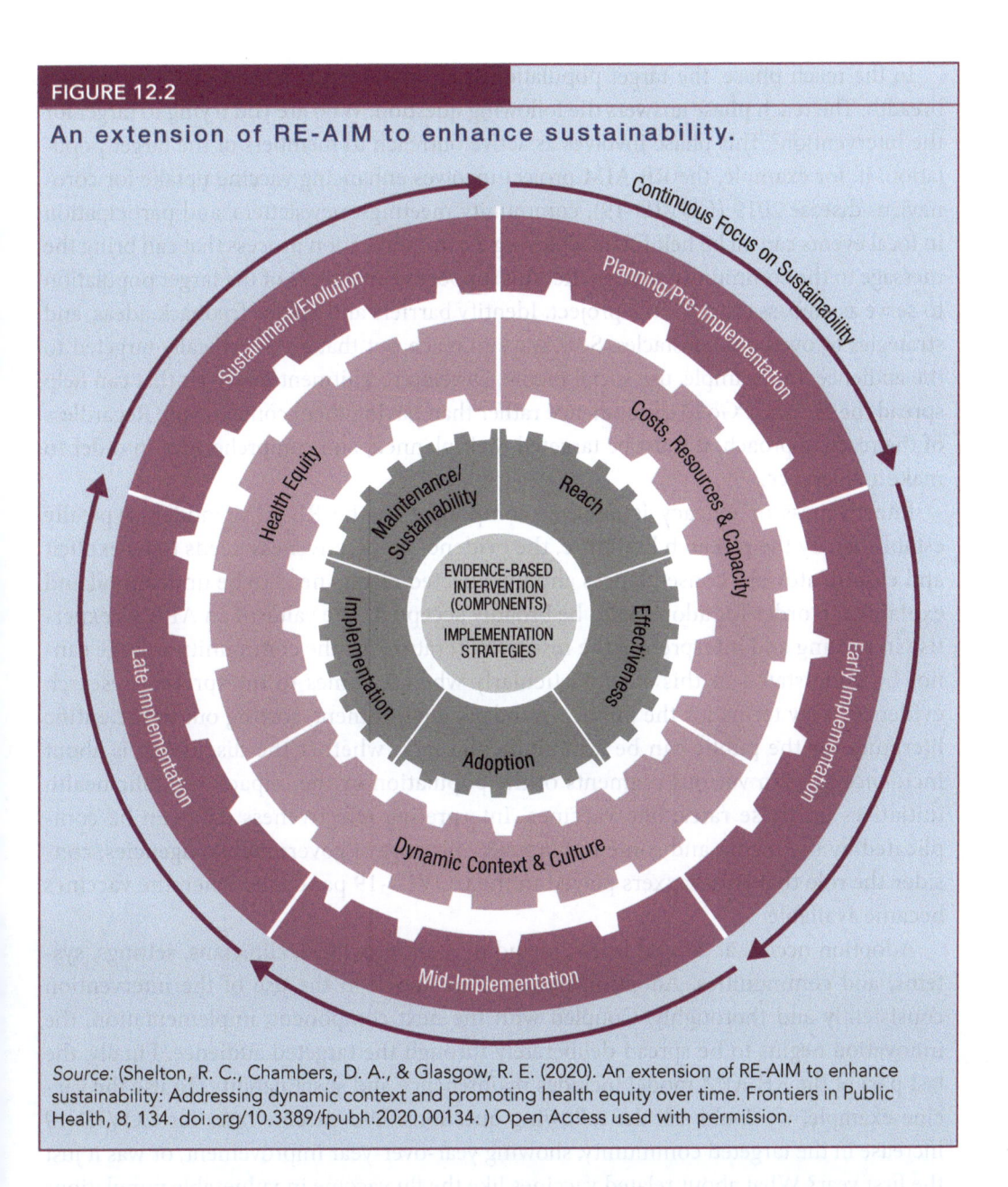

FIGURE 12.2
An extension of RE-AIM to enhance sustainability.

Source: (Shelton, R. C., Chambers, D. A., & Glasgow, R. E. (2020). An extension of RE-AIM to enhance sustainability: Addressing dynamic context and promoting health equity over time. Frontiers in Public Health, 8, 134. doi.org/10.3389/fpubh.2020.00134.) Open Access used with permission.

beyond the skill set and abilities of a single APRN. Although it may be difficult for individual APRNs in a small practice setting to see a path to national change that will filter down to their practice, membership in professional organizations and the use of more sophisticated models might be just what is needed.

The RE-AIM model is focused on five key concepts: *reach, adoption, implementation, effectiveness,* and *maintenance.* These components may be approached sequentially or in parallel. Regardless of the approach, it must be comprehensive and includes deliberate and complete planning (Glasgow et al., 1999). The PRISM model works in concert with the RE-AIM model. The PRISM model is the practical robust implementation and sustainability model which provides context and works in concert with the targeted RE-AIM outcomes (Figure 12.2).

In the reach phase, the target population is clearly identified, in terms of scope and breadth. The reach phase answers the following question: Who are you trying to target for the intervention? This phase involves as active outreach to members of the target population. If, for example, the RE-AIM project involves enhancing vaccine uptake for coronavirus disease 2019 (COVID-19), community meetings, newsletters, and participation in local events can all be helpful in achieving a communication process that can bring the message to the community at large. Recruit supportive members of the target population to serve as ambassadors for the project. Identify barriers and ask for feedback, ideas, and strategies to overcome obstacles. Seek ways to reach out that are specifically targeted to the audience, for example, use social media. Develop recruitment materials that can help spread the message. Go to the audience rather than having them come to you. Regardless of the reach approach, it must be targeted, well-planned, and comprehensive in order to make a difference.

Effectiveness or efficacy is another component in the RE-AIM model. Typically established by the research literature, the evidence of effectiveness needs to be explicit and clear. Untoward consequences and unexpected results need to be understood and explained in order for adoption to be broadly accepted. The value of an APRN's expertise in reading and interpreting the research literature for the community at large cannot be understated in this step, particularly when it comes to interpreting research evidence in lay terms for the public. In today's environment, sorting out the scientific literature for the public can be a monumental task, whether the discussion is about incidence rates in various segments of the population or the impact of public health initiatives on those rates, like vaccines. Interpreting effectiveness data can be complicated by the media and some individuals' mistrust of governmental agencies; consider the role that anti-vaxxers played in the COVID-19 pandemic when the vaccines became available.

Adoption occurs at several levels, including staff, providers, clinicians, settings, systems, and communities. Adoption indicates an uptick in the use of the intervention consistently and thoroughly. Coupled with the next component, implementation, the innovation begins to be spread deliberately through the targeted audience. Finally, the last part of the RE-AIM model includes maintenance and sustainability. To use the vaccine example, we could ask the following questions: Did vaccine rates for COVID-19 increase in the targeted community, showing year-over-year improvement, or was it just the first year? What about related vaccines like the flu vaccine in vulnerable populations and early childhood disease vaccines uptake? These questions are not only pertinent but essential and ongoing measurement is needed to see the successful spread of the innovation. One could easily consider vaccine administration a self-care health promotion behavior. However, in order to achieve uptake in the entire population, the cooperation of managed care organizations, pharmacies, providers, and the community at large clearly comes into play.

Since these models were promulgated in 1999, they have been used extensively with great success. PubMed reports 1,212 results when searched for RE-AIM; of these, there were 256 in 2022. These numbers have increased steadily since the initial launch of the RE-AIM framework in 1999. Tschampl et al. (2023) used the RE-AIM model to launch a mobile approach to providing substance abuse care management to bring resources to patients who must deal with barriers to office-based care. Researchers at the University of Pittsburgh used the RE-AIM framework to design and successfully implement a weight management intervention that includes increased activity and mobility among community-based seniors (Liu et al., 2023). Poole et al. (2023) used a qualitative research approach within the RE-AIM framework to better understand how to increase workplace participation in smoking cessation programs. All three studies used the RE-AIM model and the innovations are intended to have a global reach.

There have been successes using the RE-AIM and PRISM frameworks. However, many of these problems have a complexity in realizing global change. Consider the role of legislation, policy, and regulation, as well as professional organizations, in broadly influencing population health. Although RE-AIM and PRISM provide a roadmap, there is no reason to expect that implementing change on a massive scale to address a global problem is linear. Consider the problem of the opioid crisis in the United States. Awareness of the problem has been spread through the media, including social media, and prevention techniques have escalated. However, the mortality rate related to opioid overdose continues to escalate. Similarly, the incidence of obesity and overweight is a problem in the United States as well as a global one.

THE OPIOID CRISIS

Though the problem had existed for a long time, in 2017, the U.S. opioid crisis was declared a public health emergency (Centers for Medicare and Medicaid Services [CMS], 2022). The opioid crisis has been characterized by increasing mortality rates, which continue to escalate (National Institute on Drug Abuse, 2023). Efforts to gain control of this complex public health problem are multifaceted and interdisciplinary. Reports have been detailed with some sponsored by the U.S. government and some through grant funding (Congressional Budget Office, 2022; Humphreys et al., 2022).

The CMS launched a roadmap summarizing the escalating opioid problem and detailing prevention, treatment, and data as specific areas of focus. Six areas of influence are summarized. For example, in 2020, Medicare began coverage for methadone as medication-assisted treatment (MAT) and acupuncture for chronic back pain. Best practices have been adopted. One example is that 87% of drug management programs for Medicare Part D have adopted opioid overutilization policies and have at least one naloxone product available in Part D formularies. In addition, CMS has made nationwide Medicaid data on substance use disorder widely available. Access has improved in 28 Medicaid demonstration projects. Awareness has been created through a marketing campaign to providers to compare their prescribing practices to peers. These strategies and accomplishments to date are only a few sponsored by one governmental agency (CMS, 2022).

Healthcare professionals like APRNs and other providers, frontline nurses, social workers, behavioral health specialty providers, primary care providers, addiction specialists, pharmacists, pharmacy providers, and emergency medical technicians across the spectrum of healthcare have been actively involved in shaping legislation, advancing treatment solutions, and crafting regulation to prevent deaths related to opioid use to curb this escalating crisis. Pharmaceutical companies have been held liable for financial damages as a result of lawsuits for various violations (Haffajee & Mello, 2017). In fact, between 2004 and 2017, 12 major state and federal lawsuits included judgments holding various companies liable for damages totaling over $980,000,000, including $20,000,000 in Canada. The criminal justice system has been implicated for negative contribution to the problem. In short, addressing the opioid crisis has required countless hours of coordinated strategy, policy development, legislation, regulation by multiple governmental entities, education, and data tracking.

Consider the legislative agenda. An internet search on *opioid crisis legislation* revealed over two million hits. The amount of legislation proposed or passed at the federal and state levels over the past 5 years is staggering and ranges from laws curtailing prescribing practices to enhancing mental health and addiction services, as well as holding pharmaceutical corporations accountable for false advertising (Haffajee & Mello, 2017). The legislative agenda at the state level is just as powerful. For example, in New Jersey, in 2021 the governor signed into law P.L.2021, c.152, the Overdose Prevention Act, to encourage the widespread distribution of all FDA-approved forms of naloxone, a powerful reversal agent for opioid overdose (New Jersey Harm Reduction Coalition, 2023). In California, Assembly Bill (AB) 2760 mandates that patients be given a prescription for naloxone when prescriptions for opioids are written for high overdose risk patients (Duan et al., 2022).

Professional organizations contribute to raising awareness, providing evidence-based tools, sponsoring policy, and actively campaigning for legislation. The American Association of Nurse Practitioners (AANP) has done extensive advocacy work on a variety of topics. The *Point of Care Tools* include the opioid use disorder (OUD) tool (AANP, 2023). In the OUD point of care tool, links are provided to over 25 related organizations and government agencies and two helplines are cited along with links to their websites. Examples include Prescribe to Prevent, Substance Abuse and Mental Health Services Administration (SAMHSA), CDC Overdose Prevention, and the National Institute on Drug Abuse (NIDA) and AANP.

SUMMARY

Lewin's Change Model, Rogers' Diffusion of Innovations Theory, and the RE-AIM framework provide ample tools and a road map for change, whether localized, in a private practice, or more global (Glasgow et al., 1999; Lewin, 1951; Rogers, 2003). These models have been used successfully in healthcare, specifically in nursing, and have shown to be effective in implementing, disseminating, and sustaining changes in the service of improving outcomes. An APRN interested in program implementation will benefit from the use of these models and the tools that accompany them.

END-OF-CHAPTER RESOURCES

EXERCISES

EXERCISE 12.1 Provide one example of an intervention that demonstrated success in one venue but failed to demonstrate measurable outcomes when applied at the entire organization. Use Lewin's model as per the example in Box 12.1 to identify driving forces, the desired state, and restraining forces.

EXERCISE 12.2 As nurse manager, you launched a successful falls reduction campaign on your 36-bed medical-surgical unit. When you presented your results for the past year to the Practice Council, the Chief Nursing Officer (CNO) asked you to replicate your success on six other medical-surgical units that are like yours in terms of patient characteristics and staffing. Explain how you would use the Institute for Healthcare Improvement's (IHI) Seven Spreadly Sins (the dos and don'ts of program implementation) and any project management tool as a framework.

EXERCISE 12.3 The community coalition that you are working with has set a goal to increase vaccine uptake for people who live in the community. What information do you need before you develop a plan? You know that a multilevel approach will be needed to achieve an effective and sustainable change. Use the RE-AIM model to apply a brief description of *reach, adoption, implementation, effectiveness,* and *maintenance* to begin to consider the problem. You can learn more about RE-AIM from the website, RE-AIM.org/resources-and-tools, specifically, the use of YouTube videos, PowerPoint decks, graphics, and explanations about both RE-AIM and PRISM. Provide just one or two examples for each of the five concepts in RE-AIM.

EXERCISE 12.4 Obesity and overweight have reached epidemic proportions in the United States. As a practicing APRN in a primary care setting, you have observed this phenomenon for years and have seen firsthand the impact of this problem on the incidence and management of type 2 diabetes and hypertension. Although frustrating, you cannot help but wonder about what brought about this crisis and what prevention techniques have the potential to resolve the problem. What had been done to date and what more could be done from a policy perspective? Please include national policy implications, the legislative agenda at both the national and state level, the role of professional/provider specialty organizations, and the use of the RE-AIM framework to effect change.

A robust set of instructor resources designed to supplement this text is located at http://connect.springerpub.com/content/book/978-0-8261-4377-8. Qualifying instructors may request access by emailing textbook@springerpub.com.

REFERENCES

American Association of Colleges of Nursing. (2021). *AACN Essentials*. AACN. Retrieved 2/22/2023 from https://www.aacnnursing.org/DNP/DNP-Essentials

American Association of Nurse Practitioners. *Links and downloads opiod-related overdose prevention*. AANP. Retrieved 4/18/2023 from https://rise.aanp.org/PointOfCare/?_gl=1*8hfwuv*_gcl_aw*R0N-MLjE2ODE4NTM0NzYuRUFJYUlRb2JDaE1JclkzOHRiQzBfZ0lWY1kxYkNoMWpWUWt6RUFB-WUFTQUFFZ0piMVBEX0J3RQ..#/lessons/6m_70LxkN2I_AOICrm5ik4GHehy8npom

American Association of Nurse Practitioners. (2023). *Opiod use disorder (OUD) point of care tool*. AANP. Retrieved 4/18/2023 from https://rise.aanp.org/PointOfCare/#/

American Diabetes Association Professionals. (2023). *Practice guidelines resources*. ADA. Retrieved 3/16/2023 from https://professional.diabetes.org/content-page/practice-guidelines-resources

ASQ. (2023a). *Failure mode and effects analysis (FMEA)*. ASQ adapted from The Quality Toolkit. Retrieved 3/29/2023 from https://asq.org/quality-resources/fmea

ASQ. (2023b). *What is a GANTT chart?* ASQ. Retrieved 3/29/2023 from https://asq.org/quality-resources/gantt-chart

Balas, E. A., & Chapman, W. W. (2018). Road map for diffusion of innovation in health care. *Health Affairs, 37*(2), 198–204. https://doi.org/10.1377/hlthaff.2017.1155

Bauer, M. S., Damschroder, L., Hagedorn, H., Smith, J., & Kilbourne, A. M. (2015). An introduction to implementation science for the non-specialist. *BMC Psychology, 3*(1), 32. https://doi.org/10.1186/s40359-015-0089-9

Bauer, M. S., & Kirchner, J. (2020). Implementation science: What is it and why should I care? *Psychiatry Research, 283*, 112376. https://doi.org/https://doi.org/10.1016/j.psychres.2019.04.025

Berwick, D. M. (2003). Disseminating innovations in health care. *JAMA, 289*(15), 1969–1975. https://doi.org/10.1001/jama.289.15.1969

Centers for Medicare and Medicaid. (2022). *Ongoing emergencies and disasters*. CMS. Retrieved 4/18/2023 from https://www.cms.gov/about-cms/agency-information/emergency/epro/current-emergencies/ongoing-emergencies#:~:text=On%20Thursday%20October%2026%2C%202017,is%20a%20national%20health%20emergency.%E2%80%9D

Dingfelder, H., & Mandell, D. (2011). Bridging the research-to-practice gap in autism intervention: An application of diffusion of innovation theory. *Journal of Autism & Developmental Disorders, 41*(5), 597–609. https://doi.org/10.1007/s10803-010-1081-0

Duan, L., Lee, M.-S., Adams, J. L., Sharp, A. L., & Doctor, J. N. (2022). Opioid and naloxone prescribing following insertion of prompts in the electronic health record to encourage compliance with California State Opioid Law. *JAMA Network Open, 5*(5), e229723. https://doi.org/10.1001/jamanetworkopen.2022.9723

Glasgow, R. E., Vogt, T. M., & Boles, S. M. (1999). Evaluating the public health impact of health promotion interventions: The RE-AIM framework. *American Journal of Public Health, 89*(9), 1322–1327. https://doi.org/10.2105/ajph.89.9.1322

Haffajee, R. L., & Mello, M. M. (2017). Drug companies' liability for the opioid epidemic. *New England Journal of Medicine, 377*(24), 2301–2305. https://doi.org/10.1056/NEJMp1710756

Hilton, K., & Anderson, A. (2018). *White paper: IHI psychology of change framework to advance and sustain improvement*. Retrieved 3/18/2023, from https://www.ihi.org/resources/Pages/IHIWhitePapers/IHI-Psychology-of-Change-Framework.aspx

Humphreys, K., Shover, C. L., Andrews, C. M., Bohnert, A. S. B., Brandeau, M. L., Caulkins, J. P., Chen, J. H., Cuéllar, M.-F., Hurd, Y. L., Juurlink, D. N., Koh, H. K., Krebs, E. E., Lembke, A., Mackey, S. C., Larrimore Ouellette, L., Suffoletto, B., & Timko, C. (2022). Responding to the opioid crisis in North America and beyond: recommendations of the Stanford—*Lancet* Commission. *The Lancet, 399*(10324), 555–604. https://doi.org/10.1016/S0140-6736(21)02252-2

Hussain, S. T., Lei, S., Akram, T., Haider, M. J., Hussain, S. H., & Ali, M. (2018). Kurt Lewin's change model: A critical review of the role of leadership and employee involvement in organizational change. *Journal of Innovation & Knowledge, 3*(3), 123–127. https://doi.org/https://doi.org/10.1016/j.jik.2016.07.002

Institute for Healthcare Improvement. (2023). *IHI psychology of change framework*. IHI. Retrieved 3/18/2023 from https://www.ihi.org/resources/Pages/IHIWhitePapers/IHI-Psychology-of-Change-Framework.aspx

Lewin, K. (1951). Field theory in social science. In D. Cartwright (Ed.), *Selected theoretical papers*. Harper & Row.

Lien, A. S., & Jiang, Y. D. (2017, May). Integration of diffusion of innovation theory into diabetes care. *Journal of Diabetes Investigation, 8*(3), 259–260. https://doi.org/10.1111/jdi.12568

Liu, X., Kieffer, L. A., King, J., Boak, B., Zgibor, J. C., Smith, K. J., Burke, L. E., Jakicic, J. M., Semler, L. N., Danielson, M. E., Newman, A. B., Venditti, E. M., & Albert, S. M. (2023). Program factors affecting weight loss and mobility in older adults: Evidence from the mobility and vitality lifestyle program (MOVE UP). *Health Promotion Practice, 0*(0). https://doi.org/10.1177/15248399231162377

MindTools. (2022). *SWOT analysis*. Emerald Works Limited. Retrieved 3/29/2023 from https://www.mindtools.com/amtbj63/swot-analysis

Mohammadi, M. M., Poursaberi, R., & Salahshoor, M. R. (2018). Evaluating the adoption of evidence-based practice using Rogers's diffusion of innovation theory: A model testing study. *Health Promotion Perspectives, 8*(1), 25–32. https://doi.org/10.15171/hpp.2018.03

National Institute on Drug Abuse. (2023). *Drug overdose death rates*. U.S. Department of Health and Human Services; National Institutes of Health. Retrieved 4/18/2023 from https://nida.nih.gov/research-topics/trends-statistics/overdose-death-rates

New Jersey Harm Reduction Coalition. (2023). *Naloxone access; getting naloxone where it is needed most*. New Jersey Harm Reduction Coalition. Retrieved 4/18/2023 from https://njharmreduction.org/naloxone-access/

NIH National Cancer Institute. (2022). *Implementation science practice tools*. Retrieved 3/16/2023 from https://cancercontrol.cancer.gov/is/tools/practice-tools

Poole, N. L., Nagelhout, G. E., Magnée, T., de Haan-Bouma, L. C. I., Barendregt, C., van Schayck, O. C. P., & van den Brand, F. A. (2023). A qualitative study assessing how reach and participation can be improved in workplace smoking cessation programs. *Tobacco Prevention and Cessation, 9*, 07. https://doi.org/10.18332/tpc/161589

RE-AIM. (2023a). *Improving public health relevance and population health impact: What is PRISM?*. RE-AIM. Retrieved 3/30/2023 from https://RE-AIM.org/learn/prism/

RE-AIM. (2023b). *Improving public health relevance and population health impact: What is RE-AIM?* RE-AIM. Retrieved 3/30/2023 from https://RE-AIM.org/learn/what-is-RE-AIM/

Rew, L., Cauvin, S., Cengiz, A., Pretorius, K., & Johnson, K. (2020). Application of project management tools and techniques to support nursing intervention research. *Nursing Outlook, 68*(4), 396–405. https://doi.org/https://doi.org/10.1016/j.outlook.2020.01.007

Rogers, E. (2003). *Diffusion of innovations* (5th ed.). Free Press.

Scarbrough, H., & Kyratsis, Y. (2022). From spreading to embedding innovation in health care: Implications for theory and practice. *Health Care Management Review, 47*(3), 236–244. https://journals.lww.com/hcmrjournal/Fulltext/2022/07000/From_spreading_to_embedding_innovation_in_health.8.aspx

Scott, S. D., Plotnikoff, R. C., Karunamuni, N., Bize, R., & Rodgers, W. (2008). Factors influencing the adoption of an innovation: An examination of the uptake of the Canadian Heart Health Kit (HHK). *Implementation Science, 3*(1), 41. https://doi.org/10.1186/1748-5908-3-41

Setswe, G., & Zungu, L. (2022). Embracing implementation science in nursing and midwifery to translate evidence-based interventions into policies and clinical practice. *Africa Journal of Nursing & Midwifery, 24*(2), 1–6. https://doi.org/10.25159/2520-5293/12431

Shelton, R. C., Chambers, D. A., & Glasgow, R. E. (2020). An extension of RE-AIM to enhance sustainability: Addressing dynamic context and promoting health equity over time. *Frontiers in Public Health, 8*, 134. https://doi.org/10.3389/fpubh.2020.00134

Shirey, M. R. (2008). Project management tools for leaders and entrepreneurs. *Clinical Nurse Specialist: The Journal for Advanced Nursing Practice, 22*(3), 129–131. https://login.proxy.libraries.rutgers.edu/login?url=https://search.ebscohost.com/login.aspx?direct=true&db=c8h&AN=105745201&site=ehost-live

Tidd, J., & Bessant, J. (2023). *Innovation portal*. John Wiley and Sons Ltd. Retrieved 3/29/2023 from http://www.innovation-portal.info/toolkits/browse-tools-by-category/

Tschampl, C. A., Regis, C., Johnson, N. E., Davis, M. T., Hodgkin, D., Brolin, M. F., Do, E., Horgan, C. M., Green, T. C., Reilly, B., Duska, M., & Taveras, E. M. (2023). Protocol for the implementation of a statewide mobile addiction program. *Journal of Comparative Effectiveness Research, 12*(5), e220117. https://doi.org/10.57264/cer-2022-0117

White, K., Dudley-Brown, S., & Terhaar, M. F. (2021). *Translation of evidence into nursing and healthcare* (3rd ed.). Springer.

Williamson, K. M., Nininger, J., Dolan, S., Everett, T., & Joseph-Kemplin, M. (2021). Opportunities in chaos: Leveraging innovation to create a new reality in nursing education. *Nursing Administration Quarterly, 45*(2), 159–168. https://doi.org/10.1097/NAQ.0000000000000464

CHAPTER 13

IMPLICATIONS OF GLOBAL HEALTH IN POPULATION-BASED NURSING

SUZANNE WILLARD AND VERA KUNTE

CORE COMPETENCIES IN GLOBAL HEALTH

In 2021, the American Association of Colleges of Nursing (AACN) refined their *Essentials for Professional Nursing Education,* presenting the expected competencies for both entry-level and advanced-level nursing practice. The new *Essentials,* which include 10 domains and eight interrelated concepts, are addressed throughout this book for multiple advanced practice registered nursing roles. Particularly relevant to global health issues are Domain 3: Population Health and Domain 7: Systems-Based Practice. Within these domains, there is an emphasis on the concepts of diversity, equity and inclusion, ethics, health policy, and the social determinants of health (AACN, 2021).

Global health has been defined as "…the goal of improving health for all people by reducing avoidable diseases, disabilities, and deaths" (Institute of Medicine, 2009, p. 18) and an "area for study, research, and practice that places a priority on improving health and achieving equity in health for all people worldwide" (Koplan et al., 2009, p. 1994). These definitions highlight the multinational, multidisciplinary, and equity-oriented nature of this emerging field. There is no shortage of those speaking out on models of competency for global health, and many echo those of public health. The AACN formed an interdisciplinary collaboration with the Association of Schools and Programs of Public Health (ASPPH) to develop global health competencies. This partnership led to the publication of the Global Health Competency Model in 2011. An updated version of the competencies, Global Health Concentration Competencies for the Master of Public Health Degree, was released in 2018 (Jacobsen et al., 2019). The toolkit for the ASPPH

This chapter is a revision of the chapter that appeared in the third edition of this textbook, authored by Lucille A. Joel and Irina McKeehan Campbell, and we thank them for their original contribution.

competencies is at s3.amazonaws.com/ASPPH_Media_Files/Docs/GH-competencies-Toolkit.pdf.

The Consortium of Universities of Global Health (CUGH) has identified 11 domains in defining competencies for global health education and professional development (CUGH, 2023):

1. Global Burden of Disease
2. Globalization of Health and Healthcare
3. Social and Environmental Determinants of Health
4. Capacity Strengthening
5. Collaboration, Partnering, and Communication
6. Ethics
7. Professional Practice
8. Health Equity and Social Justice
9. Program Management
10. Sociocultural and Political Awareness
11. Strategic Analysis

The second edition of the *CUGH Global Health Education Competencies Toolkit* may be accessed at www.cugh.org/online-tools/competencies-toolkit.

As public health is global health and global health is local health, there is much overlap in the various models defining the desirable competencies. The domains in the ASPPH and the CUGH global health models clearly align with the AACN *Essentials,* particularly as they all relate to health equity, social justice, ethical practice, and social determinants of health.

Healthcare delivery to individuals and populations often involves working with programs that cross political and national borders. Global health is an extension of population health. Diseases can affect people across geographical boundaries and specific population aggregates, such as mothers and children or those who have hepatitis or are HIV positive. This was acutely evident in the coronavirus disease 2019 (COVID-19) pandemic which underscored the importance of global health by demonstrating how rapidly disease can be transmitted across international borders. By implementing the global health domains in nursing practice, APRNs can play a focal role in developing models of care that link population health with health policy, contain infectious diseases, and eliminate health disparities. For example, ICAP (formerly called the International Center for AIDS Care and Treatment Programs) at Columbia University supports large-scale evidence-based programs to strengthen healthcare systems and improve services for communicable and noncommunicable diseases, especially HIV, malaria, and TB in over 40 countries. The ICAP global team includes many APRNs; Susan Strasser, PhD, APN, FAAN, is a senior director at ICAP and is also a pediatric nurse practitioner. Her work focuses on improving acute and chronic healthcare as well as management and mitigation of disease outbreaks. Most recently, to protect vulnerable frontline workers during infectious disease outbreaks, Dr. Strasser was involved in a successful collaborative project that provided rapid COVID-19 training to healthcare staff in 11 African countries (Tsiouris et al., 2022).

This chapter explores the implications, benefits, and barriers of practicing global health for the APRN. The following areas are discussed:

- How geography, climate, and demographic factors influence the causes, transmission, and outcomes of communicable and noncommunicable diseases
- Global health competencies
- Effects of multilevel contexts of global health, population, and individual health
- Relationships between global health competencies and interdisciplinary collaboration
- Health initiatives of pivotal international agencies, such as the United Nations (UN) and the World Health Organization (WHO)
- Global health educational opportunities that exist for advanced practice registered nurses (APRNs)

CHANGING AMERICAN DEMOGRAPHIC LANDSCAPE

From 1975 until 2022, nearly 3.5 million refugees have been admitted to the United States. The United States annually sets a cap on how many refugees will be accepted. In 2022, that cap was raised and admissions have increased over the previous years (Migration Policy Institute [MPI], 2023). Immigrants, including refugees and migrant workers, have changed the demographic landscape of the United States. The U.S. population is becoming more culturally diversified and mobile, as ever greater numbers of people come to the United States seeking a better quality of life than the one they left behind. The global economy also has affected this movement, with increases seen in corporate, business, student, and academic exchanges. APRNs, who often work on the front lines of primary and preventive care, will increasingly encounter people from other countries. APRNs can work with existing stakeholders and international programs to provide optimal health services to both citizens and noncitizens in the United States.

The U.S. Immigration and Nationality Act (INA), derived from the post-World War II United Nation (UN) 1951 Convention, defines a *refugee* as "someone who: is located outside of the U.S.; is of special humanitarian concern to the U.S.; demonstrates that they were persecuted or fear persecution due to race, religion, nationality, political opinion, or membership in a particular social group" (U.S. Citizenship and Immigration Services [USCIS], 2022). As of mid-2022, there are 32.5 million refugees globally, with 72% originating from Syria, Venezuela, Ukraine, Afghanistan, and Sudan (UNHCR, 2023). Many refugees who are presently in other countries will seek entry into the United States.

The Homeland Security Act of 2002 dismantled the Immigration and Naturalization Service (INS) and separated the agency into three components within the Department of Homeland Security (DHS). The Homeland Security Act created the USCIS to enhance the security and efficiency of national immigration services by focusing exclusively on the administration of benefit applications. The law also formed the Immigration and Customs Enforcement (ICE) and Customs and Border Protection (CBP) to oversee immigration enforcement and border security.

The INA has regulated immigration into the United States through a variety of laws since 1921. The Act was amended in 1965 as the Hart–Celler Act. This Act made changes to the immigration quota system based on country and nationality. It was designed to maintain the same ethnic proportion in the United States as was reflected in the 1920 Census. Asians were excluded from immigration by amendments to the Act in 1924. In 1965, immigration criteria replaced nationality or country-of-origin quotas with requirements for employable skills and reuniting families with connections in the United States. The United States has more immigrants than any other country in the world. The population of immigrants is also very diverse, with just about every country in the world represented among U.S. immigrants. Since 1965, when U.S. immigration laws replaced a national quota system, the number of immigrants living in the United States has increased exponentially. According to the Current Population Survey, in September 2022, there are nearly 47.9 million immigrants living in the United States, making up almost 14.6% of the nation's population (Camarota & Zeigler, 2022). This represents a more than fourfold increase since 1960, when 9.7 million immigrants lived in the United States, comprising 5.4% of the total U.S. population, falling just shy of the all-time record of 14.8% posted in 1890 (Budiman et al., 2020).

Since the creation of the federal Refugee Resettlement Program in 1980, more than three million refugees have resettled in the United States—more than any other country. The largest origin group of refugees are from areas of economic needs, conflict, and political upheaval, notably Mexico, the Democratic Republic of the Congo, followed by Bhutan, Burma (Myanmar), and now the Ukraine. A common denominator of these countries is that they have experienced or are experiencing internal strife, such as wars and political or religious persecutions. California, Texas, and New York have resettled nearly a quarter of all refugees admitted. However, most immigrants live in just 20 major metropolitan areas, with the largest populations residing in New York City, Los Angeles, and Miami. The unauthorized immigrant population in the United States increased rapidly from 1990, reaching a peak of 12.2 million in 2007 (Lopez et al., 2021). In recent years, their numbers have largely stabilized, with an estimated 11 million unauthorized immigrants living in the country in 2019 (MPI, n.d.). The number of immigrants from contiguous countries like Nicaragua, Ecuador, Peru, San Salvador, and Columbia has continued to grow. They usually utilize a variety of methods to travel overland, many of which are considered dangerous and have resulted in numerous deaths. Despite limited employment opportunities, unauthorized immigrants are increasingly likely to be long-term U.S. working residents. Two thirds of adult unauthorized immigrants have lived in the country for more than 10 years, more than half have a high school or higher education, and almost half have incomes at or above 200% of the federal poverty level (MPI, n.d.).

As of December 2022, there are nearly 600,000 young adults who are active recipients of the Deferred Action for Childhood Arrivals (DACA) program residing in the United States (KFF, 2023). The program was created by presidential executive order in 2012 to protect eligible immigrants who came to the United States illegally as children from being deported. Many political leaders have worked hard to end the program. However, it has been kept alive by many court challenges. The bipartisan Dream Act of 2023 (S.365), if passed, will provide a pathway to citizenship for certain non-U.S. nationals (defined as Dreamers) who entered the United States before age 18 and have grown up here. A summary of S.365 may be viewed at www.congress.gov/bill/118th-congress/senate-bill/365.

Temporary Protected Status (TPS) is offered to immigrants from designated countries where natural disasters, war, or violence make it unsafe to return. As of 2023, nearly 700,00 persons from 16 countries are either receiving or are eligible for TPS. Designated countries include South Sudan, Sudan, Syria, Venezuela, Afghanistan, Cameroon, and, more recently, the Ukraine (Pew Research Center, 2023).

Immigrants in the United States, as a whole, have lower levels of education than the U.S.-born population. In 2021, immigrants were less likely than U.S.-born individuals to have completed high school (19% versus 27%) but were as likely to have a college degree or more, with rates at 34% versus 35% (Ward & Batalova, 2023). This is explained by the higher numbers of better-educated immigrants since 2017. Education levels vary by the country of origin, and recent adult immigrants from India (80%), United Arab Emirates (78%), and Saudi Arabia (77%) were the most likely to have a bachelor's degree or more. Among Venezuelans, the fastest-growing U.S. immigration group, more than half of all adults hold at least a bachelor's degree. Immigrants from Guatemala (8%), Mexico (9%), and El Salvador (9%) were the least likely to have a bachelor's degree or higher. Literacy is an important issue. Among immigrants ages 5 and older, Spanish is the most commonly spoken language. However, there are many dialects and languages. Some 43% of immigrants in the United States speak Spanish at home (Ward & Batalova, 2023).

In 2021, immigrants comprised 17.4% of the civilian labor force, contributing billions in annual tax dollars (Bureau of Labor Statistics [BLS], 2021). Among less-educated workers, immigrants earned less than native workers with the same education level. Immigrants were twice more likely to be employed in the service industry, construction, and maintenance occupations and less likely than U.S.-born workers to be employed in professional and management-related occupations. Immigrants were also disproportionately affected by the COVID-19 pandemic. Not only were they more likely to occupy hazardous frontline jobs deemed essential during the crisis, but they also faced higher unemployment rates than the U.S.-born individuals during that same time. In short, most immigrants are working, often in low-paying jobs that are in high need, particularly in the service industry.

Such diversity in the population, with an increased rate of mobility across international borders, presents challenges for the APRN in all practice settings. The APRN needs to know the populations that they serve, from their customs to their ability to access healthcare. Some of the biggest barriers to utilizing APRNs in immigrant health and in providing care to foreign-born individuals are language, cultural beliefs, and the ability to develop therapeutic relationships (Giwa et al., 2020). APRNs need to be familiar with federal policies that bar hospitals from asking about citizenship before providing services. The 1986 Emergency Medical Treatment and Active Labor Act (EMTALA), which is part of the Consolidated Omnibus Budget Reconciliation Act (COBRA), stipulates that hospitals deliver emergency healthcare to everyone, regardless of national origin, legal status, or ability to pay (EMTALA, 2018). Such care is uncompensated at the hospital and state level unless Medicaid funds are appropriated for various population health programs to cover charity care. While undocumented immigrants are entitled to a basic education, they are ineligible for federally funded benefits like social security, Medicare, and Medicaid (Biggerstaff & Skorma, 2020). It is important for the APRN to become familiar with local, community, state, and federal organizations that provide services for immigrant populations. For example, the American Immigration Lawyers Association, a not-for-profit group that advocates for fairness and justice in immigration law, may provide resources to tackle any legal issues that arise. By integrating the AACN concepts of ethics, equity, compassionate care, and social justice in their nursing practice, the APRN can improve health outcomes for vulnerable immigrant populations.

Twenty-first-century advances in communication, trade, transportation technologies, and scientific exchanges bring health issues from other continents to the threshold of the American urban and community hospital. These advances are accompanied by national security concerns, as was acutely evident with the recent COVID-19 pandemic as well as the 2014 Ebola outbreak in West Africa. APRN population-based practice has daily relevance as people bring their national, environmental, socioeconomic, and cultural contexts with them whenever they visit their healthcare provider. APRNs who encounter individuals from other countries need to understand and become familiar with programs or policies addressing the complex global factors influencing the context of individual and population health.

Health as an International Phenomenon

Individual health is embedded in the larger socio-ecological context of the global community. Not only does each individual's health status affect others, but also the health of one group in a society can influence the welfare of other groups. The importance of maintaining health in populations and the lack of preparedness for managing global health security were highlighted in the current era of rapid-spreading pandemics. APRNs need a good understanding of epidemiology, including methods of disease transmission and how to prevent transmission. The spread of infectious disease across borders reveals the importance of applying evidence-based knowledge to treat and prevent disease at both national and international levels. In the early days of the COVID-19 pandemic, before the availability of the vaccine, there was an increased awareness of the need to educate the public on methods to limit transmission such as masking, social distancing, and quarantine. For example, APRNs working in long-term care facilities had to embrace multiple roles, but mitigating the spread of COVID-19 was central to their practice (McGilton et al., 2021). Later, COVID-19 vaccine hesitancy and denial stressed the need for APRNs to reassure the public about the safety and efficacy of vaccination. Just as the introduction of medical advances and evidence-based healthcare practices can positively affect a nation's health, the spread of infectious diseases can affect it adversely.

Article 25 of the Universal Declaration of Human Rights (UDHR) stipulates that all people have the right to a standard of living that guarantees health (UN, n.d.a). This article was adopted by the UN Charter of 1948. In 1960, the UDHR further specified health as the highest attainable standard of physical, social, and mental well-being rather than as solely the absence of disease. Health, according to the UDHR, is achievable through the promotion of maternal and child health, reduction of mortality and morbidity, improvements in environmental sanitation, and the provision of adequate medical services. The UN reaffirmed health as an intrinsically valuable end by emphasizing that poor health is caused primarily by poverty and environmental conditions. The adoption of the Sustainable Development Goals by the UN advocates and supports the global issue of equity by protecting the planet, ending poverty, and ensuring good health for all (UN, n.d.b.).

The human rights movement in health, which raised the issue of equity in health status, tied universal access to comprehensive medical and health services for different social groups. Universal access implies the availability of services to all individuals and groups. Evaluating the distinctions between individual medical care and public healthcare becomes important as a means of monitoring health status, measured by indicators of equity and quality of care. Equity in access does not automatically lead to equity in health status. Equity in health status among social groups is constrained by the macro-social process of the delivery of healthcare, as well as by the sociocultural, economic, and political arrangements of the community in which the delivery system functions. Global health programs have initiated various strategies to resolve these social determinants of health, increase access to basic health services, and achieve equity in outcomes. Essentially, equity in outcomes is the only true measure of equity in health status.

SOCIAL DETERMINANTS OF HEALTH

The social determinants of health are the conditions in which people are born, grow, live, work, and age. These circumstances are shaped by the distribution of money, power, and resources at global, national, and local levels. The social determinants of health are acutely responsible for health inequities—the unfair and often avoidable differences in health status seen within and between countries.

There are many conceptual frameworks for social determinants of health crafted by public and private entities, among them the CDC, the WHO, the European Union, and more. In fact, they all contain the multifactorial components of population health that impact health outcomes. Common themes focus on empowerment, interprofessional collaborations, and education. The framework is presented in Figure 13.1.

Inherent in these frameworks are the interactions between these social determinants, their influence on inequities, and the sociopolitical and economic influences on health and well-being. The status of the health of a nation is an international phenomenon that is embedded within the larger socio-ecological, cultural, and political context of the global community. Arguably, the United States is the most technologically advanced country in the world, with internationally renowned medical centers and cutting-edge treatment modalities that are grounded in the tenets of Western medical scientific research. Yet among civilized nations, its healthcare outcomes, especially for preventable diseases and access to health services, lag far behind those of its counterparts with regard

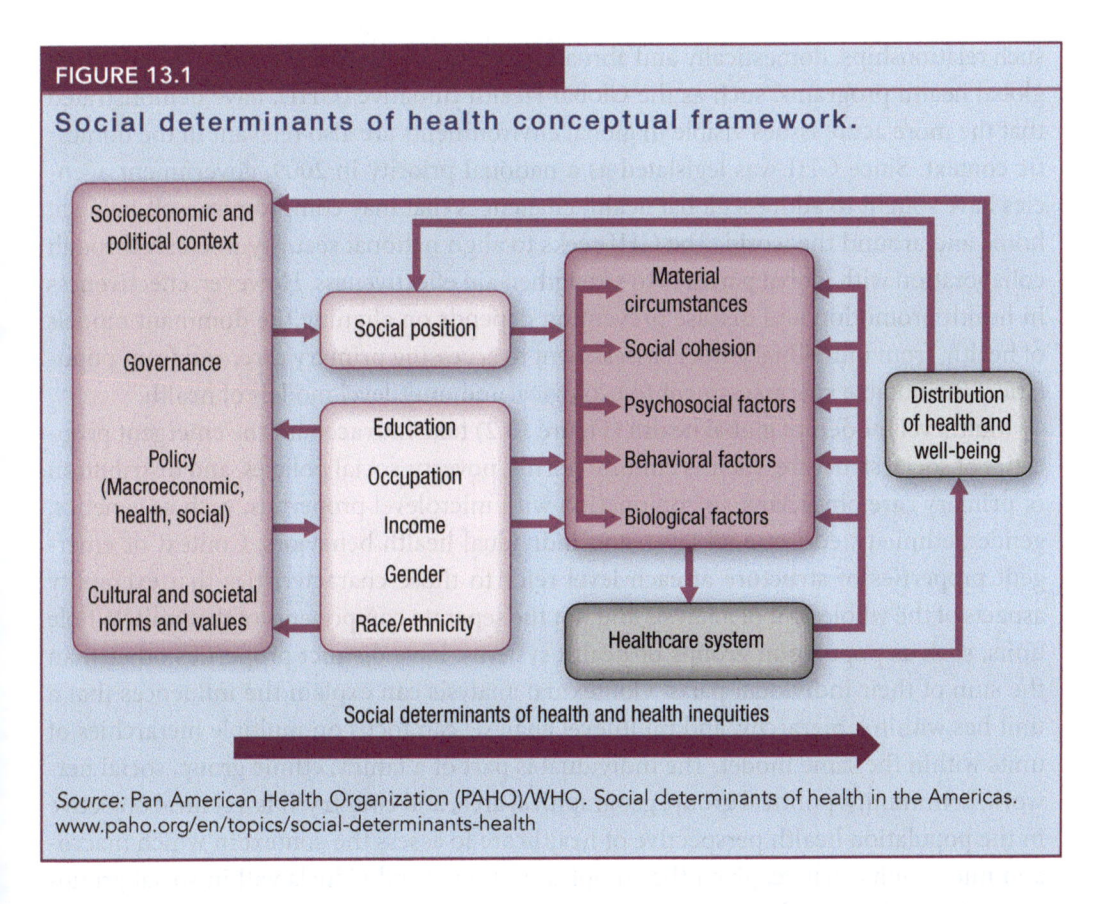

FIGURE 13.1

Social determinants of health conceptual framework.

```
Socioeconomic and
political context
                                      Material
                                      circumstances
                    Social position
                                      Social cohesion
Governance
                                                              Distribution
                                      Psychosocial factors   of health and
                    Education                                well-being
Policy                                Behavioral factors
(Macroeconomic,     Occupation
health, social)
                    Income            Biological factors

                    Gender
Cultural and societal
norms and values    Race/ethnicity    Healthcare system
```

Social determinants of health and health inequities →

Source: Pan American Health Organization (PAHO)/WHO. Social determinants of health in the Americas. www.paho.org/en/topics/social-determinants-health

to multiple indicators. According to the Commonwealth Fund (2023), when compared to the 38 high-income countries from the Organization for Economic Co-operation and Development (OECD), healthcare spending was the highest, life expectancy was the lowest, and maternal and infant mortality rates were the highest in the United States.

MULTILEVEL MODEL OF GLOBAL HEALTH

The growth of population-based nursing not only illustrates the need for further documentation of ethnocultural variation in health outcomes but also provides an equally important mandate to translate clinical research into culturally competent programs. Population health is an emerging paradigm, differentiated from global health not only by scope but also by a focus on which groups are susceptible or at greater risk for specific diseases. Global health, on the other hand, provides a broader perspective on the extent to which the complex relations of macrostructural factors of health determine the distribution of population-level and individual-level health outcomes. Macrofactors of salience explain how the environment, education policy, information technology, ethnic diversity and health disparity, geographical and socioeconomic factors, and inequities affect disease transmission and the delivery of health services across national borders.

To promote a greater understanding of the links among individual health, population health, and global health, the U.S. government has developed programs that address such relationships, domestically and abroad. The best practices and lessons learned from global health programs, such as the Global Health Initiative (GHI), have demonstrated that the more acute issues visible in global environments are also relevant in the domestic context. Since GHI was legislated as a national priority in 2009, government agencies have sought to address global health challenges that may compromise well-being at home and around the world. The GHI seeks to align national security interests through collaboration with global partners to strengthen aid effectiveness. However, effectiveness in health promotion and disease prevention depends on aligning the dominant models of health, from individual clinical assessment to accessing primary care, and from population attributable risk assessment to ecological and multilevel models of health.

Multilevel models of global health (Figure 13.2) take into account the emergent properties of social structure, such as cultural norms, poverty, social policies, and distribution of primary care physicians, in conjunction with microlevel properties, such as genetics, gender, ethnicity, educational level, and individual health behaviors. Context or emergent properties of structure at each level refer to those characteristics that exemplify aspects of the whole unit of analysis and not the separate components of that unit. Whole units, such as population groups or health systems, have distinct properties other than the sum of their individual parts. Contextual analysis can explain the influences that a unit has within a hierarchy, and multilevel analysis can focus on multiple hierarchies of units within the same model. The individual is part of a family, ethnic group, social network, community, political group, geographical area, and country. It is a central objective in the population health perspective of healthcare to assess the context in which macro- and micro-units change, given the complex nesting of individuals within social groups and cultures (Naik et al., 2019).

Global health intervention differs from medical intervention foremost in its emphasis on the socio-environmental context of individual health status. Second, global health recognizes that a continuous distribution in health status, such as blood pressure, characterizes populations. Third, global health programs are not restricted by focusing solely on the clinical designation of individuals as potential cases for treatment, with or without disease.

A clearer understanding of global health identifies the differences in individual health, while retaining the ethnocultural context experienced by people. The multilevel model of population and global health enables the identification of health differences among individuals and among social groups. It also identifies specific structural conditions in the community that affect the health of people living there. Last, it separates the structural and ethnocultural determinants of health from the effects of individual psychosocial and health behaviors on health outcomes. For example, health disparity is part of the community context within which people live; country of origin, ethnicity, and cultural values are group characteristics. But ethnocultural factors are almost always measured at the individual level, a misspecification of the research model. The domain of preventive strategies in community health is the at-risk population as a whole and that of clinical medicine is the at-risk individual.

A multilevel evaluation of global health, therefore, gauges negligible and high-risk factors at both the population level and the individual level. As abundant research has

FIGURE 13.2

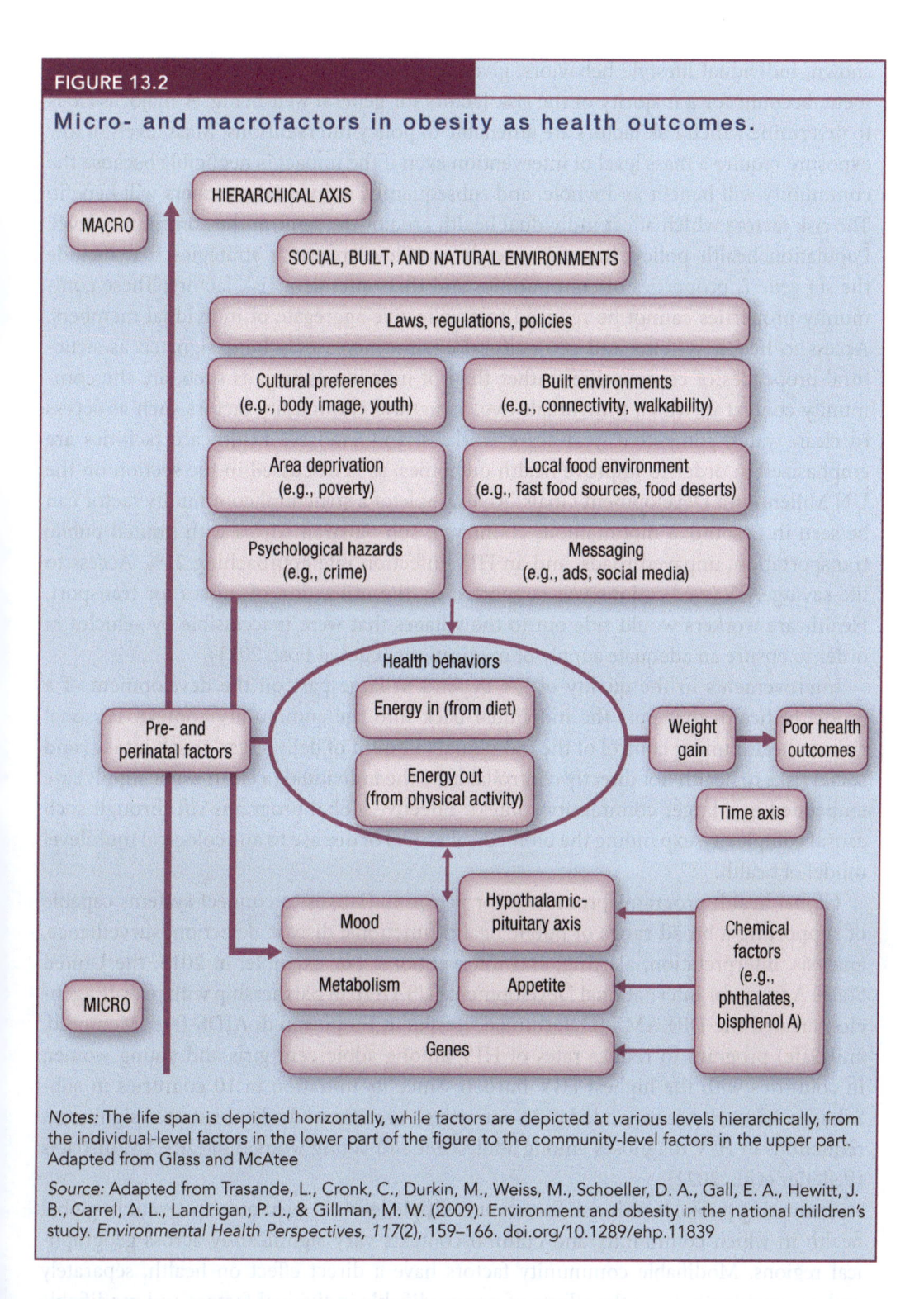

Micro- and macrofactors in obesity as health outcomes.

MACRO

HIERARCHICAL AXIS

SOCIAL, BUILT, AND NATURAL ENVIRONMENTS

Laws, regulations, policies

- Cultural preferences (e.g., body image, youth)
- Built environments (e.g., connectivity, walkability)
- Area deprivation (e.g., poverty)
- Local food environment (e.g., fast food sources, food deserts)
- Psychological hazards (e.g., crime)
- Messaging (e.g., ads, social media)

Pre- and perinatal factors

Health behaviors
- Energy in (from diet)
- Energy out (from physical activity)

→ Weight gain → Poor health outcomes

Time axis

- Mood
- Hypothalamic-pituitary axis
- Metabolism
- Appetite
- Genes

Chemical factors (e.g., phthalates, bisphenol A)

MICRO

Notes: The life span is depicted horizontally, while factors are depicted at various levels hierarchically, from the individual-level factors in the lower part of the figure to the community-level factors in the upper part. Adapted from Glass and McAtee

Source: Adapted from Trasande, L., Cronk, C., Durkin, M., Weiss, M., Schoeller, D. A., Gall, E. A., Hewitt, J. B., Carrel, A. L., Landrigan, P. J., & Gillman, M. W. (2009). Environment and obesity in the national children's study. *Environmental Health Perspectives, 117*(2), 159–166. doi.org/10.1289/ehp.11839

shown, individual lifestyle behaviors, given a specific level of socioeconomic development, account for a majority of the risk factors for general well-being. A major issue is to determine which risk factors are amenable to policy interventions. Mass levels of low exposure require a mass level of intervention even if the impact is negligible because the community will benefit as a whole, and subsequently, individual members will benefit. The risk factors which affect individual health are not the same at the community level. Population health policy, therefore, needs multilevel research strategies that include the *sui generis* properties of communities and their attendant risk factors. These community properties cannot be reduced to a collective aggregate of individual members. Access to health systems and geo-cultural environments may be designated as structural properties of communities rather than of individuals and, as such, are the community context in which individuals live. Structural community factors such as access to clean water, competent healthcare workers, and available healthcare facilities are emphasized in order to improve health outcomes, as is discussed in the section on the UN Millennium Development Goals. An example of a structural community factor can be seen in Lesotho, a mountainous country in sub-Saharan Africa with limited public transportation, unpaved roads, and an HIV infection rate approaching 25%. Access to life-saving HIV medications was supported by the utilization of horses for transport. Healthcare workers would ride out to the villages that were inaccessible by vehicles in order to ensure an adequate supply of medications (Global Post, 2011).

Improvements in the quality of life depend in large part on the development of a model of health that puts the individual back into the community context. Personal risks to health under control of the individual (amount of daily sugar or salt intake) and social risks to health not directly controllable by the individual (a clean water supply) are embedded in a larger community context. Effective global programs sift through such causal complexity, expanding the biomedical model of disease to an ecological multilevel model of health.

Global health programs promote information initiatives to connect systems capable of supporting a broad range of public health functions: disease detection, surveillance, analysis, interpretation, alerting, and interventions. For example, in 2015, the United States Agency for International Development (USAID), in partnership with private agencies, created the DREAMS (Determined, Resilient, Empowered, AIDS-free, Mentored, and Safe) program to reduce rates of HIV among adolescent girls and young women in countries with the highest HIV burden. Since its initiation in 10 countries in sub-Saharan Africa, it has expanded to 16 countries. A recent study demonstrated significant reductions in HIV diagnoses among adolescent and young women in DREAM districts (Pelletier et al., 2022).

Evaluating public health risk factors at multiple levels is even more relevant in global health in which community and cultural contexts vary significantly across geographical regions. Modifiable community factors have a direct effect on health, separately and independently from the effects of nonmodifiable individual factors and modifiable individual lifestyle practices. Individual behavioral solutions may be sought for population-level issues, when attributing or generalizing individual characteristics to the group. In designing or implementing large-scale health programs, it is important to be aware that both individual and community contextual factors, including geographical locators, should be systematically included in public health education and research to design effective programs.

National Global Health Initiatives

U.S. global health efforts, under the umbrella of USAID, is focused on investments in strengthening health systems and innovation. Its three strategic priorities for global health are preventing maternal and child deaths, controlling the HIV epidemic, and combatting infectious diseases (USAID, n.d.). The U.S. administration has allocated resources and funding to increase access to health services in global programs as a measure of diplomacy and to ensure national security. A poll conducted by the Kaiser Family Foundation (KFF) (Kates et al., 2019) found that more than half of the U.S. public believes that the United States should play a leading (14%) or major (43%) role in improving health for people in developing countries. USAID has bipartisan support in Congress, which has a longstanding tradition of working in unison for humanitarian causes. Response to any disease outbreak requires surveillance, evaluation, and implementation of control measures. The George W. Bush administration initiated two extremely successful programs, the President's Emergency Fund for AIDS Relief (PEPFAR) and the U.S. President's Malaria Initiative (PMI). PEPFAR provides education, medications, and support for HIV programs worldwide. The program not only supports HIV prevention, care, and treatment but also addresses concomitant problems like tuberculous and cervical cancer. For more information on this program, go to www.hiv.gov/federal-response/pepfar-global-aids/pepfar. PMI supports programs in 24 countries in Africa and in three areas of the Greater Mekong region in Southeast Asia, which represents 80% of the global malarial burden. Since its inception, PMI has prevented two billion infections and saved 11.7 million lives. More information can be found at www.pmi.gov.

Although infectious diseases still abound and new outbreaks of diseases like COVID-19, mpox, Ebola, severe acute respiratory syndrome (SARS), and H1N1 threaten national security, vaccine-preventable diseases have been nearly eliminated in the United States. One of the keys to controlling an infectious outbreak is effective communication and the implementation of evidence-based practice. The failure to do so was evident in the early responses to the COVID-19 pandemic which led to thousands of preventable deaths. Limited knowledge of this novel yet serious disease led to the spread of misinformation and disinformation about the disease. Supposed therapies, unsupported by evidence, were often touted in the United States and abroad by elected officials as well as by healthcare providers. In the United States, President Trump discouraged medical experts from providing scientific, evidence-based information. In other countries such as Tanzania, the then president refused to provide COVID-19 data to the WHO, proclaiming that there was no COVID-19. Undeterred, local leaders, aware that the disease was among them, quietly advocated protective and preventive measures (Carlitz et al., 2021). The COVID-19 vaccinations were developed very rapidly, thanks to the pressure and support from the Trump administration. Unfortunately, the rapid pace of the development and approval of the vaccine, amid often confusing and conflicting messaging from leadership, has contributed to vaccine hesitancy and vaccine skeptics.

APRNs have a role in shaping public opinion and have many opportunities to improve population health through health promotion, education, and research. Public health programs and health education, for example, have successfully contained HIV, and many preventive programs in the United States today focus on chronic diseases. Until the 20th century, communicable diseases were the singular cause of mortality, but chronic diseases now top the list. The smallpox vaccine was responsible for preventing nearly two million annual deaths around the world by 1980. In the 1950s, polio crippled about 35,000 children in the United States annually but was largely eradicated through vaccination by 1979. Polio is currently spreading in the war-torn countries of Syria, Djibouti, Eritrea, Ethiopia, and Somalia (Centers for Disease Control and Prevention [CDC], 2022). More recently, critical investments have led to the development of vaccines for both Ebola and COVID-19. Such quick collaboration among national groups underscores the critical role that the United States plays in global health, as well as the interconnections between national security and public health. In July 2022, as cases were reported worldwide in places where the disease was not endemic, the WHO declared mpox (previously known as monkey pox) a "public health emergency of international concern" (PHEIC). This allowed countries to abide by WHO recommendations and institute public health emergencies at home. Efforts to stem this epidemic came from local, national, and international agencies collaborating with the WHO on surveillance, infection prevention and control, and the targeted distribution of an effective vaccine. Organizations such as the American Public Health Association, the Association of Nurses in AIDS Care, and the International AIDS Society provided educational resources to their memberships. More than 87,000 thousand cases (30,000 in the United States) were reported through May 2023, when the WHO finally declared the outbreak to be over.

Since its inception in 1990, the *Healthy People* framework has outlined national health goals for individuals and communities across the United States to improve their health and well-being. The first global health goal appeared in *Healthy People 2020*: "to improve public health and strengthen U.S. national security through global disease detection, response, prevention, and control strategies." *Healthy People 2030* includes a more explicit global health goal "to improve health by preventing, directing and responding to public health events worldwide" (*Healthy People 2030*, n.d.).

Due to the drop in cases, COVID-19 is at this time the fourth leading cause of death in the United States (Figure 13.3); it was the third leading cause of death in 2020 and 2021 (Figure 13.4). The pandemic and its aftermath demonstrate how the *Healthy People 2030* connections between American health status and global developments are relevant. Diseases prevented with vaccinations are the cause of one of every five deaths among children younger than 5 years in underdeveloped countries. *Healthy People 2030* and the Institute of Medicine (IOM) advocate a focal role for the United States in increasing the global capacity for establishing an infectious disease surveillance system to protect U.S. national security and to prevent the cross-border spread of diseases.

FIGURE 13.3

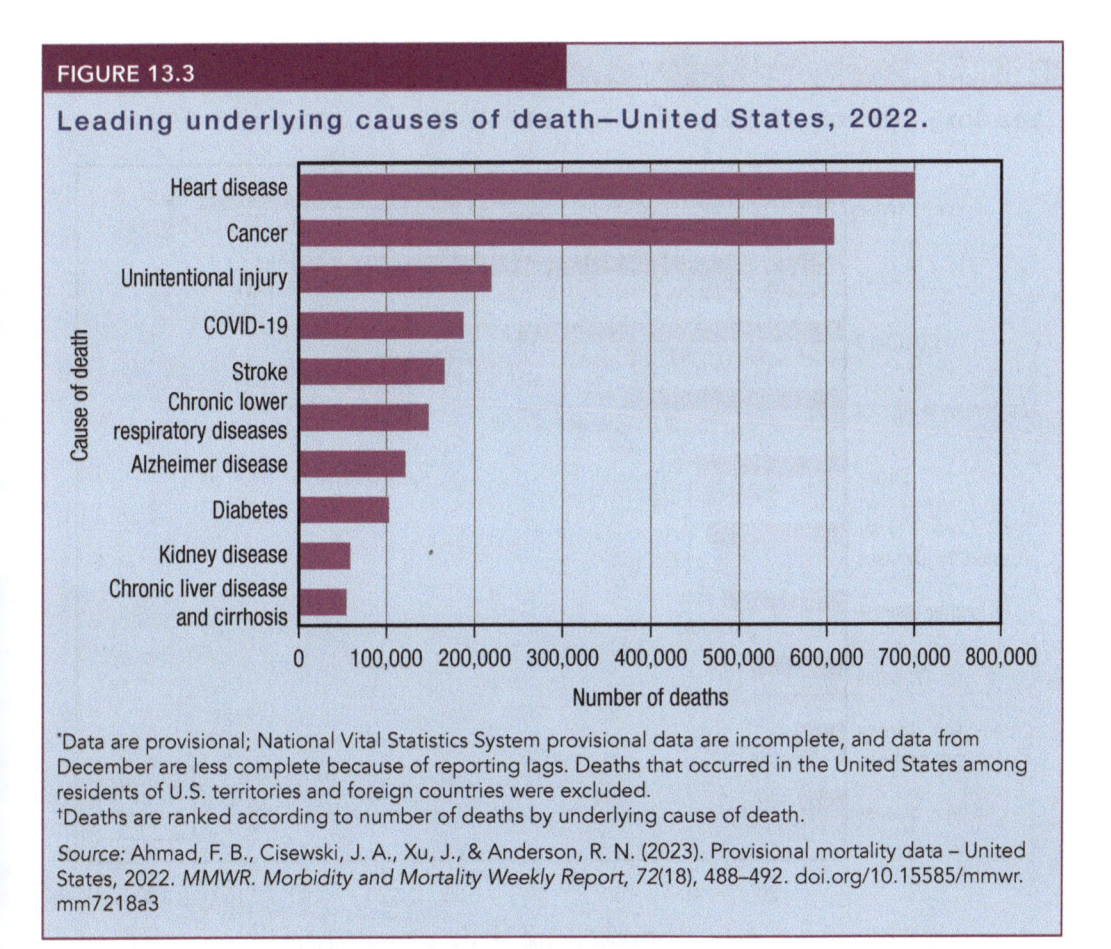

Leading underlying causes of death—United States, 2022.

Cause of death	Number of deaths (approx.)
Heart disease	~700,000
Cancer	~600,000
Unintentional injury	~225,000
COVID-19	~190,000
Stroke	~165,000
Chronic lower respiratory diseases	~145,000
Alzheimer disease	~120,000
Diabetes	~100,000
Kidney disease	~55,000
Chronic liver disease and cirrhosis	~55,000

*Data are provisional; National Vital Statistics System provisional data are incomplete, and data from December are less complete because of reporting lags. Deaths that occurred in the United States among residents of U.S. territories and foreign countries were excluded.
†Deaths are ranked according to number of deaths by underlying cause of death.

Source: Ahmad, F. B., Cisewski, J. A., Xu, J., & Anderson, R. N. (2023). Provisional mortality data – United States, 2022. *MMWR. Morbidity and Mortality Weekly Report, 72*(18), 488–492. doi.org/10.15585/mmwr.mm7218a3

Many U.S. government agencies provide funding, human resources, and technical support to international health agencies and initiatives, including the UN's *Millennium Development Goals* (MDGs), WHO *Global Polio Eradication Initiative*, PEPFAR, PMI, neglected tropical diseases (such as Ebola), and tobacco use. The U.S. administration's health strategy recognizes communicable diseases as a leading cause of mortality globally. The CDC has invested heavily to help partner countries improve health outcomes through strengthened health systems, with a particular focus on eradicating vaccine-preventable diseases and improving the health of women, newborns, and children.

The COVID-19 pandemic serves as an example of how important it is for the United States to work with multiple organizations to protect the health of the American people. On March 11, 2020, the WHO declared COVID-19 a pandemic. The pandemic quickly exposed the level of worldwide unpreparedness to deal with such an outbreak and had a devastating impact on the economy and educational and health systems in the United States. In short order, public life came to a halt as businesses, schools, and institutions were shuttered. Social distancing and masking guidelines were imposed, travel bans and restrictions went into effect, robust screening was instituted, and proof of being COVID-19-free was required for entry as well as exits in countries around the world. Yet, the United States fared worse than most countries, reporting one of the highest number

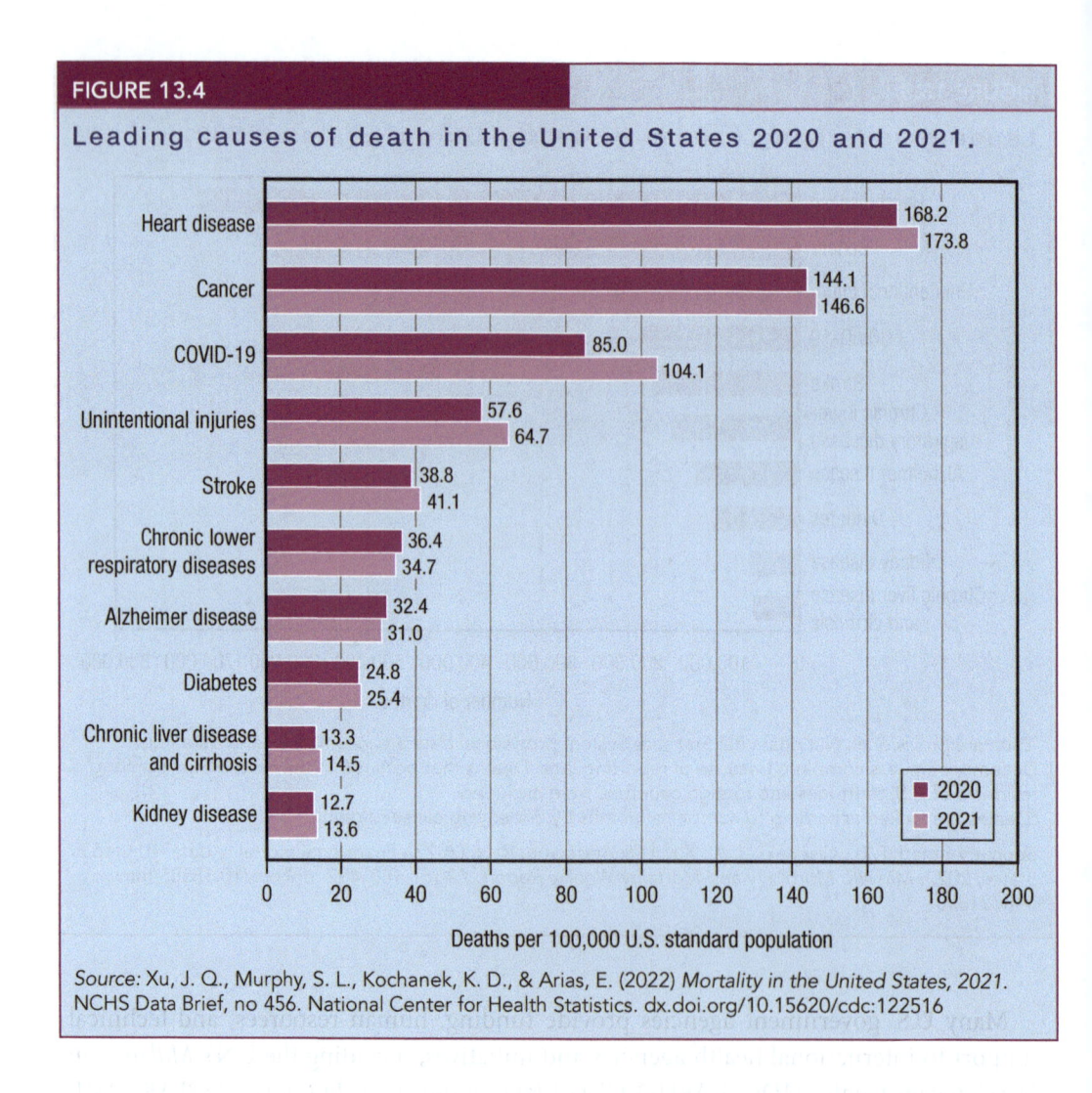

FIGURE 13.4

Leading causes of death in the United States 2020 and 2021.

Cause	2020	2021
Heart disease	168.2	173.8
Cancer	144.1	146.6
COVID-19	85.0	104.1
Unintentional injuries	57.6	64.7
Stroke	38.8	41.1
Chronic lower respiratory diseases	36.4	34.7
Alzheimer disease	32.4	31.0
Diabetes	24.8	25.4
Chronic liver disease and cirrhosis	13.3	14.5
Kidney disease	12.7	13.6

Deaths per 100,000 U.S. standard population

Source: Xu, J. Q., Murphy, S. L., Kochanek, K. D., & Arias, E. (2022) *Mortality in the United States, 2021.* NCHS Data Brief, no 456. National Center for Health Statistics. dx.doi.org/10.15620/cdc:122516

of cases and deaths, due to the slow, uneven, decentralized response to the pandemic. In response to the resultant economic crisis, the Trump Administration signed the Coronavirus Aid, Relief, and Economic Security (CARES) Act, which provided funds to individuals, families, businesses, and local and state governments including the CDC. The biggest success was the rapid development of effective vaccines fueled by government funding and public-private partnerships. The CDC and professional associations invested in developing education programs for health practitioners to ensure the safety of clinicians, updating protocols on patient treatment, and monitoring as needed. In association with the Smithsonian Institution, the CDC has published an online "*CDC Museum COVID-19 Timeline*" at www.cdc.gov/museum/timeline/covid19.html.

In 2022, the Biden Administration released the National COVID-19 Preparedness Plan with four key goals:

1. Protect against and treat COVID-19.
2. Prepare for new variants.

3. Prevent economic and educational shutdowns.
4. Continue to vaccinate the world.

On May 5, 2023, the WHO declared COVID-19 was no longer a global health emergency, and on May 11, the United States expired the federal Public Health Emergency for the disease, lifting all COVID-19 travel restrictions.

THE UNITED STATES AND THE GLOBAL HEALTH GAP

Mortality differences among nations have been associated with various theories of health disparities between populations and countries, some of which are dependent on policy. This is an extensive list that includes socioeconomic transformation, environmental pollution, lack of an adequate social safety net, relative poverty, socioeconomic deprivation, historical and generational effects of a political heritage, regional disparities, and psychosocial stress. Other perspectives emphasize individual lifestyle such as poor health practices and violent behavior.

Average income is weakly related to mortality within wealthier countries, such as the United States. However, the relative distribution of income, rather than average income, is more strongly associated with differences in death rates within wealthy countries. This is because the uneven distribution and concentration of resources leads to a relative deprivation of some population sectors. It has been long thought that the quality of life is higher in regions with more egalitarian distributions of income, such as Scandinavia, where relative deprivation is less pronounced. An international comparison of U.S. health status with those of other high-income countries demonstrates that the United States has lower health outcomes on several indicators including infant mortality and low birth weight, injuries and homicides, adolescent pregnancy, sexually transmitted infections, HIV and AIDS, drug-related deaths, obesity, diabetes, heart disease, chronic lung disease, and disability. For example, the maternal death rate in the United States is several times higher than other high-income countries (23.8 deaths per 100,000 live births), and with Black women, the risk is three times higher than for White women. While social determinants have been considered a reason, more recently, the impact of stress and stressors on women's lives is being seen as a driver of this phenomenon (Hill et al., 2022). The most alarming recent trend is the rise in pediatric all-cause mortality rate, with an increase of 10.7% in 2020 and an additional 8.3% in 2021 (Woolf et al., 2023). The authors attribute this critical increase to firearms (50% of the increase) and to "man-made pathogens" (i.e., bullets, drugs, and automobiles).

In a comparison of the healthcare systems of 11 high-income countries across 71 performance measures, the Commonwealth Fund (2021) ranked the U.S. healthcare system last. There were four features that distinguished top-performing countries from the United States. The top performers provide universal coverage and remove cost barriers, invest in primary care systems, reduce administrative burdens, and invest in social services. Despite outspending other comparable nations on healthcare, the United States still lags on healthcare outcomes (Table 13.1). Those that can afford it receive high-quality care, but low-income and vulnerable populations lack access to affordable care,

TABLE 13.1 Healthcare System Performance Rankings of 11 High-Income Countries

	AUS	CAN	FRA	GER	NETH	NZ	NOR	SWE	SWIZ	UK	US
OVERALL RANKING	3	10	8	5	2	6	1	7	9	4	11
Access to care	8	9	7	3	1	5	2	6	10	4	11
Care process	6	4	10	9	3	1	8	11	7	5	2
Administrative efficiency	2	7	6	9	8	3	1	5	10	4	11
Equity	1	10	7	2	5	9	8	6	3	4	11
Healthcare outcomes	1	10	6	7	4	8	2	5	3	9	11

Data: Commonwealth Fund analysis.

Source: Schneider, E. C., et al., Mirror, mirror 2021 — reflecting poorly: health care in the U.S. compared to other high-income countries. Commonwealth Fund. doi.org/10.26099/01DV-H208

especially preventive services. This renders a sicker population with a high disease burden of chronic illnesses. A sicker population with no access to affordable care explains the high death toll of COVID-19 and the subsequent drop in the life expectancy at birth in the United States. In 2021, the U.S. life expectancy dropped to 76.1 from 77 in 2020 (CDC, 2022). See Figure 13.5.

AMERICAN NATIONAL SECURITY AND GLOBAL HEALTH

Although Americans have a comparatively poorer health status than peer countries, federal initiatives, such as *Healthy People 2030*, try to address these health disparities. *Healthy People 2030* includes the global health goal of strengthening U.S. national security and protecting the well-being of its people by preventing, detecting, and responding to public health events worldwide. The U.S. government, through USAID and the CDC, actively collaborates with global health agencies like the UN and the WHO, participating in global, regional, and country-specific public health programs. In addition, PEPFAR and PMI are two successful programs that have significantly impacted the incidence and prevalence of HIV/AIDS and malaria. The U.S. Department of Health and Human Services (HHS) launched the GHI in 2009 to integrate multiple government programs with global partners, as well as to cooperate with the WHO in health promotion and disease prevention efforts.

The Foreign Assistance Act of 1961, supported by President Kennedy, formed the USAID from several post-World War II foreign assistance programs. The mission of USAID is to work with governmental and nongovernmental agencies, as well as the military, providing foreign assistance to resolve and prevent instability or active conflicts around the world. USAID works to ensure domestic security by investing in health systems, democratic institutions, and agricultural advances (USAID, n.d.). It has spearheaded U.S. technical and financial aid to increase health and economic self-sufficiency in the developing world through polio eradication, family planning

FIGURE 13.5

Life expectancy in the United States at birth and at age 65 for years 2020 and 2021.

Category	2020	2021
At birth, Both sexes	77.0	76.4
At birth, Male	74.2	73.5
At birth, Female	79.9	79.3
At age 65, Both sexes	18.5	18.4
At age 65, Male	17.0	17.0
At age 65, Female	19.8	19.7

Note: Access data table at www.cdc.gov/nchs/data/databriefs/db456.pdf

Source: Xu, J. Q., Murphy, S. L., Kochanek, K. D., & Arias, E. (2022) *Mortality in the United States, 2021.* NCHS Data Brief, no 456. National Center for Health Statistics. dx.doi.org/10.15620/cdc:122516

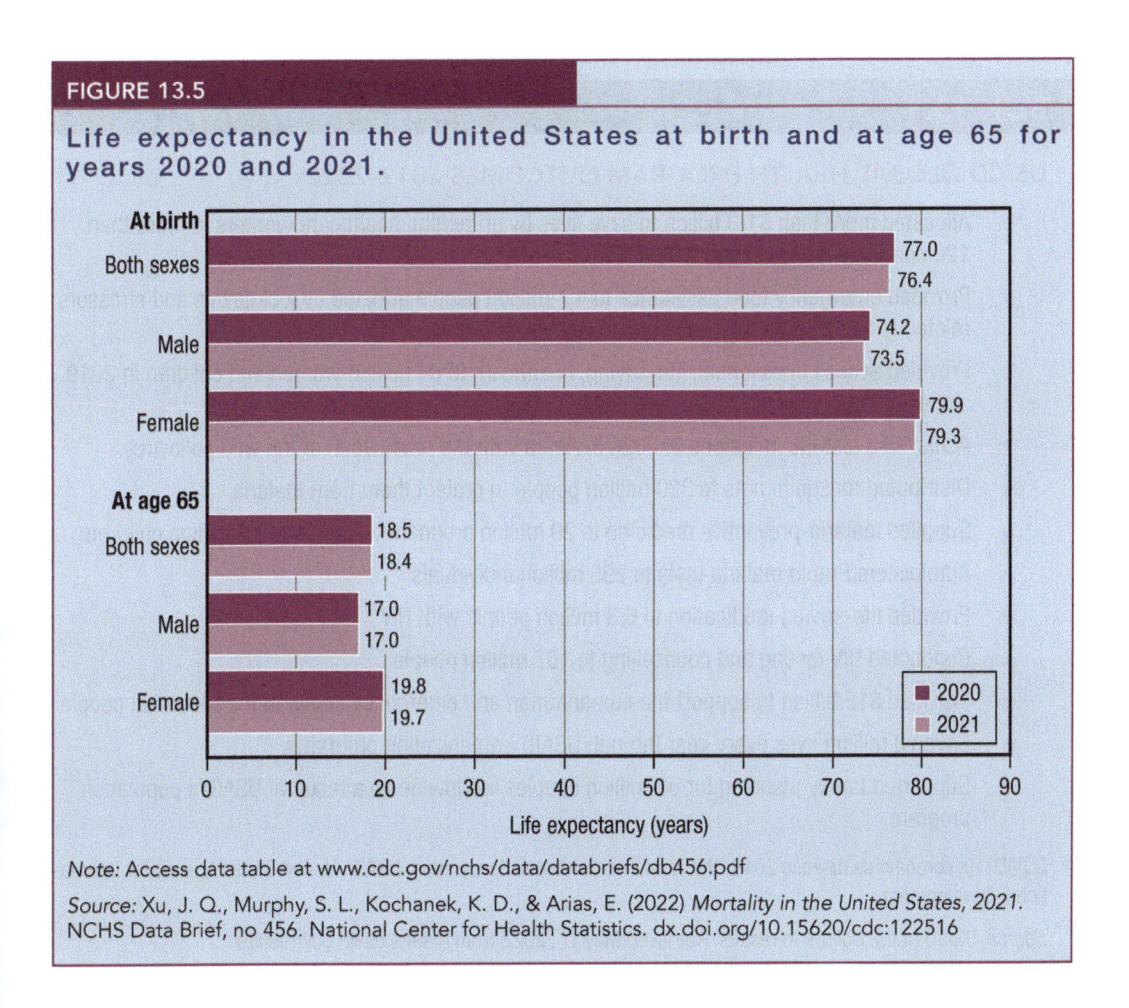

(FP), and maternal and child health programs. Historically, USAID has focused primarily on preventing hunger, promoting women's education and health, and population planning around the world as a means to curtail political conflicts. These efforts have also entailed supporting free market economic growth, nongovernmental organizations (NGOs), and antipoverty programs. USAID, as the main government agency tasked with ending extreme poverty and building democracy abroad, has been responsible for helping to rebuild former war zones such as Afghanistan and Iraq by building social safety nets with healthcare and education programs in the region (USAID, n.d.). Box 13.1 enumerates some of the successful results USAID has achieved through investments in global health.

APRNs should be aware that U.S. global health initiatives fluctuate over time due to differing views and political philosophies. For example, although the United States is the largest donor to FP and reproductive health (RH) in the world, funding particulars are impacted by U.S. policies. For example, the Mexico City policy was first issued by President Reagan in 1984. This policy required foreign NGOs to certify that they would not perform or actively promote abortion as a method of FP with their own non-U.S. funds as a condition of receiving U.S. FP assistance (prior to this, only U.S. funding could not be used). The Mexico City policy was rescinded by President Clinton, reinstated

> ### BOX 13.1
>
> #### USAID GLOBAL HEALTH PROGRAM OUTCOMES 2019–2022
>
> - Allocated more than $1.3 billion to save lives by protecting healthcare workers in more than 120 countries during COVID-19 pandemic
> - Provided emergency food assistance to 4.7 million people affected by lockdowns and stressors related to COVID-19
> - Provided access to essential, life-saving, healthcare to 84 million women and children in 2019 alone
> - Achieved a historic milestone in 2020 in Africa with the eradication of the wild poliovirus
> - Distributed mosquito nets to 320 million people to protect them from malaria
> - Supplied malaria-preventive medicine to 20 million pregnant women and 14 million children
> - Administered rapid malaria tests to 295 million individuals
> - Provided life-saving medication to 6.3 million people with HIV
> - Conducted HIV testing and counselling to 167 million people
> - Provided $15 billion to support the humanitarian and emergency needs of the Ukrainian people
> - Saved 3 million lives every year through USAID immunization programs
> - Supported family planning for 50 million couples worldwide as a result of USAID's population program
>
> COVID-19, coronavirus disease 2019; HIV, human immunodeficiency virus; USAID, United States Agency for International Development.
>
> *Source*: USAID (n.d.). Dollars to results. Retrieved May 15, 2023 from results.usaid.gov/results

by President G. W. Bush, and again rescinded by President Obama. In 2017, President Trump reinstated the policy and dramatically expanded it, renaming it the "Protecting Life in Global Health Assistance" (PLGHA). This policy extended the restrictions to almost all U.S. global health assistance, including support for PEPFAR; PMI; maternal and child health programs; and even water, sanitation, and hygiene programs. Because it now strictly restricted agencies from even "mentioning" abortion, it quickly became known as the "global gag rule." It had a worldwide devastating effect not only on women's health but also on healthcare access and services in general. In 2021, President Biden rescinded the Mexico City policy (KFF, 2021).

THE WORLD HEALTH ORGANIZATION

In 1945, diplomats throughout the world met to form the UN. A key discussion point was the need to set up a global health organization. The WHO was created in 1946 to find solutions for post-World War II Europe. Any member country of the UN can be a member of the WHO. The WHO, recognizing that international collaboration could control infectious diseases better than any single country, spearheaded the establishment of International Health Regulations (IHR) which delineates the legal framework for global public health security (WHO, 2023a). The WHO defines *global public health security* as "the activities required, both proactive and reactive, to minimize the danger and impact of acute public health events that endanger people's health across geographical regions and international boundaries" (WHO, 2023b).

The IHR provides an overarching legal framework that defines countries' rights and obligations in handling public health events and emergencies that have the potential to cross borders. The goals of the IHR are to promote a collective defense against the international spread of disease and population health emergencies by addressing diplomatic, political, economic, trade, and business interests. The IHR also lists diseases for mandatory reporting by all countries (e.g., polio, smallpox, etc.); specifies responses to radioactive, nuclear, or chemical emergencies; encourages global cooperation in science and technology; and recommends increased workforce and laboratory capacity.

The WHO manages global disease registries, databases, and classification of diseases that are used by members, including the United States. In order to maintain comparable definitions of health indicators, the WHO, with the agreement of member countries, developed Nomenclature Regulations in 1967. The regulations standardize nomenclature with respect to morbidity and mortality and established globally consistent coding, age groupings, territorial regions, and languages for the compilation and publication of health information. All members of the WHO have agreed to use the same nomenclature to collect and publish annual data.

The *International Classification of Diseases (ICD)* standardizes diagnostic categories and is used globally to track the incidence and prevalence of disease; in the United States, it is also used to consistently code billing for services. The 11th revision of the *ICD* (ICD-11) came into effect in January 2022 and is available for use at icd.who.int/en. The WHO included the International Classification for Nursing Practice (ICNP) in 1996; it was last updated in 2022. The ICNP is a classification system that improves communication among nurses from different countries through standard language. It describes nursing practice in institutional and noninstitutional environments. The ICNP is designed to enable comparisons of nursing data across countries. It includes nursing diagnoses, nurse-sensitive patient outcomes, and nursing interventions. It also facilitates international nursing research and the promulgation of health policy (ICN, 2023).

The ICNP is copyrighted by the International Council of Nurses (ICN), which ensures the integrity of the classification system. The ICN maintains collaboration with other systems of classification to facilitate cross mapping of vocabularies and interoperability. The ICN indicates that it has a number of formal agreements to best represent the nursing domain and promote semantic interoperability. The International Health Terminology Standards Development Organization (IHTSDO) and the ICN engaged in a formal agreement to ensure that nursing requirements are adequately captured within the Systematized Nomenclature of Medicine-Clinical Terms (SNOMED CT). Under its agreement with ICN, SNOMED International now manages, produces, releases, and distributes ICNP as part of SNOMED CT. ICN retains ownership of ICNP and continues to define and revise its content. The ICNP 2022 codes mapped with SNOMED CT may be downloaded from www.icn.ch/what-we-do/projects/ehealth/icnp-download/icnp-download.

BOX 13.2

THE UNITED NATIONS MILLENNIUM DEVELOPMENT GOALS FOR IMPROVING THE HEALTH STATUS OF COUNTRIES

1. Eradicate extreme poverty and hunger.
2. Achieve universal primary education.
3. Promote gender equality and empower women.
4. Reduce child mortality.
5. Improve maternal health.
6. Combat HIV/AIDS, malaria, and other diseases.
7. Ensure environmental sustainability.
8. Develop a global partnership for development.

Note: The MDGs came to an end in 2015 and are now superseded by the SDGs.

Source: From World Health Organization. (2023c). *Millennium development goals (MDGs).* Retrieved from www.who.int/news-room/fact-sheets/detail/millennium-development-goals-(mdgs)

THE UNITED NATIONS MILLENNIUM DEVELOPMENT GOALS

The MDGs (Box 13.2) and targets were articulated by the UN Millennium Declaration of 2000 and was signed by 189 countries, including 147 heads of state and governments and at least 23 international organizations. The MDGs included eight goals that reaffirmed the commitment of individual nations to a collective responsibility for human dignity, equality, and equity (UN General Assembly, 2000). The goals and targets were interrelated, and members agreed to achieve the MDGs by 2015. UN members provided financial support to achieve MDG-targeted outcomes by the set date.

The eight MDGs, which ranged from halving extreme poverty rates to halting the spread of HIV/AIDS and providing universal primary education, formed a blueprint agreed to by all the world's countries and all the world's leading development institutions. They galvanized unprecedented efforts to meet the needs of the world's poorest. The WHO worked with its partners to follow the prescriptions of the UN MDGs by organizing global strategies and setting priorities to improve health status across countries. *The Millennium Development Goals Report 2014*, approved in New York on July 7, 2014, summarized the assessment of global and regional progress toward meeting the MDGs. In comparison with the initial 2000 assessment, UN member countries reported significant improvement across all goals by 2014, but continued work was required to fully meet the 2015 and post-2015 development agenda. Since the achievement of the MDGS in 2015, the UN continues to work with governments, civil society, and other partners to carry on with an ambitious post-2015 development agenda.

> **BOX 13.3**
>
> **THE UNITED NATIONS SUSTAINABLE DEVELOPMENT GOALS**
> 1. No poverty
> 2. Zero hunger
> 3. Good health and well-being
> 4. Quality education
> 5. Gender equality
> 6. Clean water and sanitation
> 7. Affordable and clean energy
> 8. Decent work and economic growth
> 9. Industry, innovation, and infrastructure
> 10. Raise your voice against discrimination
> 11. Sustain cities and communities
> 12. Responsible production and consumption
> 13. Climate action
> 14. Life below waters (clean oceans)
> 15. Life on land (environmental protection)
> 16. Peace, justice, and strong institutions (use your right to elect your county and community leaders)
> 17. Partnerships for the goals (SDGs in action)
>
> SDG, sustainable development goals.
>
> *Source:* United Nations (n.d.b). *The 17 goals.* Retrieved May 17, 2023 from sdgs.un.org/goals

SUSTAINABLE DEVELOPMENT GOALS AND PLANETARY HEALTH

As the MDGs era came to a conclusion in 2015, the UN launched the bold and transformative 2030 Agenda for Sustainable Development, with 17 Sustainable Development Goals (SDG) at its core (Box 13.3). It was adopted by all UN Member States in September 2015. Included in these SDGs or Global Goals are a series of ambitious objectives and targets to end extreme poverty and hunger, fight inequality and injustice, and tackle climate change by 2030. This echoes the concept that global health is not an island but a part of a matrix for the sustainability of the planet. The new Agenda calls on all countries, developed and developing, to begin efforts to achieve 17 SDGs by 2030. "The seventeen sustainable development goals are our shared vision of humanity and a social contract between the world's leaders and the people," said UN Secretary-General Ban Ki-moon. "They are a to-do list for people and planet, and a blueprint for success" (UN, n.d.c).

The SDGs acknowledge that climate change is a threat to human health and that safeguarding planetary health is a global health priority. Our natural life support systems such as fresh water, arable land, clean air, and clean oceans are changing, and this impacts our health and drives the global burden of disease. The Rockefeller-Lancet Commission (Whitmee et al., 2015) warned that the degradation of these natural systems threatens health gains made in the last century. Based on this report, the Planetary Health Alliance (PHA) was founded in 2016. PHA defines *planetary health* as "a solutions-oriented, transdisciplinary field and social movement focused on analyzing and addressing the effects of human disruptions to the Earth's natural systems on human health and all life on Earth" (PHA, n.d.). PHA is currently composed of over 350 universities, organizations, and government agencies from over 60 countries committed to addressing global environmental change and its impact on human health. PHA disseminates the latest planetary health research; develops educational resources; and provides planetary health information and solutions to the general public, private sector, and policymakers.

The world paused in 2020 with the COVID-19 pandemic. Many saw the pandemic as a turning point, serving as a moment of transition for humanity. In 2021, PHA issued the São Paulo Declaration on Planetary Health, a call to action that outlines the work needed to optimize the health and well-being of all people and the planet (Meyers et al., 2023). The declaration charts a path forward to support a more equitable and resilient post-pandemic world. There is a push to reimagine the way we design and live within nature and with each other and in communities. Such a paradigm shift requires immediate attention and participation of every sector, every community, and every individual.

These declarations all advocate for patient-centered policies, including public access to health services as a human right and the integration of solutions and services within communities. The planetary health framework is reflected in the AACN *Essentials* which call for an understanding of the impact of climate change on population health and promoting advocacy efforts to ensure social and environmental justice and equitable health outcomes for all (AACN, 2021 Domain 3b, 35, 36). Planetary changes affect the health of vulnerable populations disproportionately. The poor and people of color are more likely to be living in spaces with commercial hazards and higher levels of soil, water, and air pollution (LeClair & Potter, 2022). Besides advocating for clean water, clean air, and food security for their vulnerable patients, the APRN should also advocate for public health infrastructure and policies that will protect the air, water, food, and green spaces for all (Kurth & Potter, 2022). In addition to implementing green strategies in their own practice, APRNs should assume leadership roles in transitioning institutions to reduce waste and energy consumption. It is important to educate patients and communities about the connection between a sick planet and sick patients. And as proposed in *the Essentials*, the APRN should foster population health by creating action plans and strengthening patient preparedness for public health emergencies.

WORLD HEALTH ORGANIZATION COLLABORATING CENTERS

The WHO has a network of over 800 collaborating centers each with a unique focus. WHO Collaborating Centers (CCs) are institutions such as universities, laboratories, research institutes, hospitals, ministries, or national academies which are designated by the Director-General to carry out activities in support of the Organization's programs.

> **BOX 13.4**
>
> **WHO EVALUATION TERMS OF REFERENCE OUTPUTS BETWEEN U.S. SCHOOLS OF NURSING COLLABORATING CENTERS AND THE WHO**
>
> - Health workforce information and knowledge base strengthened, and country capacities for policy analysis, planning, implementation, information sharing, and research built up
> - Technical support provided to member states, with a focus on those facing severe health workforce difficulties in order to improve the production, distribution, skill mix, and retention of the health workforce
> - Human resource policies and practices in place to attract and retain top talent, promote learning and professional development, manage performance, and foster ethical behavior
> - Management and organization of integrated, population-based health service delivery through public and nonpublic providers and networks improved, reflecting the primary healthcare strategy; scaling up coverage, equity, quality, and safety of personal and population-based health services; and enhancing health outcomes
>
> WHO, World Health Organization.
>
> *Source:* From World Health Organization. (n.d.d.). *World Health Organization Collaborating Centres*. Retrieved from apps.who.int/whocc/List.aspx?cc_code=USA&

For the Americas, the Pan American Health Organization (PAHO) collaborates with the WHO to establish a robust group of centers that focus on a variety of subjects. Each PAHO/WHO CC cooperates with a specified technical area, according to terms of reference to carry out research, assisting in the development of PAHO/WHO guidelines, gathering and analyzing data, disseminating information, providing training courses, standardizing terminology, or providing technical advice to the Organization to provide more information about nursing.

The WHO has formed CCs with select schools of nursing in the United States (WHO, n.d.b). These CCs bring together experts to solve problems in nursing; to address chronic and communicable diseases, nutrition, mental health, and other areas; and to share data, outcomes, and resolutions with UN member countries. The U.S. schools of nursing have agreed to produce a variety of outputs as part of their collaboration agreement with the WHO (Box 13.4). The U.S. schools of nursing WHO CCs each focus on such specific themes as clinical training in health promotion, nursing knowledge implementation and dissemination, international nursing development in primary healthcare, and clinical training in home care nursing.

These collaboration initiatives (Table 13.2) promote the work of U.S. nurses in (a) international NGOs focusing on health, (b) best practices in achieving the MDGs and SDGs, (c) capacity building of nursing human resources, (d) capacity building in nursing education for primary care, (e) training in disease prevention methods, and (f) supporting nurse educational programs in home care and self-management of chronic diseases (WHO, n.d.d.). These issues are important for the APRN to consider when planning effective health delivery programs focusing on the individual and

TABLE 13.2 WHO Collaborating Centers With Schools of Nursing (Active [Variable] 2023–2027)

INSTITUTION	TITLE	TERMS OF REFERENCE
University of Pennsylvania Philadelphia, PA	WHO Collaborating Center for Nursing and Midwifery Leadership	• Support PAHO/WHO's efforts to increase knowledge and understanding of maternal health and mortality. • Support PAHO/WHO to build capacity in nursing education. • Support PAHO/WHO to strengthen nursing research under the leadership of PAHO/WHO.
University of Alabama at Birmingham Birmingham, AL	WHO Collaborating Center for International Nursing	• Support PAHO/WHO's efforts to strengthen the quality of nursing education and practice based on Universal Access to Health, Universal Health Coverage, and Primary Health Care. • Support the Organization in its activities to strengthen the availability and dissemination of knowledge resources that build capacity and leadership for nurse and midwife educators.
Columbia University New York, NY	WHO Collaborating Center for Advanced Practice Nursing	• Support the Organization's efforts to strengthen human resources through the training of advanced practice nursing. • Support the Organization's efforts to strengthen human resources through the development of nursing and midwifery research and training. • Support the Organization's efforts to build capacity of human resources for health development with expanded knowledge and application of digital health in nursing and midwifery.
University of Michigan Ann Arbor, MI	WHO Collaborating Center for Research and Clinical Training in Health Promotion Nursing	• Support PAHO/WHO in disseminating experiences about evidence-based practices of health promotion related to maternal home strategies and nurse and midwifery personnel. • Provide technical support to PAHO/WHO in strengthening and building nursing capacity in training, quality of care, and communication of data related to the profession.
New York University New York, NY	WHO Collaborating Center in Gerontological Nursing Education	• Support PAHO/WHO in building interprofessional workforce capacity using the ICOPE guidelines to strengthen health system-based integrated care for older persons including promoting healthy aging, managing chronic disease, teaching self-care for older persons, and other priority issues for healthy aging identified by PAHO/WHO. • Support PAHO/WHO in building the capacity of interprofessional providers to document and assess data about the implementation and outcomes of ICOPE evidence-based practices that can inform decisions about services to address aging and the health of older adults. • Support PAHO/WHO to increase the capacity of the healthcare workforce to meet dependence of care needs of older adults living in the communities.

(continued)

TABLE 13.2 WHO Collaborating Centers With Schools of Nursing (Active [Variable] 2023–2027) *(continued)*

INSTITUTION	TITLE	TERMS OF REFERENCE
University of Miami Miami, FL	WHO Collaborating Center for Nursing Human Resources Development and Patient Safety	• Support PAHO/WHO in its efforts to develop and strengthen nursing education leadership competencies, with a focus on training program development in nursing and patient safety. • Support the dissemination of information and share knowledge regarding patient safety to enhance nursing workforce development and technical expertise under the direction of PAHO/WHO. • Support the development and strengthening of nursing workforce development, patient safety, and health disparities.
University of North Carolina Chapel Hill, NC	WHO Collaborating Center in Quality and Safety Education in Nursing and Midwifery	• Support the Organization in its efforts to strengthen nursing, interprofessional training, and collaborative practice activities with a focus on leadership and quality of care. • Support in the development and dissemination of training, best practices, and research to inform evidence-based practice and collaboration in nursing and midwifery quality of care under the leadership of PAHO/WHO.

ICOPE, Integrated Care for Older People; PAHO, Pan American Health Organization; WHO, World Health Organization.

Source: From World Health Organization. (n.d.d). *World Health Organization Collaborating Centres.* Retrieved from apps.who.int/whocc/Default.aspx

community levels and ensuring that a safety net includes culturally competent health interventions.

The U.S. Surgeon General's Goals of 2000 identified three broad areas that influence population health status and that require public policy and nursing intervention: (a) health practices or health promotion (decreasing risk factors, personal habits such as smoking, lack of physical exercise, poor diet, alcohol abuse), (b) ecological factors or health protection (decreasing occupational and environmental toxic exposures, decreasing accidents), and (c) medical care factors or preventive health services (increasing access to services such as prenatal care, infant programs, FP, hypertension control) (Campbell, 2004). These goals are reiterated in the macropopulation health indicators of *Healthy People 2030* and the SDGs of the UN, and progress has already been made in measuring and addressing these concepts of health inequity and inequality. The APRN can further contribute to the monitoring of inequity in health, as a part of population health practice. With nurse leadership, the lessons learned from the application of effective health strategies in different countries can be shared with interprofessional teams in the United States and international communities.

IMPLICATIONS FOR ADVANCED PRACTICE NURSING

The number of advanced practice nursing programs and APRNs has grown exponentially in the last few decades, both nationally and globally. Nursing has become increasingly more active in global health programs by expanding interprofessional and interdependent collaborations. Global health is an essential component in APRN education and practice. Many schools of nursing have formed GHIs to strengthen culturally sensitive nursing education domestically. APRNs work as educators, policymakers, and clinicians in a variety of communities, with different cultural and ethnic groups, as well as with populations that spend extended time in other countries, such as veterans (National League for Nursing [NLN], 2022). Such programs promote a deeper understanding, in APRN practice, of the complex political, economic, and social factors that affect an individual's health in a community context.

The WHO declared 2020 the Year of the Nurse and Midwives to acknowledge the important work that nurses do globally and to recognize the 200th birthday of Florence Nightingale. The year-long effort celebrated the work of nurses and midwives, highlighted the challenging conditions they often face, and advocated for increased investments in the nursing and midwifery workforce. The WHO decision was made in 2019, well before the onset of COVID-19, which thrust the profession into the pandemic front lines. The impact of COVID-19 was acutely felt by nurses, especially newly graduated nurses and new APRNs. Nurses were faced with challenges in providing care as well as personal concerns of bringing the virus home. This epidemic claimed more nurses' lives than lives of other healthcare workers. The stressful situations not only affected their personal health but also their mental health. The pandemic highlighted the need for advanced practice nurses as well, as many states instituted emergency measures to expand the role of the nurse practitioner (Stucky et al., 2021). Although the opportunity to practice at the top of their license is only temporary, there is a push to convince the public and the authorities that a nationwide fully independent practice authority will lead to a more efficient and effective healthcare system. Unsurprisingly, the existence of the advanced practice nurse role is more prevalent in countries with low physician density, suggesting that greater professional autonomy for nurses could be a policy response to mitigate physician shortages.

In the future, nurses, including APRNs, will find themselves more and more often in the position of being asked to form strategic partnerships with public and private organizations to strengthen health systems and to deliver culturally competent healthcare. The NLN formed the International Nursing Education, Services, and Accreditation (INESA) joint task force with the NLN Accreditation Commission (NLNAC). This evolved into the Accreditation Commission for Education in Nursing (ACEN). INESA coordinates exchanges between nurse educators from the United States and around the world and supports the Nursing Education Network of the ICN (NLN, 2022). INESA also promotes educating nurses as an ethnic and culturally diverse workforce to meet the challenge of a worldwide nursing shortage and increased migration across nations. The ACEN serves as a consultant on accreditation issues of nursing education programs in different countries (ACEN, n.d.).

International activities have expanded for nursing faculty to include curriculum development, international collaboration in research, presentations and publications, consulting in hospital administration, and clinical expertise. Applying U.S. models, concepts, and theories of nursing practice in other nations are not appropriate or feasible, given varying cultural values and beliefs. Many nursing interventions, practices, licensure requirements, and policies are context specific and cannot be transferred across cultures. However, there are concepts in advanced practice that are global in nature. This would include lifelong learning philosophies and acknowledgments that nurses are vital to positive health outcomes. Medical treatments are not stand-alone products. Interprofessional efforts which are central to APRN practice are core values of quality health care.

APRNs, as primary care providers, should develop awareness of political and cultural issues that influence individual behaviors, lifestyle, risk factors, and clinical care (Liu et al., 2022). The multilevel global health model for APRN practice emphasizes cultural sensitivity in engaging in comparative effectiveness programs and interdisciplinary, interprofessional educational interchanges (Merritt & Murphy, 2019). APRNs can play a leadership role in implementing transcultural changes in healthcare; disseminating science within nursing practice; and collaborating with global partners, such as the WHO.

SUMMARY

The APRN is well positioned to contribute to the scientific international discourse on subjects related to national and global health initiatives. This chapter has discussed global health core competency models developed by CUGH and the ASPPH in collaboration with the AACN and has explained the interrelationship of these models to the AACN *Essentials*. It is well recognized that the health of a nation is predicated on its ability to have far-reaching influence on the health status of populations around the world. Although U.S. healthcare expenditures are now nearly 20% of the GDP, healthcare outcomes have not improved with rising healthcare costs. Fragmentation of care, lack of access, third-party payer systems, hospital administrative costs, and expense of health-related technologies all have been cited as reasons for the escalating cost of healthcare in this country. Furthermore, with the increase in the immigrant population within the United States and the resultant heightened cross-national border transmission of disease, advanced nursing practice programs must address and include global healthcare concepts within their curricula.

Moving beyond the notion that health outcomes are singularly related to the behaviors of the individual, research supports changing the focus of the discussion on health outcomes to include social determinants of health and factors associated with the contextual environment in which the individual resides. The constructs of social determinants of health, MDGs, and SDGs serve to provide a useful framework upon which the APRN can design and implement strategies to address the multifactorial, sociopolitical, economic, ecological, and cultural underpinnings that influence and shape population health. Similarly, the theoretical construct for the Multilevel Model of Global Health supports the approach to analyze and evaluate risk factors and treatment effectiveness at both the individual and community levels. Enhanced knowledge and understanding of the impact of GHIs on health outcomes for communities around the world provides the APRN with the tools needed to contribute to the national and international dialogues related to population health.

END-OF-CHAPTER RESOURCES

EXERCISES

EXERCISE 13.1 You are the executive director for a nurse-managed clinic in an underserved community. A large segment of the community population consists of immigrants and refugees. As the APRN in this leadership role, what resources would you use to develop policies and procedures for provision of vaccinations for COVID-19? What strategies would you implement to develop evidence-based guidelines for practice?

EXERCISE 13.2 As the program director for an APRN doctoral program of study, you are asked to develop the syllabus for a course on population and global health. Develop the course description, objectives, and weekly topical outline for a course titled "Current and Emerging Trends in Population-Based Global Health."

EXERCISE 13.3 As an APRN, you have been requested to present a paper at a national nursing conference on the design, implementation, and evaluation of a community health clinic. The audience consists of advanced practice clinicians and academicians. List the objectives for the presentation. How would you include the eight recommendations of the IOM Report "The Future of Nursing"? Develop the outline for the presentation to include concepts related to social determinants of health, healthcare access, data collection, and analyses and healthcare outcome evaluation.

EXERCISE 13.4 One of the important components of the role of the APRN is to influence public policy and to interface with lawmakers and elected officials in the design and implementation of rules and regulations impacting the health of a nation. Toward that end, how might you develop guidelines for a public policy brief on a current health issue?

> **SPRINGER PUBLISHING CONNECT** A robust set of instructor resources designed to supplement this text is located at http://connect.springerpub.com/content/book/978-0-8261-4377-8. Qualifying instructors may request access by emailing textbook@springerpub.com.

REFERENCES

Accreditation Commission for Education in Nursing. (n.d). *Mission purpose goals.* Retrieved May 15, 2023 from https://www.acenursing.org/about/mission-purpose-goals/

American Association of Colleges of Nursing. (2021). *The Essentials: Core competencies for professional nursing education.* https://www.aacnnursing.org/Portals/42/AcademicNursing/pdf/Essentials-2021.pdf

Biggerstaff, M., & Skomra, T. (2020). Nurses as immigrant advocates: A brief overview. *Online Journal of Issues in Nursing, 25*(2). https://doi.org/10.3912/OJIN.Vol25No02PPT69

Budiman, A., Tamir, C., Mora, L., & Noe-Bustamante, L. (2020, August 20). *Facts on U.S. immigrants, 2018. Statistical portrait of the foreign-born population in the United States.* Pew Research Center. https://www.pewresearch.org/hispanic/2020/08/20/facts-on-u-s-immigrants-trend-data/

Bureau of Labor Statistics. (2022, May 18). *Foreign-born workers: Labor force characteristics — 2021.* Retrieved May 15, 2023 from https://www.bls.gov/news.release/pdf/forbrn.pdf

Camarota, S. A., & Zeigler, K. (2022, October 27). *Foreign-born population hits nearly 48 million in September 2022*. Center for Immigration Studies. https://cis.org/Report/ForeignBorn-Population-Hits-Nearly-48-Million-September-2022

Carlitz, R., Yamanis, T., & Mollel, H. (2021). Coping with denialism: How street-level bureaucrats adapted and responded to COVID-19 in Tanzania. *Journal of Health Politics, Policy and Law, 46*(6), 989–1017. https://doi.org/10.1215/03616878-9349128

Centers for Disease Control and Prevention. (2022, December 8). *Mortality in the United States, 2021*. Retrieved May 14, 2023 from https://www.cdc.gov/nchs/products/databriefs/db456.htm

Consortium of Universities for Global Health. (2023). *Global health competencies toolkit*. Retrieved May 10, 2023 from https://www.cugh.org/online-tools/competencies-toolkit/

Examination and treatment for emergency medical conditions and women in labor. 42 USC § 1395dd. (2018). Retrieved May 15, 2023 from https://www.govinfo.gov/app/details/USCODE-2021-title42/USCODE-2021-title42-chap7-subchapXVIII-partE-sec1395dd

Giwa, O., Salami, B. O., & O'Rourke, T. (2020). A scoping review of nurse practitioner roles in immigrant health. *Journal for Nurse Practitioners, 16*(6), 428–432. https://doi.org/10.1016/j.nurpra.2020.03.012

Global Post (2011, December 21). *Lesotho horses help fight HIV*. Retrieved May 15, 2023 from https://theworld.org/stories/2011-12-22/lesotho-horses-help-fight-hiv

Healthy People 2030. (n.d.). *Global health*. Retrieved May 15, 2023 from https://health.gov/healthypeople/objectives-and-data/browse-objectives/global-health

Hill, L., Artiga, S., & Ranji, U. (2022, Nov 1). *Racial disparities in maternal and infant health: Current status and efforts to address them*. https://www.kff.org/racial-equity-and-health-policy/issue-brief/racial-disparities-in-maternal-and-infant-health-current-status-and-efforts-to-address-them/

Institute of Medicine. (2009). *The U.S. commitment to global health recommendations for the public and private sectors*. National Academies Press. https://www.ncbi.nlm.nih.gov/books/NBK23794/#a2001902dddd00040

International Council of Nurses. (2023) *Who we are*. Retrieved May 15, 2023 from https://www.icn.ch/who-we-are

Jacobsen, K. H., Zeraye, H. A., Bisesi, M. S., Gartin, M., Malouin, R. A., & Waggett, C. E. (2019). Master of public health global health concentration competencies: preparing culturally skilled practitioners to serve internationally, nationally, and locally. *American Journal of Public health, 109*(9), 1189–1190. https://doi.org/10.2105/AJPH.2019.305208

Kates, J., Michaud, J., Kirzinger, A., Wu, B., & Brodie, M. (2019, April 24). *Where does public opinion stand on the U.S. role in global health?* Retrieved May 16, 2023, from https://www.kff.org/global-health-policy/poll-finding/where-does-public-opinion-stand-u-s-role-global-health/

KFF. (2021, January 28). *The Mexico city policy: An explainer*. https://www.kff.org/global-health-policy/fact-sheet/mexico-city-policy-explainer/

KFF. (2023, April 13). *Key facts on deferred action for childhood arrivals (DACA)*. https://www.kff.org/racial-equity-and-health-policy/fact-sheet/key-facts-on-deferred-action-for-childhood-arrivals-daca/

Koplan, J. P., Bond, T. C., Merson, M. H., Reddy, K. S., Rodriguez, M. H., Sewankambo, N. K., & Wasserheit, J. N. (2009). Towards a common definition of global health. *The Lancet, 373*(9679), 1993–1995. https://doi.org/10.1016/S0140-6736(09)60332-9

Kurth, A., & Potter, T. (2022). The public health crisis is planetary-and nursing is crucial to addressing it. *American Journal of Public Health, 112*(S3), S259–S261. https://doi.org/10.2105/AJPH.2022.306877

LeClair, J., & Potter, T. (2022). Planetary health nursing. *The American Journal of Nursing, 122*(4), 47–52. https://doi.org/10.1097/01.NAJ.0000827336.29891.9b

Liu, T. T., Chen, M. Y., Chang, Y. M., & Lin, M. H. (2022). A preliminary study on the cultural competence of nurse practitioners and its affecting factors. *Healthcare, 10*(4), 678. https://doi.org/10.3390/healthcare10040678

Lopez, M. H., Passel, J. S., & Cohn, D. (2021, April 13). *Key facts about the changing U.S. unauthorized immigrant population*. Pew Research Center. https://www.pewresearch.org/short-reads/2021/04/13/key-facts-about-the-changing-u-s-unauthorized-immigrant-population/

McGilton, K. S., Krassikova, A., Boscart, V., Sidani, S., Iaboni, A., Vellani, S., & Escrig-Pinol, A. (2021). Nurse practitioners rising to the challenge during the coronavirus disease 2019 pandemic in long-term care homes. *The Gerontologist, 61*(4), 615–623. https://doi.org/10.1093/geront/gnab030

Merritt, L. S., & Murphy, N. L. (2019). International service-learning for nurse practitioner students: Enhancing clinical practice skills and cultural competence. *The Journal of Nursing Education, 58*(9), 548–551. https://doi.org/10.3928/01484834-20190819-10

Migration Policy Institute. (2023). *U.S. annual refugee resettlement ceilings and number of refugees admitted, 1980–present.* https://www.migrationpolicy.org/programs/data-hub/charts/us-refugee-resettlement

Migration Policy Institute. (n.d.). *Unauthorized immigration population profiles.* Retrieved May 10, 2023 from https://www.migrationpolicy.org/programs/us-immigration-policy-program-data-hub/unauthorized-immigrant-population-profiles

Naik, Y., Baker, P., Ismail, S. A., Tillmann, T., Bash, K., Quantz, D., Hillier-Brown, F., Jayatunga, W., Kelly, G., Black, M., Gopfert, A., Roderick, P., Barr, B., & Bambra, C. (2019). Going upstream—An umbrella review of the macroeconomic determinants of health and health inequalities. *BMC Public Health, 19*(1), 1678–1678. https://doi.org/10.1186/s12889-019-7895-6

National League for Nursing. (2022). *Mission and strategic plan.* Retrieved May 15, 2023 from https://www.nln.org/about/about/mission-and-strategic-plan

Osingada, C. P., & Porta, C. M. (2020). Nursing and sustainable development goals (SDGs) in a COVID-19 world: The state of the science and a call for nursing to lead. *Public Health Nursing, 37*(5), 799–805. https://doi.org/10.1111/phn.12776

Pelletier, A. R., Derado, J., Maoela, L., Lekhotsa, T., Sechache, M., & Nkuatsana, K. (2022). Impact of the DREAMS program on new HIV diagnoses in adolescent girls and young women attending antenatal care - Lesotho, 2015–2020. *MMWR. Morbidity and mortality weekly report, 71*(2), 48–51. https://doi.org/10.15585/mmwr.mm7102a3

Pew Research Center. (2023). *How temporary protected status has expanded under the Biden administration.* https://www.pewresearch.org/short-reads/2023/04/21/biden-administration-further-expands-temporary-protected-status-to-cover-afghanistan-cameroon-ukraine/

Planetary Health Alliance (n.d.). *Planetary health.* Retrieved May 17, 2023. https://www.planetaryhealthalliance.org/planetary-health

Stucky, C. H., Brown, W. J., & Stucky, M. G. (2021). COVID-19: An unprecedented opportunity for nurse practitioners to reform healthcare and advocate for permanent full practice authority. *Nursing Forum, 56*(1), 222–227. https://doi.org/10.1111/nuf.12515

The Commonwealth Fund. (2021, August 4). *Mirror, mirror 2021: Reflecting poorly. Healthcare in the U.S. compared to other high-income countries.* https://www.commonwealthfund.org/publications/fund-reports/2021/aug/mirror-mirror-2021-reflecting-poorly

The Commonwealth Fund. (2023, January 31). *U.S. health care from a global perspective, 2022: Accelerating spending, worsening outcomes.* https://www.commonwealthfund.org/publications/issue-briefs/2023/jan/us-health-care-global-perspective-2022

Trasande, L., Cronk, C., Durkin, M., Weiss, M., Schoeller, D. A., Gall, E. A., Hewitt, J. B., Carrel, A. L., Landrigan, P. J., & Gillman, M. W. (2009). Environment and obesity in the national children's study. *Environmental Health Perspectives, 117*(2), 159–166. https://doi.org/10.1289/ehp.11839

Tsiouris, F., Hartsough, K., Poimbouef, M., Raether, C., Farahani, M., Ferreira, T., Kamanzi, C., Maria, J., Nshimirimana, M., Mwanza, J., Njenga, A., Odera, D., Tenthani, L., Ukaejiofo, O., Vambe, D., Fazito, E., Patel, L., Lee, C., Michaels-Strasser, S., & Rabkin, M. (2022). Rapid scale-up of COVID-19 training for frontline health workers in 11 African countries. *Human Resources for Health, 20*(1), 43–43. https://doi.org/10.1186/s12960-022-00739-8

UNHCR The UN Refugee Agency. (2023). *Refugee data finder.* Retrieved May 18, 2023 from https://www.unhcr.org/refugee-statistics/

United Nations. (n.d.a). *The universal declaration of human rights.* Retrieved from http://www.un.org/en/documents/udhr

United Nations. (n.d.b). *The 17 goals.* Retrieved May 17, 2023 from https://sdgs.un.org/goals

United Nations. (n.d.c). *We can end poverty.* Retrieved May 17, 2023 from http://www.un.org/millenniumgoals

United States Agency for International Development. (n.d.). *Global health.* Retrieved May 16, 2023 from https://www.usaid.gov/global-health

U.S. Citizenship and Immigration Services. (2022, October 26). *Refugees.* Retrieved May 10, 2023 from http://www.uscis.gov/humanitarian/refugees-asylum/refugees

Ward, N. & Batalova, J. (2023, March 14). Frequently requested statistics on immigrants and immigration in the United States. *Migration Policy Institute.* Retrieved May 15, 2023 from https://www.migrationpolicy.org/article/frequently-requested-statistics-immigrants-and-immigration-united-states

Whitmee, S., Haines, A., Beyrer, C., Boltz, F., Capon, A. G., de Souza Dias, B. F., Ezeh, A., Frumkin, H., Gong, P., Head, P., Horton, R., Mace, G. M., Marten, R., Myers, S. S., Nishtar, S., Osofsky, S. A., Pattanayak, S. K., Pongsiri, M. J., Romanelli, C., ... Yach, D. (2015). Safeguarding human health in the anthropocene epoch: report of the Rockefeller Foundation—Lancet Commission on planetary health. *The Lancet, 386*(10007), 1973–2028. https://doi.org/10.1016/S0140-6736(15)60901-1

Woolf, S. H., Wolf, E. R., & Rivara, F. P. (2023). The New crisis of increasing all-cause mortality in US children and adolescents. *JAMA: the Journal of the American Medical Association, 329*(12), 975–976. https://doi.org/10.1001/jama.2023.3517

World Health Organization. (2023a). *International health regulations.* Retrieved May 17, 2023 from https://www.who.int/health-topics/international-health-regulations#tab=tab_1

World Health Organization. (2023b). *Health security.* Retrieved May 17, 2023 from https://www.who.int/health-topics/health-security#tab=tab_1

World Health Organization. (2023c). *Millennium development goals (MDGS).* Retrieved from https://www.who.int/news-room/fact-sheets/detail/millennium-development-goals-(mdgs)

World Health Organization. (n.d.d.). *World Health Organization Collaborating Centres.* Retrieved May 17, 2023 from http://apps.who.int/whocc/List.aspx?cc_code=USA&

Xu, J. Q., Murphy, S. L., Kochanek, K. D., & Arias, E. (2022) *Mortality in the United States, 2021.* NCHS Data Brief, no 456. National Center for Health Statistics. https://dx.doi.org/10.15620/cdc:122516

INDEX

AACN (American Association of Colleges of Nursing), 2, 265
AAFA (Asthma and Allergy Foundation of America), 173
AAN (American Academy of Nursing), 191
ABN (call abandonment rate), 226
absolute risk reduction (ARR), 79
ACA (Affordable Care Act), 3, 252, 266–267
Accountable Care Organization (ACO), 213, 252–253
   applicant to meet requirements, 253
accreditation, 245–260, 330
   offers healthcare providers opportunity to qualify and quantify, 260
   program, 236
Accreditation Commission for Education in Nursing (ACEN), 330
accrediting bodies, 247
   Commission on Accreditation of Rehabilitation Facilities (CARF), 247
   Community Health Accreditation Partner (CHAP), 248, 250
   Det Norske Veritas (DNV; formerly DNV-GL), 247
   Healthcare Facilities Accreditation Program (HFAP), 248
   The Joint Commission (TJC), 247
   National Committee for Quality Assurance (NCQA), 247
   Public Health Accreditation Board (PHAB), 248
   Utilization Review Accreditation Commission (URAC), 247
ACEN (Accreditation Commission for Education in Nursing), 330
ACIP (Advisory Committee on Immunization Practices), 3

ACO (Accountable Care Organization), 213, 252–253
ACS (American Cancer Society), 8, 173
actuarial method, 85, 87
administrative data, 54, 230–232, 234, 235
advanced practice nursing, implications for, 330–331
advanced practice registered nurses (APRNs), 6, 14–16, 21, 130
   academic preparation of the DNP-educated, 258
   committed a type I error, 108
   creating the plan, 258–259
   creativity in improving patient outcomes, 178
   discovers breastfeeding rates, 81
   eliminate potentially confounding factor (gender), 96
   evaluates credibility and trustworthiness, 143
   needs to be aware of both publication bias and citation bias, 111
   outcomes research in, 15
   plans to compare the patients' SLE knowledge, 134
   plans to evaluate an intervention to reduce burden, 95
   postulates that a wellness program based on PAR strategies, 134
   professional APRN competencies, 266
   role in program accreditation, 258
   sample nurse-sensitive clinical quality measures in DM, CM, and H&W programs, 224
   targets specific groups and designs interventions at multiple levels, 23
   use WWSs to make observations, 277

advanced practice registered nurses (APRNs) (cont.)
  working in a community-based clinic with a Hispanic population, 51
  works in a community that has been hard-hit by COVID-19, 24
Advisory Committee on Immunization Practices (ACIP), 3
Affordable Care Act (ACA), 3, 252, 266–267
  legislation, 3
Agency for Healthcare Research and Quality (AHRQ), 124
age-specific mortality, 83
age-specified death rate, 79
aggregate- or community-based care, 23
aggregates, defined, 7
AHA (American Heart Association), 173, 246
AHRQ (Agency for Healthcare Research and Quality), 124
alcohol, 7–8, 11, 13, 14, 28, 50, 51, 57, 114, 329
  leading cause of cancer, 8
alcohol use disorder (AUD), 7
alternative explanations, 116
Alzheimer's disease, 7
ambulatory health, 245
ambulatory-sensitive conditions (ASCs), 226
American Academy of Nursing (AAN)
  created the Edge Runners Initiative, 191
American Association of Colleges of Nursing (AACN), 2, 265
  identify 10 domains of educational content for nursing education, 245–246
  professional APRN competencies, 266
  role in improving population health in many settings, 35
American Cancer Society (ACS), 8, 173
American Civil War, 1
American Heart Association (AHA), 173, 246
American Nurses Association (ANA), 6, 15, 137
  ANA-recognized terminology and data set, 163
  developed Nursing's Safety and Quality Initiative, 52
  incorporated the ANCC as a subsidiary nonprofit organization, 255
  nursing work in burn care and prevention, 265

American Nurses Credentialing Center (ANCC), 124
  manages the Magnet® designation program, 201, 255
  requiring data entry for accreditation by programs, 124
American Public Health Association, 137, 316
American Red Cross, 1
American Society of Anesthesiologists (ASA), 149
ANA (American Nurses Association), 6, 15, 137
analytic epidemiology, 92
ANCC (American Nurses Credentialing Center), 124
antagonism, 114
antipoverty programs, 321
APRNs (advanced practice registered nurses), 6, 14–16, 21, 130
AR (attributable risk), 93
ARR (absolute risk reduction), 79
Arts and Humanities Citation Index, 137
ASA (American Society of Anesthesiologists), 149
ASA (average speed of answer), 226
ASCs (ambulatory-sensitive conditions), 226
Association of Nurses in AIDS Care, 316
Association of Schools and Programs of Public Health (ASPPH), 304
Asthma and Allergy Foundation of America (AAFA), 173
attributable risk (AR), 93
AUD (alcohol use disorder), 7
autonomy, 29–35, 225, 330
average speed of answer (ASA), 226

Baby Friendly Hospital Initiative (BFHI), 257
balanced scorecard (BSC) model, 217
barriers, 52, 59, 149, 150, 154, 164, 167–171, 186, 195, 198, 206, 218, 259, 282, 290, 292, 294, 298, 299, 308, 319
  patient factors, 170
  social media, use of, 169–170
  technical issues, 170–171
behavioral health (BH), 221, 245, 247, 254, 257, 267, 299

behavioral risk factor surveillance system, 45–46
beneficence, 29, 30, 32
best practices concept, 131, 185–187, 258, 299, 312, 327, 329
BFHI (Baby Friendly Hospital Initiative), 257
BH (behavioral health), 221, 245, 247, 254, 257, 267, 299
bias, 79, 107–109
  citation, 111
  contamination, 110
  exclusion, 109
  information, 110–112, 136, 231
  lead time, 84–85
  measurement, 110
  misclassification, 110
  overdiagnosis, 85
  publication, 111
  recall, 111, 123, 231
  reporting, 111
  selection, 109, 119
  volunteer, 109
  withdrawal, 109, 121
biostatistics, 14, 69, 256
bipartisan Dream Act of 2023, 308
Black and Hispanic infants, statistically significant decline in mortality, 5
blinding, 114–115
blogs, 166
BMI (body mass index), 44, 51, 148, 167, 177, 213
body mass index (BMI), 44, 51, 148, 167, 177, 213
Breakdown on Insurance Coverage for Children and Adults in 2022, 5

CAHPS (Consumer Assessment of Healthcare Providers and Systems), 228
call abandonment rate (ABN), 226
call center metrics, 226
cardiac patient education toolkit, 295
cardiovascular disease (CVD), 7, 9, 21, 176
CARF (Commission on Accreditation of Rehabilitation Facilities), 247
case-control studies, 94–96, 119, 122, 123, 125, 132
  calculation of OR in, 95, 123

case fatality percent, 83
case fatality rate (CFR), 79, 83
case management (CM), 211, 220, 247
case reports, 90–91
case series, 90–91
case studies
  APRN as coordinator for organ transplant program, 164
  APRN describing problem of nonventilator hospital-acquired pneumonia (NVHAP), 122
  APRN design current technology in a health system to make information available, 177
  APRN reviews and evidence-based, school-based asthma education program, 49
  APRN working as a PCP in a large medical practice for patients live with PD, 72–73
  collaborative community effort to improve awareness in the Lee County, 281–283
  use of IOWA model to improve post-stroke care transitions for, 152–153
  to work with a team to identify opportunities for improving delivery of, 206
catheter-associated urinary tract infections (CAUTIs), 250
causality, 116–117
CAUTIs (catheter-associated urinary tract infections), 250
CBP (Customs and Border Protection), 306
CCM (Chronic Care Model), 150
CDC (Centers for Disease Control and Prevention), 27
CEA (cost-effective analysis), 28
censorship, 86
Centers for Disease Control and Prevention (CDC), 27
  addressing health improvement greater impact when shared responsibility of, 269
  as community health improvement navigator, 274
  demonstrating that by tying reimbursement to quality, improvements, 214
  developed HRQOL tool, 27

Centers for Disease Control and Prevention (CDC) (*cont.*)
  estimated cigarette smoking, 73
  estimates money spent on healthcare related to diseases, 251
  Health Insurance Coverage, 5
  Internet resources support population-based nursing, 174
  polio currently spreading in war-torn countries, 316
  published an online "*CDC Museum COVID-19 Timeline*", 318
Centers for Medicare and Medicaid Services (CMS), 4, 124, 152, 199, 213, 247, 248, 268
  ACOs demonstrate same type of improvement in similar measures as Medicare Advantage health plans, 226
  ACOs designed under the Affordable Care Act (ACA), 252
  ACO the applicant meeting requirements, 253
  adopted use of HEDIS in its STAR rating program for, 223
  began to limit reimbursement to hospitals, 234
  CMS Innovation Center, 253
  functions under aegis of the U.S. Department of Health and Human Services (DHHS), 214
  Healthcare Common Procedure Coding System (HCPCS) codes, 230
  HIPAA continues to influence data management processes and, 234
  impact on healthcare in the United States since Medicare legislation in, 235
  mandated use of an agreed-upon set of questions, 227
  pharmacy measures to patients dually eligible for both Medicare and Medicaid, 226
  pharmacy programs, hemodialysis programs and, 228
  recognizes the value of self-reported data and, 232
  roadmap summarizing escalating opioid problem, 299
  source of community-level indicators, 279
  survey form by, 228
  ties reimbursement to certain key quality indicators, 199
central line-associated bloodstream infections (CLABSIs), 214, 250
Centre for Reviews and Dissemination (CRD), 140
cerebrovascular diseases, 7
certification programs, 236
cessation of exposure, 117
CFCS (conditions for coverage), 249
CFR (case fatality rate), 79, 83
CHA (community health assessment), 248, 250, 264, 269–270
Change Model, 291, 295
CHAP (Community Health Accreditation Partner), 248, 250
chat rooms, 169
checklists, 161
chest x-ray, 26
childhood obesity, 29
CHNA (community health needs assessment), 266–267
Chronic Care Model (CCM), 150
chronic conditions, 13–15, 191, 194, 223, 226, 232
chronic liver disease, 7
chronic lower respiratory diseases, 7
CHWs (community health workers), 52
cirrhosis, 7
citation bias, 111
CLABSIs (central line-associated bloodstream infections), 214, 250
claims data, 230
climate change, 325
Clinical Care Classification, 161
clinical quality, 223–224
  CM programs, 223
  common disease states managed by DM programs, 223
  STAR rating, 224
clinical questions, 131
clinical stage of disease, 71
CM (case management), 211, 220, 247
CMS (Centers for Medicare and Medicaid Services), 4, 124, 152, 199, 213, 247, 248, 268

INDEX   341

CMS STARs (Medicaid Services Five-Star Quality Rating System), 213
COBRA (Consolidated Omnibus Budget Reconciliation Act), 308
Cochrane page, 135
cohort designs, 93, 121
cohort studies, 93–94, 121
    calculation of attributable risk (AR), 93
    calculation of relative risk (RR), 93
collaboration, 22, 197, 274, 280, 310
    AACN formed an interdisciplinary collaboration ASPPH to develop, 304
    among community members, 22
    among healthcare agencies and, 266
    in critical investments led to development of vaccines for, 316
    facilitates deliberation and decision making, 256
    fosters bidirectional communication, deep understanding, and, 264
    foundation for, 265–268
    and hospital investment in community health, 267
    ICN maintains collaboration with other systems of classification to facilitate, 323
    IHI's Pathways to Population Health (P2PH) describe, 213
    initiatives promote the work of U.S. nurses in, 327–329
    needed for IRS compliance for 501(c)(3) hospitals under, 268
collaboration/community partnership, 280–281
Commission on Accreditation of Rehabilitation Facilities (CARF), 247
commitment, 31, 76, 151, 187, 196, 197, 253, 324
Commonwealth Fund, 4, 311, 319, 320
communication, 32, 50, 53, 57, 60, 185, 197, 204, 205, 271, 274, 281, 295, 298, 305, 309, 315. *See also* social media
    APRNs role in, 159–160
    basic questions engaging in strategies to, 205
    devices routinely integrated into care delivery process, 159
    ICNP classification system that improves, 323
    nonverbal communication, 205
    from nurse to PCP, 237
    patient-centered, 60
    verbal communication, 205
community, 7, 22
community advisory boards, 236–237
community-based prevention, 28
community engagement, foundation for, 265
community guide topics, and outcome examples, 50–51
community health, 21–22, 255
Community Health Accreditation Partner (CHAP), 248, 250
community health assessment (CHA), 264, 269–270
    assessment methods, 274
    assessment tools, 271–272
    CDC community health improvement navigator, 274
    community health assessment toolkit, 273
    community tool box, 272–273
    conducting assessment, 270–271
    county health rankings, 273–274
    disease and health reports, 278, 280
    focus groups, 274–275
    health department vital statistics, 278, 280
    Healthy People 2030, 272
    key informant interviews, 275–276
    participant observation, 277–278
    secondary data sources and, 278
    sources of community-level indicators, 279
    surveys, 276–277
    U.S. Census data, 278
    walking survey, 277
    windshield survey, 277
community health assessment compliance, 267–268
community health needs assessment (CHNA), 266–267
community health programs, evaluation framework for, 188, 190
community health workers (CHWs), 52
community resources, 184
comparative databases, 235–236
competence, 197
conditions for coverage (CFCS), 249

conditions of participations (COPs), 249
confounder, variable, 112
confounding, 112–113
congestive heart failure, 7, 220, 246
consequences, positive and negative, awareness of, 197
Consolidated Omnibus Budget Reconciliation Act (COBRA), 308
Consolidated Standards of Reporting Trials (CONSORT), 120
　guidelines, 120
　website, 120
CONSORT (Consolidated Standards of Reporting Trials), 120
Consortium of Universities of Global Health (CUGH), 305
　domains in defining competencies for, 305
Consumer Assessment of Healthcare Providers and Systems (CAHPS), 228
contamination bias, 110
coordination, 54, 59, 60, 151, 197, 204, 218–220, 224, 252–253
COPs (conditions of participations), 249
core business processes, 228–230
Coronavirus Aid, Relief, and Economic Security (CARES) Act, 318
coronavirus disease 2019 (COVID-19), 7, 21, 47, 117, 147–148, 166, 170, 172, 326, 330
　APRN works in a community that has been hard-hit by, 24
　Black and Hispanic people, disproportionately affected by, 60
　death toll and life expectancy at birth, 320
　development of vaccines for both Ebola and, 316
　drop in cases, 316
　emphasis on autonomy became an issue during, 35
　immigrants disproportionately affected by, 308
　impact of county-level SDOH on, 48
　leading underlying causes of death—United States, 2022, 317
　long-term outcomes, 44
　mistrust of governmental agencies on the use of vaccine, 298
　National COVID-19 Preparedness Plan, 318–319
　obesity puts people at risk for, 82
　produced many unanticipated and unprecedented changes in healthcare delivery and, 194
　refused to provide COVID-19 data to the WHO, 315
　testing center located at an international airport overbilled Medicare, 252
　training to healthcare staff in, 306
　underscored the importance of global health by demonstrating, 305
　USAID global health program outcomes 2019–2022, 322
　vaccine hesitancy and denial stressed the need for APRNs to, 309
　WHO declared COVID-19 a pandemic, 317
correlation studies, 91
cost-effective analysis (CEA), 28
cost-effectiveness ratio, 29
cost-saving intervention, 28
COVID-19 (coronavirus disease 2019), 7, 21, 47, 117, 147–148, 166, 170, 172, 326, 330
CRD (Centre for Reviews and Dissemination), 140
Crimean War, 1
cross-sectional studies, 91–92
crude death rate, 79
crude rates, standardization of, 82
CUGH (Consortium of Universities of Global Health), 305
Cumulative Index to Nursing and Allied Health Literature (CINAHL), 135–136
customer satisfaction, 226–228
Customs and Border Protection (CBP), 306
CVD (cardiovascular disease), 7, 9, 176

data, sources of, 192. *See also specific type entries*
　assembling a team, 196–197
　consumer and societal trends and demands, 194–195
　identifying key stakeholders, 195–196
　justification, 198–200
　organization level data, 193–194
　population-level data, 192–193

INDEX

databases, 123–124, 125, 132
    Cumulative Index to Nursing and Allied Health Literature (CINAHL), 135–136
    National Database of Nursing Quality Indicators® (NDNQI®), 52
data collection, 115–116
data editing, 124
data sources, 230–232
data to target populations, 7
death in the United States, causes of, 7
Deferred Action for Childhood Arrivals (DACA) program, 307
Department of Homeland Security (DHS), 306
Department of Justice (DOJ), 252
descriptive epidemiology, 76–80, 90
Det Norske Veritas (DNV), 246–248, 251
    acute care hospital accredited through, 246
    disease-specific care certifications, 254
Det Norske Veritas (DNV; formerly DNV-GL), 247
DHS (Department of Homeland Security), 306
differential misclassification, 110
diffusing innovation, tools for, 296
digital divide term, 167
DIN (disease impact number), 80
disease impact number (DIN), 80
disease management (DM) program, 134, 151, 211, 220, 246
Disease-Specific Care (DSC) Certification Program, 254
DNV (Det Norske Veritas), 246–248, 251
Doctor of Nursing Practice (DNP)-educated nurses, 258
DOJ (Department of Justice), 252
Donabedian framework, 42, 52, 212, 214–216
double-blind, 115
DREAMS (Determined, Resilient, Empowered, AIDS-free, Mentored, and Safe) program, 314

Ebola, 309, 315–317
EBP (evidence-based practice), 15, 36, 51, 53, 62, 69, 76, 107, 119, 125, 130, 150, 191, 251, 269, 290, 315, 328–329
ED (emergency department), 94, 193, 212

education, 8, 12, 16, 24–25, 40, 46, 48, 52, 58, 62, 113, 134, 149–151, 163, 166, 175, 184, 193, 256, 265, 271, 278, 281, 296, 308
effect size, 97
E-health, 177
EHR (electronic health records), 35, 160–161, 168, 215, 217, 224, 231–233, 237, 294
Electronic alerts, 177
electronic health records (EHRs), 35, 160–161, 168, 215, 217, 224, 231–233, 237, 292, 294
electronic medical record (EMR), 232
electronic resources, 173
email, 169
emergency department (ED), 94, 193, 212
Emergency Medical Treatment and Active Labor Act (EMTALA), 308–309
EMR (electronic medical record), 232
EMTALA (Emergency Medical Treatment and Active Labor Act), 308–309
epidemiological triangle, 75
epidemiology, 14, 14. 69, 69, 75, 76, 83, 86, 92, 94, 114, 187, 309
    analytic, 92
    descriptive, 76–78, 100
errors in measurement, 107–108
The Essentials of Doctoral Education for Advanced Practice Nurses, 265
establishing program need, 191–192
    common elements or themes, 191
ethics, 22, 29–35, 61, 76. 111, 118, 120, 140, 165, 169, 178, 188, 304, 305, 309, 327
ethnicity, 7
evidence. *See also* evidence-based practice (EBP)
    assessment, 137
    based care, 2, 6, 40, 130, 131, 253
    based prevention education, 8
    defined, 130
    integration into practice, 149–150
    levels with revisions to 2008 hierarchy, 142
    types of, 132
evidence-based practice (EBP), 15, 36, 51, 53, 62, 69, 76, 107, 119, 125, 130, 150, 191, 251, 269, 290, 315, 328–329
    models of, 150–151, 153–154
    online resources for, 139
    tool for, 140

e-Wellness program, 144
exclusion bias, 109

Facebook, 169
failure mode and effects analysis (FMEA), 295
Farr, William, 1
Federal agencies, 62
federally qualified health centers (FQHCs), 253
Federal Refugee Resettlement Program, 1980, 307
50 Edge Runners models, 191
FMEA (failure mode and effects analysis), 295
FQHCs (federally qualified health centers), 253
framework or model of change, 186
　12-step process, 186–187
Frontier Nursing Service (FNS), 1
functional health patterns, definition of, 162
The Future of Nursing (2010), IOM seminal work, 245

Gantt chart, 295
GDP (gross domestic product), 3–4, 331
geographical location, 7
GHI (Global Health Initiative), 312
global health, 304
　American national security and, 320–322
　first global health goal appeared in *Healthy People 2020*, 316
　leading causes of death in the United States 2020 and 2021, 318
　leading underlying causes of death—United States, 2022, 317
　multilevel model of, 311–315
　the United States and global health gap, 319–320
Global Health Initiative (GHI), 312
Gordon's functional health patterns, 161
governmental programs, 248
　Accountable Care Organization (ACO), 252–253
　centers for medicare and medicaid services, 248–251
　state designations, 251–252
gross domestic product (GDP), 3–4, 331

HACs (hospital-acquired conditions), 250
Hart-Celler Act, 306, 307
HCAHPS (Hospital Consumer Assessment of Healthcare Providers and Systems), 227, 292
health. *See also* community health assessment (CHA); global health
　as international phenomenon, 309–311
　micro- and macrofactors in obesity as health outcomes, 313
　outcomes, 42
　social determinants of, 310–311
　conceptual framework, 311
health and the social environment, 10–12
Health and Wellness (H&W) program, 218, 220, 223–225, 228, 230–233
Healthcare Facilities Accreditation Program (HFAP), 248
healthcare practices, need for change in, 1
healthcare providers, improved clinical decisions by, 168
healthcare reform, 2–3, 6, 195
healthcare resources, 42
　utilization of, 224–226
healthcare system performance rankings of 11 high-income countries, 320
health disparities, 41, 55, 58–59
　examples of, 60–62
health education programs, 21
health equity, 41, 55
health impact assessment (HIA), 89–90
　calculations used in, 79–80
health information exchange (HIE), 160
Health Information National Trends Survey (HINTS)-American Sign Language survey data, 92
health insurance coverage, 4
Health Insurance Portability and Accountability Act (HIPAA), 234
Health Outcomes Survey (HOS), 228
health-related behaviors, 134

health-related quality of life (HRQOL), 27
  data, 27
Health Resources and Services Administration (HRSA), 3
Healthy Days Measures, 27
  HRQOL tool, 27
  useful at national level for, 27
Healthy People 2030, 54–55, 316
Healthy People framework, 316
HEDIS "hybrid" method, 231
HFAP (Healthcare Facilities Accreditation Program), 248
HIA (health impact assessment), 89–90
HIE (health information exchange), 160
HIPAA (Health Insurance Portability and Accountability Act), 234
HITECH (Health Information Technology for Economic and Clinical Health) Act, 233
H1N1 threaten national security, 315
Home Health Care Classification, 161
Homeland Security Act of 2002, 306
HOS (Health Outcomes Survey), 228
hospital-acquired conditions (HACs), 250
Hospital Consumer Assessment of Healthcare Providers and Systems (HCAHPS), 227, 292
HRQOL (health-related quality of life), 27
HRSA (Health Resources and Services Administration), 3
hypertension, 52

ICD (International Classification of Diseases), 230, 323
iceberg phenomenon, 71
ICE (Immigration and Customs Enforcement), 306
ICER (incremental cost-effectiveness ratio), 29
ICN (International Council of Nurses), 323
ICNP (International Classification for Nursing Practice), 161, 323
ICU (intensive care unit), 221
IHI (Institute for Healthcare Improvement), 213
IHR (International Health Regulations), 322
IHTSDO (International Health Terminology Standards Development Organization), 323

immigrants, 306
  APRNs encounter lack of available data and, 46
  Temporary Protected Status (TPS) offered to, 308
  unauthorized, 307
  undocumented, 309
  in the United States, 307–308
Immigration and Customs Enforcement (ICE), 306
Immigration and Naturalization Service (INS), 306
immunization
  educational campaigns to ensure, 117
  as primary prevention, 26, 73
implementation science, 290
incidence rate, 78, 81
incremental cost-effectiveness ratio (ICER), 29
INESA (International Nursing Education, Services, and Accreditation), 330
infant and maternal deaths, 1
infant mortality, 4
  by race and ethnicity, 5
infectious diseases, 27
influenza immunization program, 28
information, 2, 44–45. *See also* Electronic health records (EHR); health information exchange (HIE)
  aggregated data provide valuable, 125
  AHRQ's website has useful information for, 54
  APRNs and other users tailor information available from, 55, 62, 124, 130, 140, 142, 160, 280
  assist in antibiotic selection, hospital staffing, and, 117
  bias, 109–111, 136, 231
  CEA provide information on health benefits and, 28
  database provide wealth of information on, 53
  demographic, 116, 192
  on disease etiology, 76
  on the effects of childhood stress, 11
  gathered in PRECEDE steps, 187
  on geographical characteristics, 112

information (*cont.*)
   to help Americans understand risk factors for, 13
   Hispanic population gather information on factors related to, 52
   and instruction, 166
   obtained from the *MMWR*, 77
   online, 167–168, 170–173
   population-level demographics and, 45, 48
   on prevalence of childhood obesity in the United States, 82
   on preventing excessive alcohol, 8
   record patient, 124
information technology, 165, 229, 235, 311
innovative care delivery models, 191
innovative technologies, 159–160
innovative technology, enhancement for traditional cardiac rehabilitation (CR), 165
INS (Immigration and Naturalization Service), 306
Instagram, 169
Institute for Healthcare Improvement (IHI), 213
   Triple Aim initiative, 213
Institute of Medicine (IOM), 316
   for establishing an infectious disease surveillance system to protect U.S. national security, 316
intensive care unit (ICU), 221
intent-to-treat principle, 110–111
interaction, 44, 59, 61, 70, 75, 107, 114, 116, 140, 170, 176, 190, 206, 233, 310
interactive voice response (IVR), 227
   surveys, 228
Internal Revenue Service (IRS), 266
International AIDS Society, 316
International Classification for Nursing Practice (ICNP), 161, 323
International Classification of Diseases (ICD), 230, 323
International Council of Nurses (ICN), 323
International Health Regulations (IHR), 322
International Health Terminology Standards Development Organization (IHTSDO), 323
International Nursing Education, Services, and Accreditation (INESA), 330
Internet, 47, 98, 137, 144, 165–167, 169–171, 280, 300
   resources supporting population-based nursing, 174–177
   search on opioid crisis legislation, 300
IOM (Institute of Medicine), 316
Iowa Model, 150–153
Iowa Model Collaborative, 151
Iowa Model Revised, 151
IRS (Internal Revenue Service), 266
isoniazid (INH), 26
IVR (interactive voice response), 227

JBI EBP Database, 135
Johns Hopkins Nursing Evidence-Based Practice (JHNEBP) model, 151
joint venture partners, 253
justice, 11, 30, 34, 35
   criminal justice system, 300
   in immigration law, 309
   social, 31, 305, 326

Kaiser Family Foundation (KFF), 4
Kaplan–Meier curves, 88–89
Kaplan–Meier method, 87
kappa statistic, 116

language barriers, 52
lead time bias, 84
Lean Six Sigma model, 217
legislation, 3, 8, 12, 14, 74, 234, 235, 250, 265–266, 299–300. *See also* justice
Lewin's Change Model, 291–292
Lewin's stages of change, 291–292
   changing, moving, or transition, 292
   refreezing, 293
   unfreezing, 292
LHDs (local health departments), 266
licensed medical professionals, 252
life expectancy in the United States, 321
life-prolonging treatments, 26
LinkedIn, 169
literature review, tool used to assess, 145–148
local health departments (LHDs), 266

INDEX

Logical Observation Identifiers Names and Codes (LOINC®), 161
logic model, 185–186
    steps for, 185
logistic regression, 88
log rank test, 88
longer length of stay (LOS) for patient, 222
long-term acute care (LTAC), 245
long-term care hospitals (LTCHs), 226
LTAC (long-term acute care), 245
LTCHs (long-term care hospitals), 226
Lupus Foundation, 137

MACRA (Medicare Access and CHIP Reauthorization Act), 250
Magnet®, 124
Magnet Recognition Program, 175, 256
Malcolm Baldrige Award, 217
mammograms, 26
managed care organizations (MCOs), 211
marketing
    American Marketing Association define as, 205
    as component to consider in program design and development, 204
    of healthcare services, 204
    plan, profitability and sustainability of program, 205
    positioning as concept, 205–206
matched pairs, 113
MAT (medication-assisted treatment), 299
MCOs (managed care organizations), 211
measurement bias, 110
Medicaid expansions, 5
Medicaid expansion states, 5
Medicaid Services Five-Star Quality Rating System (CMS STARs), 213
Medical Library Association (MLA), 171
Medicare Access and CHIP Reauthorization Act (MACRA), 250
medication-assisted treatment (MAT), 299
medication therapy management (MTM) programs, 226
merit-based incentive payment system (MIPS), 250

methicillin-resistant *Staphylococcus aureus* (MRSA), 250
the Mexico City policy, 321
MIPS (merit-based incentive payment system), 250
misclassification bias, 110
MLA (Medical Library Association), 171
mobile health, 165
mobile telephony, 165
monitoring healthcare quality, 212
morbidity and mortality data, 46–48
mortality rates, 4, 6, 9, 47, 48, 54, 60, 70, 77, 80, 82–84, 91, 144, 165, 257, 299, 311, 319. *See also* infant mortality
mortality vs. death rates, 83
MPD (Magnet program director), 258
mpox viruses, 47

naloxone, 300
NANDA-I (North American Nursing Diagnosis Association-International), 161
NANDA-I Nursing Diagnoses, 161
National Committee for Quality Assurance (NCQA), 212, 247
National Council of State Boards of Nursing (NCSBN), 170
National COVID-19 Preparedness Plan, 318–319
National Database of Nursing Quality Indicators® (NDNQI®), 258
National Global Health Initiatives, 315–319
National healthcare objectives, 53
National health expenditure (NHE), 4
National Health Interview Survey (NHIS), 5
National Institute on Drug Abuse (NIDA), 300
National Patient Safety Goals, 214
National Quality Forum's (NQFs), 214
national trends, and healthcare reform, 235
natural disasters, 21
natural history of disease, 70
NCDs (noncommunicable diseases), 13
NCQA (National Committee for Quality Assurance), 212, 247
NCSBN (National Council of State Boards of Nursing), 170
negative predictive value (NPV), 98

348 INDEX

new technology, opportunities and barriers to using, 167–168
NGOs (nongovernmental organizations), 321
NHE (National health expenditure), 4
NHIS (National Health Interview Survey), 5
NIC (Nursing Interventions Classification), 161
NIDA (National Institute on Drug Abuse), 300
Nightingale, Florence, 1
NLN Accreditation Commission (NLNAC), 330
NLNAC (NLN Accreditation Commission), 330
NNN Linkages, 161
NNT (number needed to treat), 79–80
NOC (Nursing Outcomes Classification), 161
NOC Outcomes, 161
nonclinical disease stage, 71
noncommunicable diseases (NCDs), 13
nondifferential misclassification, 110
nongovernmental organizations (NGOs), 321
nongovernmental programs, 253
nonmaleficence, 30
North American Nursing Diagnosis Association-International (NANDA-I), 161
null hypothesis, 108
number needed to treat (NNT), 79–80
nurse-designed models of care, 191
nurse-sensitive process, 221
    sample nurse-sensitive clinical quality measures, 224
nurse-sensitive quality indicators, 52–53
nursing care data, 124
Nursing Interventions Classification (NIC), 161
Nursing Minimum Data Set, 161
Nursing Outcomes Classification (NOC), 161
nursing profession, need to transform, key messages, 15. *See also* advanced practice registered nurses (APRNs)

Obama, Barack, 2, 266
obesity, 8–10, 52
OCM (oncology care model), 250
odds ratio (OR), 95, 122
    calculation in unmatched/matched case-control study, 123

OECD (Organization for Economic Cooperation and Development), 4
Office of Minority Health (OMH), 193
Omaha system, 161
oncology care model (OCM), 250
Oncology Nursing Society (ONS), 250
online education, 167
online information, evaluating the quality of, 171–173
ONS (Oncology Nursing Society), 250
OpenNotes, software program, 161–162
operating policies and procedures, 203–204
opioid crisis, 299–300
    legislation, 300
opioid overdose, 300
opioid use disorder (OUD) tool, 300
opportunities, 168
    improved adherence to self-care, 169
    improved clinical decisions by healthcare providers, 168
    shared decision-making, 168–169
    tailored patient care, 168–169
organizational models for excellence, 215–218
Organization for Economic Cooperation and Development (OECD), 4
OR (odds ratio), 95, 122
outcomes
    classifying and categorizing, 42
    health, 42
    identifying, 48–49
    indicators at population level, 221
    monitoring, 51–52
    qualitative strategies for evaluation of program, 232, 236
    data availability, 232–234
    vaccination, 51
overcoming barriers, and challenges, 206–207
overdiagnosis bias, 85
ownership, 197

PAR (Participatory Action Research), 134
Participatory Action Research (PAR), 134
patient-centered medical home (PCMH), 221
Patient Protection, 3, 41, 265, 266
PatientsLikeMe, digital health platform, 166
pay for performance (P4P), 250

PCMH (patient-centered medical home), 221
PCPs (primary care providers), 211
PDSA (plan-do-study-act), 151, 184, 296
peer support interventions, 166
period prevalence rate, 81
Perioperative Nursing Data Set, 161, 163
Pew Internet Project, 167
PHAB (Public Health Accreditation Board), 248
PHEIC (public health emergency of international concern), 316
phone automated surveys, 228
Physical and Psychosocial Health Assessment (PPHA), 144
PICO framework, clinical questions, 131, 150
PICOT Questions, 132
PIN (population impact number), 80
Pinterest, 169
plan, do, check, act (PDCA) process, 218
plan-do-study-act (PDSA), 151, 184, 296
Planetary Health Alliance (PHA), 326
PLGHA (Protecting Life in Global Health Assistance), 322
podcasts, 137, 176, 177
Point of Care Tools, 300
point prevalence, 81
policymakers, 84
policy or practice development, 184
polio vaccines, 26
population, defining, 6–7
population-based APRNs, responsible for, 23
population-based care, 1
population-based models, 218–221
population-based practice, defined, 22
population health, IHI role in Triple Aim, 51, 52, 213, 250
population health models, 213, 220
Population Health Task Force Initiatives, 267
population impact number (PIN), 80
population strategies, in acute care, 12
population survey, 307
positive predictive value (PPV), 98
postoperative surgical site infections (SSIs), 250
power analysis, 97–98
P4P (pay for performance), 250

PPV (positive predictive value), 98
practical robust implementation and maintenance model (PRISM), 295–299
PRECEDE-PROCEED model, 187–188
  adaptations and application in outdoor active pilot study, 189–190
preclinical stage of disease, 70–71
Preemptive Pharmacogenomic Testing for Preventing Adverse Drug Reactions (PREPARE) study, 41
prevalence rate, 10, 74, 78, 81
prevention, 10, 15, 73
  community health improvement navigator, 274
  levels of, 25-26
  objective. *See Healthy People*, goal of
  primary, 26, 73–74
  secondary, 74
  strategies, 28
  tertiary, 74-75
preventive care service, 3
primary care providers (PCPs), 211
primary prevention, 26, 73–74
Princeton Survey Research Associates, 4
PRISM (practical robust implementation and maintenance model), 295–299
probability of surviving, calculation, 86
process improvement models
  characteristics and commonalities of, 219
  and tools, 218
professional organizations, 255
  American College of Surgeons (ACS), 255
  American Nurses Credentialing Center (ANCC), 255–257
  specialty organizations, 257
  World Health Organization (WHO) Baby Friendly Hospital Initiative (BFHI), 257
prognosis, 85–86
program design and implementation, 200
  impact of transitional program intended to reduce readmission rates, 202–203
  outcomes, 201–203
  SMART provides a template for writing objectives, 202
  structure, 200–201
  of program proposal outline, 201

proportional hazard models [Cox models], 88
proportionate mortality ratio, 79, 84
Protecting Life in Global Health Assistance (PLGHA), 322
provider advisory committees, 237
publication bias, 111
public health, 245
   definition, 21
   ethics, 29
      frameworks, 31–35
      methods, 35
   nurses, 21, 42, 150
   nursing, defined by APHA, 21
   programs, 26
   objectives of, 25–27
Public Health Accreditation Board (PHAB), 248
public health emergency of international concern (PHEIC), 316
PubMed, 137

QR codes, 277
quality, defined, 212–213
quality improvement (QI) models, 184
   PDSA steps, 184–185
quality of life, 11, 24, 27, 44, 46, 50, 60, 89, 99, 134–136, 136, 144–148, 193, 223, 273, 283, 306, 314, 319

random error, 108, 109
randomized controlled trials (RCTs), 96–97, 114, 120, 136
random sampling, 110
rates, 76
   calculating rates, 77–79
   case fatality rate, 79
   crude or specific, 77–78
   death rates, 77
   incidence rates, 77
   mortality, 4, 6, 9, 47, 48, 54, 60, 70, 77, 80, 82–84, 91, 144, 165, 257, 299, 311, 319
   prevalence, 78
   survival, 86
RCTs (randomized controlled trials), 96–97

reach, adoption, implementation, and maintenance model (RE-AIM), 295–300
   to enhance sustainability, extension of, 295, 297
really simple syndication (RSS), 137, 177
recall bias, 111
refugee, defines, 306
rehabilitation, 26, 164, 193, 211, 215, 226, 229, 232, 247–248
relative risk reduction (RRR), 94
relative risk (RR), 93
religion, 7, 58, 271, 306
replicate findings, 117
reporting bias, 111
reproductive health (RH), 321
research synthesis, 143
return on investment (ROI) analysis, 225
Robert Wood Johnson Foundation (RWJF), 137, 191
   white paper recommendations and nurse leaders involved in, 191–192
Rockefeller-Lancet Commission, 326
Rogers' diffusion of innovations theory, 293–295
RR (relative risk), 93
RRR (relative risk reduction), 94
RSS (really simple syndication), 137
RWJF (Robert Wood Johnson Foundation), 137, 191

SAMHSA (Substance Abuse and Mental Health Services Administration), 300
sample selection, 97
sample size, 97
SARS (severe acute respiratory syndrome), 315
scientific misconduct (fraud), 118–119
scientific plausibility, 117
screening programs, calculations used in, 80
screening test, 98
   validity, 98
secondary intervention, 26
secondary prevention, 26, 74
selection bias, 109

self-care, 136, 159, 162, 165, 166, 171, 202, 228, 298
  and behavior change, 167
  improved adherence to, 169
sensitivity, 80, 98
serious reportable events (SREs), 214
severe acute respiratory syndrome (SARS), 315
sexually transmitted infections (STIs), 47
SHADAC (State Health Access Data Assistance Center), 27
shared decision-making, 168–169
short message service (SMS) for patients, 165
significance, 97
single-blind, 115
Six Sigma approach, 216–217
social determinants of health, 24–25, 46
social media, 159, 169, 177, 277, 298, 299, 313
Social Sciences Citation Index, 137
specificity, 80, 98
specific rates, 79
SPIDER acronym, clinical questions, 131
SREs (serious reportable events), 214
standardized data definitions, 235–236
standardized language in nursing, 53
State Health Access Data Assistance Center (SHADAC), 27
statistic tests, 116
STIs (sexually transmitted infections), 47
strength of association, 116
strengths, weaknesses, opportunities, and threats (SWOT), 292, 293, 295
stroke, 7, 70, 112, 151, 164, 202, 251
  leading underlying causes of death—United States, 2022, 317
  prevention, outcome examples, 50
study design, 112, 119
  strengths and weaknesses, 119
study designs, hierarchy of, 141
subpopulations, defining, 6–7
Substance Abuse and Mental Health Services Administration (SAMHSA), 300
suicide, 12–13
survival analysis, 87
survival curve, 87
  using data, 88
survival rates, after treatment, 86

survival time, 84
susceptibility, stage of, 70
sustainable development goals
  acknowledge climate change threat to, 325–326
  2030 Agenda for, 325
  and planetary health, 325–326
SWOT (strengths, weaknesses, opportunities, and threats), 292, 293, 295
synergism, 114
systematic error, 108–110, 124. *See also* random error
Systematized Nomenclature of Medicine-Clinical Terms (SNOMED CT®), 161, 323

tailored patient care, 168–169
Take-Home Medication pack (THM) *versus* a standard paper prescription (SPP), 94
team communications, 184
TEAM model, 197
technology to obtain health information, 165–167
  information and instruction, 166
  peer support interventions, 166
  self-care and behavior change, 167
teleconferencing, 159
telemedicine strategies, 163
temporal relationship, 116
Temporary Protected Status (TPS), 308
tertiary prevention, 26, 74–75
texting, 169
The Joint Commission (TJC), 212, 246
  acute care hospital accredited through, 246
  certification program for congestive heart failure (CHF), 246
  disease-specific care certifications, 254
theory-based frameworks, 32
TikTok, 169
timeline illustrating lead time bias, 85
TJC (The Joint Commission), 212, 246
To Err Is Human, consensus report, 217
transparency, 31, 34, 120, 135, 143, 161, 167, 195
TREND checklist, 121
Triple Aim model, 250

Tumblr, 169
Twitter, 169
type 2 diabetes mellitus, 52
type I error, 108, 124
type II error, 97, 108, 124

UDHR (Universal Declaration of Human Rights), 309–310
the United Nations millennium development goals, 324
   for improving the health status of countries, 324
the United Nations sustainable development goals, 325
United States Census Bureau, 45
Universal Declaration of Human Rights (UDHR), 309–310
URAC (Utilization Review Accreditation Commission), 212, 247
U.S. Immigration and Nationality Act (INA), 306–307
U.S. Preventive Services Task Force (USPSTF), 3, 99
USAID immunization programs, 322
utilization management (UM), 211
Utilization Review Accreditation Commission (URAC), 212, 247

vaccination, 24, 30, 35, 44, 51, 57, 309, 315–316
vaccine-preventable diseases, 315
vaccines, 3, 26, 170, 298, 316
validity, 142–143
value-based purchasing (VBP), 250
variance, 97
VBP (value-based purchasing), 250
videoconferencing, 177
volunteer bias, 109

webcasts, 159
web of causation concept, 75
windshield and walking surveys (WWS), 270
withdrawal bias, 109
World Health Organization (WHO), 8, 13, 173, 257, 306, 310, 320, 322–323
   collaborating centers (CCs), 326–329
   collaborating centers with schools of nursing, 328–329
   created in 1946 to find solutions for post-World War II Europe, 322
   declared COVID-19 a pandemic, 317
   declared mpox a "public health emergency of international concern" (PHEIC), 316
   declared 2020 the Year of the Nurse and Midwives to acknowledge, 330
   defines global public health security, 323
   definition of health, 27
   development of PAHO/WHO guidelines, 327
   estimate NCDs kill people each year, 13
   evaluation terms of reference outputs, 327
   to follow prescriptions of the UN MDGs by, 324
   Global Polio Eradication Initiative, 317
   included the International Classification for Nursing Practice (ICNP), 323
   manages global disease registries, databases, and, 323
   network, 326
World War II, 216, 306, 320, 322
WWS (windshield and walking surveys), 270

Years of potential life lost (YPLL), 80, 90
YPLL (Years of potential life lost), 80, 90